Understanding Chinese Medicine

Understanding Chinese Medicine

Editor: Trinity Harper

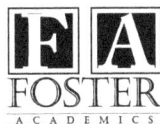

FA FOSTER
ACADEMICS

www.fosteracademics.com

www.fosteracademics.com

FA
FOSTER
ACADEMICS

Cataloging-in-Publication Data

Understanding chinese medicine / edited by Trinity Harper.
    p. cm.
Includes bibliographical references and index.
ISBN 978-1-63242-864-6
1. Medicine, Chinese. 2. Alternative medicine. 3. Traditional medicine--China. I. Harper, Trinity.
R601 .U53 2019
610.951--dc23

Foster Academics,
118-35 Queens Blvd., Suite 400,
Forest Hills, NY 11375, USA

ISBN 978-1-63242-864-6 (Hardback)

Contents

Permissions

List of Contributors

Index

Preface

The type of traditional medicine based on ancient Chinese medical practices, including qigong, tui na, herbal medicine and acupuncture, is known as traditional Chinese medicine (TCM). It is based on the belief that a body's vital energy, called qi, flows through channels, known as meridians, which have branches connected to bodily organs and functions. The Yin-Yang theory and Wu Xing theory are the main philosophies of traditional Chinese medicine. This field emphasizes that diseases are the imbalances or disharmonies in the functioning of qi, yin, yang, meridians, xue and zang-fu. This book attempts to understand the multiple branches that fall under the field of Chinese medicine and how such concepts have practical applications. It strives to provide a fair idea about this discipline and to help develop a better understanding of the latest advances within this field. The extensive content of this book provides the readers with a thorough understanding of the subject.

The researches compiled throughout the book are authentic and of high quality, combining several disciplines and from very diverse regions from around the world. Drawing on the contributions of many researchers from diverse countries, the book's objective is to provide the readers with the latest achievements in the area of research. This book will surely be a source of knowledge to all interested and researching the field.

In the end, I would like to express my deep sense of gratitude to all the authors for meeting the set deadlines in completing and submitting their research chapters. I would also like to thank the publisher for the support offered to us throughout the course of the book. Finally, I extend my sincere thanks to my family for being a constant source of inspiration and encouragement.

Editor

Will Chinese external therapy with compound Tripterygium wilfordii hook F gel safely control disease activity in patients with rheumatoid arthritis

Quan Jiang[1†], Xiao-Po Tang[1†], Xian-Chun Chen[2], Hong Xiao[1], Ping Liu[3] and Juan Jiao[1*] iD

Abstract

Background: Chinese external therapy (CET) is a topical application with mainly Chinese herb medicine therapy with thousands of years of historical implications and is a clinical routine that is commonly used for relieving joint-related symptoms in patients with arthritis in Chinese hospitals. However, there is a paucity of modern medical evidence to support its effectiveness and safety. Thus, we propose to implement a randomized, double-blinded, placebo-controlled clinical trial in patients with rheumatoid arthritis (RA) using, as the experimental intervention, topical application of a hospital-compounded gel preparation of Tripterygium wilfordii Hook F (TwHF).

Methods: This study will be an 8-week double-blinded, randomized, placebo-controlled clinical trial conducted at Guang'anmen Hospital in Beijing, China, and 168 patients with moderately active RA will be randomly assigned with a 1:1 ratio to apply a topical gel preparation containing TwHF or placebo. The primary outcome variable will be the proportion of subjects, by study group, to achieve a 20% improvement in the American College of Rheumatology criteria (ACR20) by week 8. Secondary outcome measures to be assessed at weeks 4 or 8 will include: measurement of ACR20 response rate at week 4, ACR50 response rate, the changes in DAS28 score, and joint synovitis classification assessment monitored by musculoskeletal ultrasound. Safety evaluations conducted at weeks 4, 8 and 12 will be based on spontaneous complaints by the study subjects, but special emphasis will be focused on cutaneous allergy and alterations of menstruation in premenopausal female participants. Statistical analyses will be performed using the intention to treat analysis data set.

Discussion: This proposed clinical trail is designed to evaluate the efficacy and safety of CET based on a single topically-applied agent in a relatively large patient population with RA. This study protocol gives a detailed description of the usage and dosage of the topical compound TwHF gel and the methodology of this study. In addition, it is hoped that the outcomes of this study will be viewed as supporting the generalizability of CET in the setting of inflammatory rheumatic diseases. The results of this study are expected to have important public health implications for Asian RA patients that currently utilize CET as a complimentary treatment.

Trial registration: Clinical trial gov Identifier: NCT02818361. Registrated on Jun. 15, 2016.

Keywords: Chinese external therapy, Topical application, Tripterygium, Rheumatoid arthritis

* Correspondence: jiao.juan@hotmail.com
†Equal contributors
1Rheumatism Department, Guang'anmen Hospital, China Academy of Chinese Medical Sciences, No. 5 Beixiange Street, Xicheng District, Beijing 100053, China
Full list of author information is available at the end of the article

Background

Rheumatoid arthritis (RA) is a chronic, systemic disorder characterized by persistent synovitis involving diarthrodial joints. Uncontrolled active RA can result in joint damage, disability, decreased quality of life, cardiovascular disease, and other comorbidities. Although Non-Steroid Anti-Inflammatory Drugs (NSAIDs) and steroids have been recommended by many physicians to relieve joint pain, and other symptoms related to the chronic synovitis and systemic inflammation, those drugs carry an increased potential for side effects [1] and are poorly tolerated by many patients.

For centuries in China, Chinese external therapy (CET) has been an accepted clinical approach for relieving joint-related symptoms and has been well-received by Chinese RA patients. In a narrow sense, CET is a pharmacological treatment for body surface or skin (mucosa) diseases, such as fumigation and plaster, etc.. CET has a long history that has its origins in the earliest experience of Chinese Medicine during the Chinese Qin and Han dynasties (BCE 221 to CE 220). It was observed that RA symptoms typically present as the swelling of multiple limb joints, pain, and stiffness, the main presenting clinical manifestations of active RA exist near the skin surface. CET is believed to have a rapid and favorable effect because it can be applied directly above the lesions. However, there are very few modern evidence-based data to support its effectiveness and safety in active rheumatic diseases.

Tripterygium wilfordii Hook F (TwHF), a traditional Chinese herb, has been used to relieve joint pain for a thousand years in China and its extracts have recently proven to be effective in patents with RA [2, 3]. However, the oral application of TwHF is limited for clinical use because of its high frequency of reproductive system damage [4]. In order to reduce toxicity without losing efficacy, the current study utilizes a topical rather than an oral compound THwF, hoping to thereby explore the advantages of CET. We previously conducted a 4-week double-blinded, randomized, placebo-controlled pilot clinical trial on topical compound TwHF with 70 RA patients whose joint disease was severely-active. The findings of the pilot study showed that joints pain and swelling were rapidly (within one week) reduced with the application of topical compound TwHF twice a day. Furthermore, a favorable control of the overall RA disease condition was found, as the rate of achievement rose to 20% and 50% improvement in the (ACR20 and ACR50) were 34% and 17% at week 4, using intention to treat analysis [currently awaiting publication]. The ACR20 and ACR50 response rates were found to be even higher in another study which reported responses of 58% and 20% with the TwHF group at week 6 [5]. Additionally, a previous double-blind, randomized multi-center trial found that based upon methotrexate or leflunomide, 75 out of 87 patients (90.8%) in the topical compound TwHF group and 58 out of 87 patients (69.0%) in the topical placebo-treated group reported relief from their joint pain [6].

Encouraged by the above results, we have developed the topical compound TwHF to be used as a hospital gel preparation. Thus, we plan to undertake an 8-week double-blinded randomized placebo-controlled clinical trial to further explore the safety and effectiveness of topical TwHF gel in patients with active RA.

It is important to examine whether topical treatment, with TwHF gel, as a supplement to usual care, will result in better outcomes for patients with active RA. We expect a favorable outcome for the topical compound TwHF gel that supports its efficiency. This article provides a full description of the study's design and methodology in accordance with the SPIRIT guidelines for reporting protocols for intervention trials and the CONSORT guidelines [7, 8] for reporting outcomes.

Methods

Study design

This clinical trail will be accomplished at Guang'anmen hospital, China academy of Chinese Medical Science in Beijing, China. The current study follows the guidelines of the Declaration of Helsinki for humans and has been approved by the ethic s committee of Guang'anmen Hospital (approval number: 2016–062-KY). Enrolled will be 168 patients with documented moderately active RA who will be randomized (1:1 ratio) to one of two treatment groups: the TwHF gel group and the placebo gel group. Written signed consent will be obtained from each participant before any study-related procedures are initiated.

Participants

Inclusion criteria

Eligible patients, men and women, must age from 18 to 65 years old, and must be clinically diagnosed with RA prior to screening for study entry in accordance with the 1987 revised criteria of the American College of Rheumatology [9]. Their RA disease stage must be in the moderate activity range, as defined by the criteria of the 28-joint count Disease Activity Score (DAS-28 score), ranging between 3.2 to 5.1 [10]. If patients are receiving a disease-modifying, anti-rheumatic drugs (DMARDs), those medications should be continued unchanged throughout this study, but their dosages must have been stable for at least 12 weeks prior to study entry.

Exclusion criteria

Exclusion Criteria will include: ongoing rheumatic or inflammatory joint diseases other than RA; serious medical diseases such as: hyperlipidemia, hyperglycemia, diabetes mellitus, cardiovascular diseases, gastrointestinal disease, liver disease or renal failure; patients with RA who have a prominent component of comorbid fibromyalgia syndrome, prior treatment with TwHF agents, glucocorticoids, or biological agents; skin allergies or broken skin in the areas of planned treatment with topical TwHF gel. Female patients who are pregnant, breast-feeding or who plan to become pregnant will be excluded.

Randomization

Randomization will be controlled by an independent third party, the hospital Clinical Evaluation Center, using the SAS system (Version 8.2 for Windows) to assign the eligible participants at a 1:1 ratio to receive either topical compound TwHF gel or placebo.

Blinding

This study is a double-blind and placebo-controlled design. The blinding will also be accomplished and monitored by the hospital Clinical Evaluation Center. The blinding codes record topical compound TwHF gel and the placebo as A and B, sequentially and the details of the allocation sequence will be put in sealed light-tight envelopes and maintained in the Clinical Evaluation Center. The contents of these envelopes will be unknown to the principal investigator, the study staff, and the participants. Since the packing and labeling of the treatment gels are the same, the topical compound TwHF gel and placebo gel will be masked by numeric codes from 001 to 168, which correspond with each participant's sequential enrollment number. Thus, the study researchers will enroll and evaluate study subjects but will have no influence on randomization. So the case group division is adapted to a randomized, double-blind study design.

Intervention

The ingredients for the compounding of the topical TwHF gel include: Tripterygium wilfordii Hook F, Mangxiao (Mirabilite), Chuanxiong (Rhizoma Ligustici), Ruling (Olibanum), and Moyao (M yrrh) (proportions: 4:4:2:2:1). The topical placebo gel is made of a viscous agent and sucrose which make it looks like the active preparation. Both of the gels will be prepared by the Pharmaceutical Department of Guang'anmen Hospital, and the herbs will be purchased from Beijing Fengtaijinyuan Pharmaceutical Co., Ltd. Each gel is 20 gram (g) per tube. Both the topical compound TwHF gel and the placebo gel will be applied for 1st to 5th metacarpophalangeal joints, 1st to 5th proximal interphalangeal joints, wrists, knees and ankles 10 g for 1 h, once a day from week 0 through week 4 and 10 g from week 5 through week 8.

Outcome measurements

Outcomes measurements will be assessed at baseline, at week 4, at week 8 and at the 12th week follow-up. The DAS28 joints will be assessed for swelling and tenderness by a trained staff member. All the outcome assessments will be accomplished by the same staff researcher.

The primary outcome measure will be ACR20 criteria [11] by week 8. To achieve ACR20, a patient must have a 20% or greater reduction in the number of both tender and swollen joints and a 20% or more improvement in 3 or more of the following: the physician's or patient's assessment of global health status, the patient's assessment of pain on a visual analogue scale, the patient's assessment of function using a modified version of the Health Assessment Questionnaire (HAQ), and the erythrocyte sedimentation rate (ESR) or serum C-reactive protein (CRP) level.

Secondary outcome measures will include: ACR20 assessed at week 4, ACR50 criteria assessed at weeks 4 and 8, changes at weeks 4 and 8 in DAS28, and joint synovitis classification. Since the DAS28 is a combined index to measure the disease activity in patients with RA, it can be used in combination with the European League Against Rheumatism response criteria [10]. In the present trial, the DAS28 score will be calculated, based on either the C-reactive protein (DAS28-CRP) or the erythrocyte sedimentation rate (DAS28-ESR) [10]. Changes in joint synovitis classification will be determined by serial musculoskeletal ultrasound (MUSU) focused on the total sum of synovitis classification based on the joint used gels. The MUSU synovitis classification will derive from each MUSU measurement as follows: 0 level, no doppler synovial tissue signal; level 1, three independent points or 2 successive or 1 to 2 independent dot doppler synovial tissue signals; level 2, doppler signal indicating <50% of the area representing synovium; level 3, doppler signal indicating synovium in >50% of the measured area [12].

The safety evaluation will be accomplished by a face-to-face interview at the 4th and 8th weeks and by a a telephone-interview with the remote 12th week follow-up. Adverse experiences of interest will include: manifestations of cutaneous allergy (erythema, edema, itching) and gastrointestinal stimulation due to mucous membrane damage. In addition, because of the high frequency of reproductive system damage, the safety evaluation will focus on changes in menstruation patterns among premenopausal female participants. The relevant female participants will be asked a general question about whether they have observed any change in their menstruation pattern. Irrespective of how they answer that question, a series of follow-up questions will attempt to quantify any change in the menstrual cycle (extension, shortening or no change), or in the quantity of menstrual flow (increased, reduced, or unchanged). Blood and urine routine laboratory examinations, including glutamic-pyruvic transaminase, glutamic oxalacetic transaminase, creatinine and urea nitrogen will be accomplished at baseline and on the 8th week. Quantitative changes will be addressed on the record. Professional judgments regarding the severity of any given adverse effect and any recognized relationship between the adverse effect and the study interventions will be documented if any of the above safety measures are observed to fall beyond normal clinical or laboratory ranges.

Sample size

This study is designed as a superiority trial. A previous findings showed the ACR20 response rates were 34.3% in a topical TwHF group and 12.5% in placebo group in patients with active RA [awaiting publication]. Based on the following calculation: $n = 2(u_\alpha + u_\beta)^2 2P(1-P)/(P_1-P_0)^2$ [13], it is predicted that 76 participants in each group will be needed to detect a significant (p < =0.05) with 80% power. Based upon a predicted 10% rate of drop out, we will recruit a total of 168 participants, 84 in each group.

Quality control

The identification, registration, and subsequent flow of participants in the trial will be governed by the trial standard operational protocol. The completion of the Case Report Form and compliance with the standard operation procedures will be audited. At regular intervals, a clinical research associate, will monitor the clinical trial procedures, such as compliance with the study protocol and regulatory policy. In particular, the reasons for withdrawal will be fully documented in the Case Report Form.

Data analysis

The statistical analyses will be performed using the intention to treat analysis (ITT). The safety dataset will also include all patients who received ≥1 week of topical applications. Mean ± Standard Deviation, number and percentage will be used for continuous variables and categorical variables, as appropriate. Patient movement through the study will be documented on a Consort diagram. Patient demographic characteristics will be documented in a by-group comparison table and statistically compared between topical TwHF and placebo groups using a 2-sample t test for continuous variables or Pearson 2 test for categorical variables.

All analyses will be performed using SAS system (Version 5.2.127 8.2 for Windows). *P* values less than .05 will be considered statistically significant. The primary outcome variable, the ACR20 response rate at week 8, and the secondary outcome measure, ACR20 at week 4 and ACR 50 response rate at weeks 4 and 8, will be compared between the 2 groups using the Pearson 2 test. Two-sample t tests will be performed on DAS28-CRP and DAS28-ESR at baseline and posttreatment, as well as their changes after treatment. Paired t tests will be used to compare the changes of DAS28-CRP and DAS28-ESR from baseline to posttreatment in each group. The joint synovitis classification will be compared between the 2 groups at baseline and posttreatment using Kruskal-Wallis rank sum test. Any by-group changes in the joint synovitis classification will be compared using the paired Kruskal-Wallis rank sum test.

Ethical considerations

This study has been approved by the ethics committee of Guang'anmen Hospital (approval number: 2016–062-KY). Written consent to take part in the study will be obtained from all study participants before any of the study-related procedures are initiated. Each study subject will be provided a witnessed copy of the consent document he or she signed, which also bears the signature a study investigator. They will also receive an information sheet explaining the study.

Discussion

To date, only a small number of studies have documented the effectiveness of CET using any pharmacological agent. This clinical trial is designed as a double-blinded, randomized, controlled study of TwHF-based CET in a moderate active RA population with 8 weeks of observation. Considering the main clinical features of active RA to be joint swelling, tenderness, and pain, these are the clinical manifestations monitored using validated instruments. It is anticipated that topical compound TwHF gel will also be effective in controlling the clinical manifestations of RA and safe for use by RA patients.

In animal studies, TwHF microemulsion has been observed to imeliorate the severity of a murine adjuvant-induced arthritis model and to reduce the male reproductive toxicity and hepatotoxicity [14]. It is hoped that the topical use of TwHF as a clinical application of CET in RA patients will be found to be both safe and efficacious. Although TwHF and its extracts have shown good responses in patients with RA it is currently limited to use in elderly patients because of demonstrated reproductive toxicity. Safety observations from previous studies have shown that compound TwHF applied topically can cause cutaneous reactions which are reversible with discontinuation of the topical TwHF compound. In addition, increases in serum aminotransferase and alterations in menstruation among female patients have been reported [5, 6].

There are several aspects of the current study design that are different from previous CET clinical studies using this agent. Firstly, the design of dosage adjustment in this study will demonstrate whether the period of dosage reduction will bring additional benefits to the patients. In clinical practice, patients often continue to apply the effective medicine for an additional period in order to consolidate the efficacy, though there is no evidence to support this practice. Secondly, the follow-up assessment has rarely been included in CET research. Since oral preparations of THwF have often exhibited side effects, such as gastrointestinal and menstrual disorders, special emphasis has been placed upon an 4-week follow-up (to monitor at least one menstrual cycle).

In conclusion, the successful completion of this study will contribute to the evidence base of whether TwHF compound gel is a promising complimentary treatment as a simple, inexpensive, effective and safe treatment for active RA patients. The results of this study are expected to have important public health implications which may alter the approach to management of RA in China.

Abbreviations
ACR20: 20% improvement in the American College of Rheumatology criteria; ACR50: 50% improvement in the American College of Rheumatology criteria; CET: Chinese external therapy; CRP: C-reactive protein; DAS28: 28-joint count Disease Activity Score; DAS28-CRP: DAS28 score based on C-reactive protein; DAS28-ESR: DAS28 score based on erythrocyte sedimentation rate; DMARDs: Disease-modifying, anti-rheumatic drugs; ESR: Erythrocyte sedimentation rate; G: Gram; HAQ: Health Assessment Questionnaire; ITT: Intention to treat analysis; MU SU: Musculoskeletal ultrasound; NSAIDs: Non-Steroid Anti-Inflammatory Drugs; RA: Rheumatoid arthritis; TwHF: Tripterygium wilfordii Hook F; gram: g

Acknowledgments
Sponsor: Beijing Municipal Science & Technology Commission. The authors gratefully acknowledge the Irwin Jon Russell and Wen Wang, for their insightful suggestions and comments for the study protocol and writing.

Trail status
It is anticipated that this trial will take 24 months to complete. Recruitment of subjects into the study began on Oct. 8 2016. It is anticipated that the 8-week observation of the final study subject will be completed on Aug. 30 of 2018.

Funding
This research is supported by Beijing Municipal Science & Technology Commission, Grant Number Z161100001816046. The contents of this manuscript are solely the responsibility of the authors and do not necessarily represent the official views of Beijing Municipal Science & Technology Commission.

Availability of data and materials
The clinical evaluation center of Guang'anmen Hospital is responsible for data and safety monitoring. Clinical Evaluation Center is responsible for monitoring the project including randomization, blinding, data quality checking and statistical analysis. We provide to the clinical evaluation center a number of reports including serious adverse events or death within 24 hours of knowledge of event occurrence. The members of the clinical evaluation center have no connection to any clinical investigators or any study subjects.

Authors' contributions
QJ obtained funding for the study. QJ, JJ, XT, and PL designed the randomized placebo-controlled trial. QJ, JJ, XT and HX conducted the research. XC designed and prepared the gel preparations of TwHF and pla-

cebo. JJ wrote the draft of the manuscript. All authors participated in the revision of the subsequent draft and approved the final version of the manuscript.

Ethics approval and consent to participate
We confirm that any aspect of the work covered in this manuscript that has involved RA patients has been conducted with the ethical approval approved by the ethic committee of Guang'anmen Hospital and that it follows the guideline of the Declaration of Helsinki for humans (approval number: 2016–062-KY). Written signed consent to confirm their participations and our legal rights to deal with the data out of them will be obtained from each participant before any study-related procedures are initiated.

Competing interests
We have not received any financial support or other benefits from commercial sources for the study. None of the authors have any financial interests that could create a potential conflict of interest.

Author details
[1]Rheumatism Department, Guang'anmen Hospital, China Academy of Chinese Medical Sciences, No. 5 Beixiange Street, Xicheng District, Beijing 100053, China. [2]Pharmaceutical Department, Guang'anmen Hospital, China Academy of Chinese Medical Sciences, No. 12 Fuhai Street, Daxing District, Beijing 102628, China. [3]Clinical evaluation center, Guang'anmen Hospital, China Academy of Chinese Medical Sciences, No. 5 Beixiange Street, Xicheng District, Beijing 100053, China.

References
1. Brune K, Patrignani P. New insights into the use of currently available non-steroidal anti-inflammatory drugs. J pain res. 2015;8:105-18. Ann Rheum Dis. 2015;74:1799–807.
2. Zhang W, Shi Q, Zhao LD, Li Y, Tang FL, Zhang FC, et al. The safety and effCETiveness of a chloroform/methanol extract of Tripterygium wilfordii hook F (T2) plus methotrexate in treating rheumatoid arthritis. J Clin Rheumatol. 2010;16:375–8.
3. Lv QW, Zhang W, Shi Q, Zheng WJ, Li X, Chen H, et al. Comparison of Tripterygium wilfordii Hook F with methotrexate in the treatment of active rheumatoid arthritis (TRIFRA): a randomized, controlled clinical trial. Ann Rheum Di.s 2014;73:e62.
4. Xi C, Peng S, Wu Z, Zhou Q, Zhou J. Toxicity of triptolide and the molecular mechanisms involved. Biomed Pharmacother. 2017;90:531–41.
5. Cibere J, Deng Z, Lin Y, Ou R, He Y, Wang Z, et al. A randomized double blind, placebo controlled trial of topical Tripterygium wilfordii in rheumatoid arthritis: reanalysis using logistic regression analysis. J Rheumatol. 2003;30:465–7.
6. Jiao J, Yang XP, Yuan J, Liu X, Liu H, Zhang CY, et al. EffCET of external applying compound Tripterygium wilfordii hook F.On joint pain of rheumatoid arthritis patients. Chinese Journal of Integrated Traditional and Western Medicine. 2016;36(1):29–34.
7. Chan AW, Tetzlaff JM, Altman DG, Laupacis A, Gotzsche PC, Krleza-Jeric K, et al. SPIRIT 2013 statement: defining standard protocol items for clinical trials. Ann Intern Med. 2013;158:200–7.
8. Schulz KF, Altman DG, Moher D. CONSORT 2010 statement: updated guidelines for reporting parallel group randomized trials. BMC Med. 2010; https://doi.org/10.1186/1741-7015-8-18.
9. Fransen J, van Riel PL. The disease activity score and the EULAR response criteria. Rheum Dis Clin N Am. 2009;35:745–57.
10. Arnett FC, Edworthy SM, Bloch DA, McShane DJ, Fries JF, Cooper NS, et al. The American rheumatism association 1987 revised criteria for the classification of rheumatoid arthritis. Arthritis Rheum. 1988;31:315–24.
11. American College of Rheumatology Subcommittee on Rheumatoid Arthritis Guidelines.2002. Guidelines for the management of rheumatoid arthritis: 2002 update.Arthritis Rheum. 46:328–346.

12. Szkudlarek M, Court-Payen M, Strandberg C, Klarlund M, Klausen T, Ostergaard M. Power Doppler ultrasonography for assessment of synovitis in the metacarpophalangeal joints of patients with rheumatoid arthritis: a comparison with dynamic magnetic resonance imaging. Arthritis Rheum. 2001;44:2018–23.

13. Chow SC, Shao J, Wang H. Sample size calculations in clinical research. Taylor & Francis. 2008;89

14. Wang X, Xue M, Gu J, Fang X, Sha X. Transdermal microemulsion drug delivery system for impairing male reproductive toxicity and enhancing efficacy of Tripterygium Wilfordii hook f. Fitoterapia. 2012;83:690–8.

Sheng Jiang San, a traditional multi-herb formulation, exerts anti-influenza effects in vitro and in vivo via neuraminidase inhibition and immune regulation

Tianbo Zhang[1], Mengjie Xiao[2,3], Chun-Kwok Wong[4,5], Ka-Pun Chris Mok[6], Xin Zhao[2,7], Huihui Ti[2,6*] and Pang-Chui Shaw[1,5,7*] (iD)

Abstract

Background: Sheng Jiang San (SJS), a multi-herb formulation, is used in treating high fever, thirsty and anxiety in ancient China and it is sometimes used to treat seasonal influenza nowadays. However, there is no evidence-based investigation and mechanism research to support the anti-influenza efficacy of SJS. This study aims at evaluating the anti-influenza effect of SJS and investigating its possible mechanism.

Methods: The inhibitory effect of SJS against different influenza virus strains on MDCK cells was examined. Influenza virus infected BALB/c mice were employed to evaluate the efficacy as in vivo model. Mice challenged with A/PR/8/34 (H1N1) were orally administrated 1 g/kg/day of SJS for seven days and monitored for 14 days. The survival rate, body weight changes, lung index, lung viral load, histopathologic changes and immune regulation of the mice were measured. The underlying anti-influenza virus mechanism of SJS was studied by a series of biological assays to determine if hemagglutinin, ribonucleoprotein complex or neuraminidase were targets of SJS.

Results: Results showed SJS exerted a broad-spectrum of inhibitory effects on multiple influenza strains in a dose-dependent manner. IC_{50} of SJS against A/WSN/33 (H1N1) was lower than 35 μg/ml. SJS also protected 50% of mice from A/PR/8/34 (H1N1) infection. The lung index and the lung viral load of SJS treated mice were significantly decreased compared with untreated mice. Meanwhile, SJS targeted on neuraminidase of influenza virus as SJS at 2 mg/ml inhibited 80% of neuraminidase enzymatic activity. SJS also significantly down-regulated TNF-α and up-regulated IL-2 of influenza virus induced mice.

Conclusions: Thus, SJS is a useful formulation for treating influenza virus infection.

Keywords: Sheng Jiang san, Anti-influenza activity, Neuraminidase inhibition, Immune regulation

Background

Influenza is a contagious respiratory illness causing seasonal epidemics and occasional pandemics. The death toll of influenza epidemics is between 250,000 to 500,000. The frequent reassortment of influenza virus may cause high mortality and over-burden the healthcare system [1]. For example, the outbreak of 2009 H1N1 pandemic (swine flu) caused around 185,000 of people death [2]. The most recent 2013 H7N9 is the largest annual epidemics in China also caused significant morbidity and mortality [3].

To date, two classes of anti-influenza drugs are commonly used [4]. One consists of inhibitors of the M2 ion channel, such as amantadine and rimantadine. Treatment with these drugs results in the emergence of resistant strains thus it is not recommended for general use. The other consists of neuraminidase inhibitors, such as oseltamivir, zanamivir, laninamivir and peramivir. In addition,

* Correspondence: tihuihui@gzhmu.edu.cn; pcshaw@cuhk.edu.hk
[2]State Key Laboratory of Respiratory Disease, Guangdong Provincial Key Laboratory of Molecular Target & Clinical Pharmacology, School of Pharmaceutical Sciences and The Fifth Affiliated Hospital, Guangzhou Medical University, Guangzhou 510632, People's Republic of China
[1]School of Life Sciences, The Chinese University of Hong Kong, Shatin, N.T, Hong Kong, SAR 999077, People's Republic of China
Full list of author information is available at the end of the article

ribavirin and favipiravir (T-705) show anti-viral RNA polymerase effect [5, 6]. However, resistance against these drugs has already emerged in recent years [7]. These highlight the urgent need for new anti-influenza agents.

Traditional herbal medicine remains an under-explored, yet potentially fruitful basis for antiviral discovery [8]. In ancient China, some Chinese prescriptions were used to treat Wen Bing (Warm Disease), which is considered as influenza in modern time, with influenza-like symptoms, such as high fever, thirsty and anxiety [9]. To date, these prescriptions are still used in clinics by traditional Chinese medical practitioners. Also, in South China, multi-herb drink or "cooling herbal tea" is a convenient folk treatment against normal cold or mild influenza [10]. However, the efficacy of most of these products has not been vigorously tested. There is no conclusive experimental evidence to support the clinical efficacies of these prescriptions in treating influenza. Nevertheless, researchers have begun to evaluate the therapeutic values and underlying mechanism of selected prescriptions, including Chinese patent drugs and traditional Chinese prescriptions [11–13]. For example, Lianhua Qingwen capsule [14] was shown to have broad-spectrum efficacy on a number of influenza virus strains, through regulating the immune responses after virus infection. Kang Bing Du oral liquid [15] was found to reduce the susceptibility to influenza virus via mitochondrial antiviral signaling.

Sheng Jiang San (SJS) is a famous Chinese prescription that was originally recorded in a Traditional Chinese Medicine Classic Shanghan Wenyi Tiaobian of Qing Dynasty. SJS is composed of *Rhei Radix et Rhizoma*, *Bombyx Batryticatus*, *Cicadae Periostracum* and *Curcumae Longae Rhizoma* in a ratio of 4:2:1:3 (w/w/w/w). It has been prescribed in treating "Warm Disease". In modern time, traditional Chinese medical practitioners use it to treat seasonal influenza. However, there is no proper statistics on its clinical efficacy and revelation of the anti-influenza virus mechanism. Our preliminary test showed that it could indeed inhibit influenza A/WSN/33 (H1N1) in cell culture. As a contribution to increase the clinical value and the modernization of Chinese medicine, we set forth to examine the influenza inhibitory effect of SJS.

Currently, influenza virus infected mouse model is frequently used to test the in vivo influenza therapeutic efficacy of a drug [11–16]. In this study, except examining the inhibitory effect of SJS against different influenza virus strains on Madin-Darby canine kidney (MDCK) cells, we also used influenza virus infected BALB/c mice as an in vivo model to investigate the therapeutic action of SJS. The underlying anti-influenza virus mechanisms were studied by a battery of biological assays, which

include viral absorption and release, and the function of viral polymerase complex.

Methods
Reagents
Rhei Radix et Rhizoma, Bombyx Batryticatus, Cicadae Periostracum and *Curcumae Longae Rhizoma* were purchased from Zisun Chinese Pharmaceutical Co., Ltd. (Guangzhou, China). Standard compounds of rhein, chrysophanol, emodin, aloe emodin and curcumin were purchased from Chengdu Pufeide Biotechnology Co., Ltd. (Chengdu, China). Oseltamivir was purchased from Yichang Changjiang Pharcaceutical Co., Ltd. (Wuhan, China). Minimum essential medium (MEM), Dulbecco's modified eagle medium (DMEM) and fetal bovine serum (FBS) were purchased from Life Technologies (Gibco, NY, USA). Neuraminidase inhibitors screen kit (no. P0309) was purchased from Beyotime Institute of Biotechnology Co., Ltd. (Shanghai, China). Chicken erythrocytes were purchased from Lampire Biological Laboratories (PA, USA). Tolylsulfonyl phenylalanyl chloromethyl ketone (TPCK) treated-trypsin was purchased from Sigma-Aldrich (St. Louis, MO, USA). Mouse TNF-α, IFN-α and IL-2 Enzyme-linked immunosorbent assay (Elisa) kit were purchased from Invitrogen (Carlsbad, CA, USA). Water used in this study was purified by a Milli-Q system (Millipore, MA, USA). All culture plates were obtained from Greiner (Cellstar, Germany).

Preparation of SJS extract
The identities of *Rhei Radix et Rhizoma, Bombyx Batryticatus, Cicadae Periostracum* and *Curcumae Longae Rhizoma* were confirmed by an expert at the Institute of Chinese Medicine, The Chinese University of Hong Kong, by referring to their organoleptic characteristics. The voucher specimens were kept at Li Dak Sum Yip Yio Chin R & D Centre for Chinese Medicine, The Chinese University of Hong Kong. The aqueous extract of SJS was prepared by boiling the herbs at 4:2:1:3. The four ingredients in proportion were boiled twice with deionized water for 1 h each time. The aqueous extract was filtered and concentrated by a rotary evaporator under vacuum in a 60 °C water bath. Then the concentrated extract was lyophilized into powder under vacuum of 105×10^{-3} mbar and -40 °C. The freeze-dried powder was dissolved in culture medium or water before used.

Quality control is important in Chinese prescription, as the consistency will affect the repeatability of experiments and clinical efficacy. In light of this, a large amount of freeze-dried powder of SJS was prepared only once for studies to avoid composition differences between different batches of herbs. SJS powder was analyzed by high-performance liquid chromatography (Additional file 1) and the chemical profile is shown in Additional file 2: Figure S1. By comparing with reference compounds, rhein, chrysophanol, emodin, aloe emodin and curcumin were found.

Cells, viruses and animals

MDCK cells and human embryonic kidney 293 T (293 T) cells were obtained from American Type Culture Collection and routinely cultured in MEM and DMEM, respectively, supplemented with 10% FBS and incubated at 37 °C with 5% CO_2. Influenza A/WSN/33 (H1N1) (WSN), A/PR/8/34 (H1N1) (PR8), A/GZ/GIRD07/09 (H1N1), A/HK/8/68 (H3N2), A/Aichi/2/1968 (H3N2), A/HK/Y280/97 (H9N2), A/China/24/96 (H7N3), B/Lee/1940 (Flu B) were provided by Dr. Zifeng Yang (Guangzhou Institute of Respiratory Disease, China). All in vitro tests were performed in class II biosafety cabinet.

Specific-pathogen-free Balb/c mice weighing 14–16 g were used in this study. Mice were obtained from Guangdong Medical Laboratory Animal Center (Guangzhou, China). The animal experiments were carried out according to the Guidelines of Guangdong Regulation for the Administration of Laboratory Animals. The mice were kept in biosafety level 3 housing and provided with standard laboratory diet and water ad libitum.

Cytotoxicity assay

Cytotoxic effect of SJS was assessed by 3-(4,5-dimethylthiazol-2-yl)-2,5- diphenyltetrazolium bromide (MTT) assay. MDCK cells (2×10^5) were seeded on a 96-well culture plate in MEM with 10% FBS. After overnight culture, cells were treated with different concentration of SJS in MEM. After 24 h incubation at 37 °C, MTT (5 mg/ml) in phosphate buffered saline (PBS) was freshly prepared, 10 μl of MTT solution was added to each well and the plates were incubated at 37 °C for 4 h. The medium was then removed and formazan crystal was dissolved in dimethyl sulfoxide (DMSO) (100 μl/well). Then the absorbance at 570 nm was read by a CLARIOstar multi-mode microplate reader (BMG Labtech, Germany). The 50% toxic concentration (TC_{50}) was calculated as the concentration required to decrease 50% of cell viability.

Cytopathic effect inhibition (CPE) assay

80% confluent MDCK cells in a 96-well plate were infected with 0.01 MOI of influenza virus for 1 h at 37 °C. Afterwards, the viral inoculum was removed, and cells were washed twice with PBS. 100 μl SJS at different concentration in serum-free MEM with 1 μg/ml TPCK treated-trypsin (TPCK treated-trypsin was absent when MDCK cells were infected by WSN virus) was added to the cells. After incubating at 37 °C for 48 h, 10 μl of 5 mg/ml fresh MTT solution in PBS was added to each

well and the plates were incubated at 37 °C for 4 h. The medium was then removed and formazan crystal was dissolved in DMSO (100 μl/well). Absorbance at 570 nm was read by a CLARIOstar multi-mode microplate reader (BMG Labtech, Germany). The concentration that inhibited 50% of virus-induced cytopathic effect was determined as IC_{50}.

Plaque reduction assay

Confluent MDCK cells were seeded in 6-well plates in MEM with 10% FBS. Cells were infected with around 200 pfu per well of different viral strains for 1 h at 37 °C. The inoculum was aspirated to remove unbound viral particles, followed by washing with PBS. The MDCK monolayer was then overlaid with 1% low melting agarose (Cambrex) in MEM which contained different concentration of SJS and 1 μg/ml of TPCK treated-trypsin (TPCK treated-trypsin was absent when MDCK cells were infected by WSN virus). After incubating for 72 h at 37 °C, the agarose was removed and the cell monolayers were stained with staining solution (0.25% coomassie blue, 10% acetic acid, 50% methanol). The number of plaques was counted and the percentage of plaque inhibition relative to the control (no drug treatment) was calculated.

Multicycle growth assay

80% confluent MDCK cells were seeded in a 24-well plate. After infecting with 0.001 MOI of WSN for 1 h at 37 °C, the inoculum was removed and 500 μl of SJS (500 μg/ml, 125 μg/ml, 60 μg/ml) or oseltamivir (100 μM) in MEM, or 500 μl MEM only were added to the cells and incubated at 37 °C. The supernatants were then collected at 12, 24, 48 and 72 h post infection. The virus titers were determined by plaque assay as described previously [17].

Hemagglutination inhibition assay

Twofold serial dilution of SJS was prepared in 25 μl of PBS in a 96-well U-bottom plate. WSN in 25 μl of PBS (4 HA units) was added to each dilution and mixed well, and the plate was incubated for 30 min at room temperature. Then, 50 μl of chicken erythrocytes in PBS (0.05% v/v) was added to each well and mixed thoroughly. The reaction was observed after incubating the plates at room temperature for another 30 min. Pentagalloylglucose (PGG) was used as a positive control [18] while oseltamivir was a negative control [19].

Ribonucleoprotein (RNP) reconstitution assay

2×10^6 of 293 T cells were seeded on a 6 cm dish and incubated overnight in DMEM with 10% FBS. Plasmids pcDNA3a-PB1, pcDNA3a-PB2, pcDNA3a-PA, pcDNA3a-NP, pPOL-NS-Luci (kindly provided by Dr. Ervin Fodor,

University of Oxford, UK) were transfected to 293 T cells with Lipofectamine 2000 (Invitrogen, CA, USA) to reconstitute the RNP complex. The RNP complex consisted of WSN polymerase proteins PA, PB1 and PB2, NP and a luciferase reporter gene. Plasmid pEGFP was also co-transfected to 293 T cells as an internal control to normalize the transfection efficiency. After 6 h of transfection, transfected cells were trypsinized and aliquoted into a 96-well plate. SJS at different concentration dissolved in DMEM was added into each well. After incubating for 24 h at 37 °C, the cell lysates were harvested and the luciferase activity was assayed with a luciferase reporter assay system kit (Promega, No. E1910). The luminescence was read by a CLARIOstar multi-mode microplate reader (BMG Labtech, Germany).

Neuraminidase (NA) inhibition assay
A neuraminidase inhibitors screen kit was employed to evaluate the inhibition of SJS on the NA enzymatic activity. The assay followed the instruction manual. 70 μl of reaction buffer, 10 μl of NA and 10 μl of SJS at different concentration were well mixed in a black 96-well microplate. After incubating at 37 °C for 2 min, 10 μl of substrate was added into each well, mixed thoroughly and incubated for 1 h. Fluorescence was measured with a CLARIOstar multi-mode microplate reader (BMG Labtech, Germany) at an excitation wavelength of 322 nm and an emission wavelength of 450 nm. Oseltamivir acid [19] was used as a positive control. The NA activity inhibitory percentage was calculated as follow:

$$\text{NA inhibition}\ (\%) = (F_{control} - F_{SJS})/(F_{control} - F_{blank})$$
$$\times 100\%(F : \text{Fluorescence intensity}).$$

Anti-influenza virus test in mouse model
Mice were randomly divided into vehicle group, SJS group, oseltamivir group and untreated group, with 16 mice in each group. Except the vehicle group, other groups were anaesthetized with ethyl ether and inoculated intranasally with 3 LD_{50} (50% lethal dose) of mouse-adapted PR8 virus in a volume of 50 μl. At 4 h after inoculation, SJS group and oseltamivir group were treated by gavage feeding with SJS solution (dissolved in water at a dose of 1 g/kg/day) or oseltamivir solution (dissolved in water at a dose of 90 mg/kg/day) in a volume of 200 μl, respectively. Then these two groups were administrated orally once daily for seven consecutive days. Untreated group and vehicle group were fed with water. Parameters of mice such as mortality, body weight and general conditions were monitered for consecutive 14 days.

Three mice from each group were randomly selected and sacrificed on the fourth day post-inoculation for lung index calculation, lung viral load titer and lung cytokine expression analysis. Another three mice from each group were also sacrificed on the sixth day post-inoculation for histopathologic observation. The sacrificed mice were euthanized by cervical dislocation after fully anaesthetization by inhaling diethyl ether. The remaining ten mice in each group were monitored continuously for 14 consecutive days to study their mortality and body weight changes.

Lung index
Four days after virus infection, mice were weighed and their lung tissues were extracted and washed with PBS, dried by gauze and then weighed. Lung index was calculated as follow:

$$\text{Lung index} = \text{lung weight/body weight} \times 100\%.$$

Lung viral load titer
After weighing the lung tissues, they were homogenized in MEM by a refiner (Qiagen, TissueRuptor) and centrifuged at 12000 rpm for 5 min at 4 °C. The lung homogenates were aliquoted and stored at − 80 °C. The virus titer of these homogenates were determined by plaque assay [17] on MDCK cells.

Lung cytokine expression analysis
Part of the lung homogenates was used to perform lung cytokine expression analysis with mouse cytokines Elisa kits of TNF-α, IFN-α and IL-2 (Invitrogen). The content of TNF-α, IFN-α and IL-2 were assessed according to the manufacturer's protocol. Absorbance at 450 nm was read by a spectro-photometer (Thermo Scentific).

Histopathologic observation
Six days after virus infection, lung tissues were extracted from three randomly sacrificed mice from each group. The lungs were immersed in 10% formaldehyde solution immediately and embedded in paraffin. Then the lung tissue was cut into 4 μm-thick sections. Tissue sections were stained with hematoxylin and eosin for observating the histopathologic changes under microscope.

Statistics
All statistical analyses were conducted with Graphpad Prism 6.0 (Graphpad, San Diego, CA, USA) and data were presented as mean ± SD. One-way ANOVA was used for multiple-group comparison. Differences were considered statistically significant when $p < 0.05$ (*$p < 0.05$, **$p < 0.01$, ***$p < 0.001$).

Results

Anti-influenza activity of SJS against multiple virus strains

To determine the inhibitory activity of SJS against the cytopathic effect induced by different viral strains, CPE was performed. Plaque reduction assay was also performed to confirm the antiviral efficacy of SJS on A/WSN/33 (H1N1), A/PR/8/34 (H1N1), A/GZ/GIRD07/09 (H1N1), A/Aichi/2/1968 (H3N2), A/HK/Y280/97 (H9N2) and A/China/24/96 (H7N3). B/Lee/1940 (Flu B) was only tested by CPE assay. The IC_{50} on each strain was calculated based on the results of CPE assay and is shown in Table 1. SJS had a $TC_{50} > 2$ mg/ml measured by cytotoxicity assay. The selective index (SI) of each strain was also calculated and shown in Table 1. The IC_{50} was ranging from 34.7 to 750.8 μg/ml, and SI was ranging from 2.7 to 57.7. SJS showed the best inhibitory effect on WSN virus ($IC_{50} = 34.7$ and $SI = 57.7$). According to the results of plaque reduction assay, SJS inhibited the virus strains in a dose-dependent manner. It inhibited the growth of all the seven viruses (200 pfu per well) to 100% at less than 1 mg/ml (Fig. 1a).

To evaluate the influence of SJS on viral progeny, MDCK cells were treated with SJS at 125 μg/ml and 500 μg/ml after infected with WSN virus (MOI = 0.001). The supernatant with replicated virus was collected at 12, 24, 48 and 72 h, and the viral titer at each time point was measured by plaque assay. As shown in Fig. 1b, SJS severely suppressed the WSN viral multicycle growth at 500 μg/ml. On the other hand, oseltamivir as a positive control inhibited viral production at 200 μM at 72 h. This indicated that SJS had a pronounced effect on suppressing the WSN growth.

SJS did not act on HA and RNP complex

To determine whether SJS could inhibit hemagglutinin of virus particles for binding to cell surface receptors, hemagglutination inhibition assay was performed. Influenza virus can agglutinate erythrocytes by means of hemagglutination, then erythrocytes become cross-linked and form lattice. In this assay, chicken erythrocytes

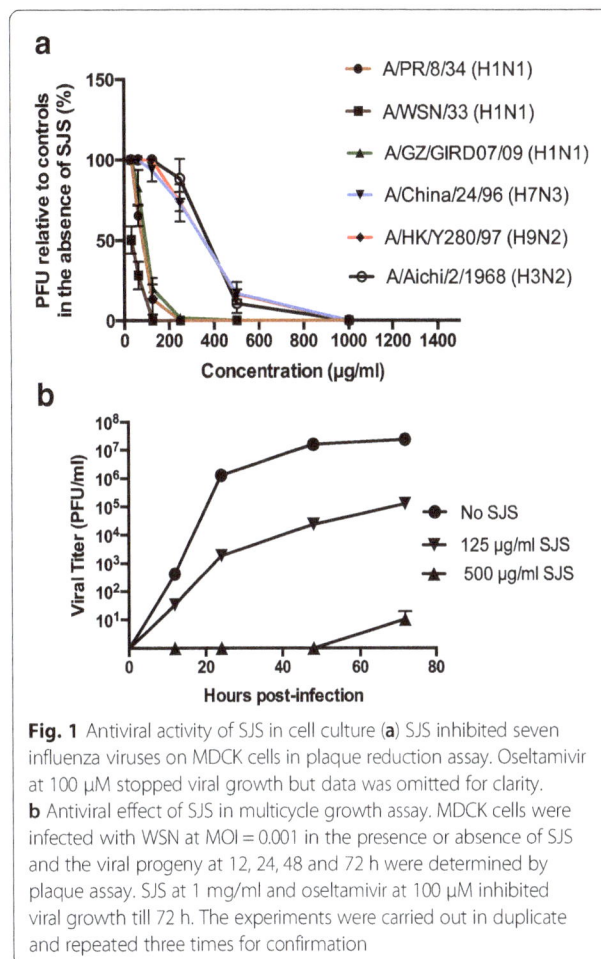

Fig. 1 Antiviral activity of SJS in cell culture (**a**) SJS inhibited seven influenza viruses on MDCK cells in plaque reduction assay. Oseltamivir at 100 μM stopped viral growth but data was omitted for clarity. **b** Antiviral effect of SJS in multicycle growth assay. MDCK cells were infected with WSN at MOI = 0.001 in the presence or absence of SJS and the viral progeny at 12, 24, 48 and 72 h were determined by plaque assay. SJS at 1 mg/ml and oseltamivir at 100 μM inhibited viral growth till 72 h. The experiments were carried out in duplicate and repeated three times for confirmation

showed a lattice appearance when treated with SJS at 63–500 μg/ml (in two-fold serial dilution) in the presence of WSN virus (4 HA units) (Fig. 2a). Chicken erythrocytes treated with the positive control PGG at 6–50 μM and WSN virus showed red spot like appearance, indicating the inhibition of hamagglutination. Oseltamivir, on the other hand, had no effect on HA. When WSN was absent, SJS and PGG treatment also showed a red spot appearance, which indicated they had no influence to chicken erythrocytes.

Influenza RNP reconstitution assay was performed to evaluate if SJS inhibited the viral RNP activity. SJS were added to 293 T cells transfected with WSN minigenomes to 250, 500 and 1000 μg/ml. Luciferase activity was measured after 24 h post-transfection. Nucleozin [16], an NP inhibitor, was used as a positive control in the assay. As shown in Fig. 2b, the luciferase activity in the presence of SJS had no obvious differences with the untreated control, while nucleozin inhibited the luciferase activity significantly.

Thus, SJS did not interfere with the absorption of WSN towards the target cells or viral polymerase activity.

Table 1 Antiviral activity of SJS against different influenza virus strain

Viral strains	IC_{50}[a] (μg/ml)	SI^b (>)
A/PR/8/34 (H1N1)	198.47	10.08
A/WSN/33 (H1N1)	34.66	57.70
A/GZ/GIRD07/09 (H1N1)	78.56	25.46
A/China/24/96 (H7N3)	371.13	5.39
A/HK/Y280/97 (H9N2)	353.55	5.66
A/Aichi/2/1968 (H3N2)	360.73	5.54
B/Lee/1940 (Flu B)	750.79	2.66

[a]Mean of the results from three independent experiments
[b]The SI (selectivity index) was calculated as the ratio of TC_{50} to IC_{50}

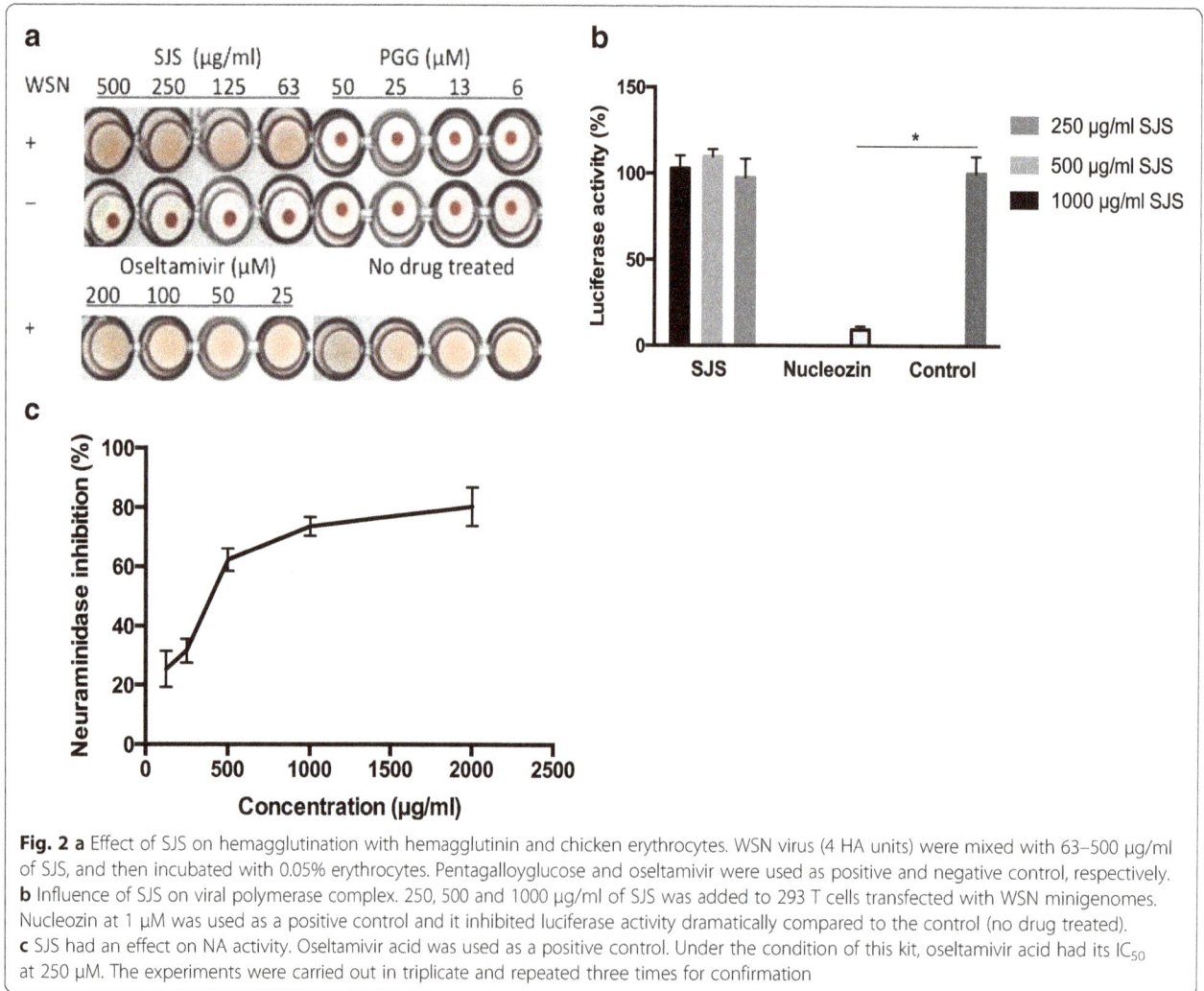

Fig. 2 a Effect of SJS on hemagglutination with hemagglutinin and chicken erythrocytes. WSN virus (4 HA units) were mixed with 63–500 µg/ml of SJS, and then incubated with 0.05% erythrocytes. Pentagalloylglucose and oseltamivir were used as positive and negative control, respectively. **b** Influence of SJS on viral polymerase complex. 250, 500 and 1000 µg/ml of SJS was added to 293 T cells transfected with WSN minigenomes. Nucleozin at 1 µM was used as a positive control and it inhibited luciferase activity dramatically compared to the control (no drug treated). **c** SJS had an effect on NA activity. Oseltamivir acid was used as a positive control. Under the condition of this kit, oseltamivir acid had its IC_{50} at 250 µM. The experiments were carried out in triplicate and repeated three times for confirmation

SJS inhibited NA activity

To explore if SJS affected NA enzymatic activity, NA inhibitory assay was conducted using a commercial neuraminidase inhibitors screen kit. Two-fold serial dilutions from 125 µg/ml to 2000 µg/ml of SJS extract were tested. NA activity was measured by fluorescence of 4-methylumbelliferone, which was the product of substrate (4-Methylumbelliferyl)-a-D-N-acetylneuraminic acid sodium salt hydrate catalyzed by the enzymatic activity of NA. Results showed that at 2 mg/ml of SJS, NA activity was inhibited up to 80% (Fig. 2(c)). Oseltamivir acid was used as a positive control and it inhibited 50% NA activity at 250 µM.

SJS improved survival rate of PR8-infected mice

To evaluate the in vivo antiviral efficacy of SJS, groups of mice were inoculated with 3 LD_{50} of mouse lung-adapted viral strain PR8 and orally administrated SJS for seven consecutive days, while vehicle group and untreated group were administrated with water instead. Vehicle control group showed normal appearance and behaviors during the 14-day observation. Mice in the untreated group all died before the 8th day post-inoculation of virus. They also showed inactive, ruffled fur and respiratory distress signs. Mice orally administrated with SJS daily had their life span prolonged. This group showed mortality on day 9 post-inoculation and up to 50% mice survived after 14 days (Fig. 3a). Besides, the average body weight of SJS group rebound on day 9 post-inoculation, similar to the positive control (oseltamivir) group (Fig. 3b). These results suggested that SJS at 1 g/kg/day had significant protective effect on mice infected with PR8 virus.

SJS reduced lung index, lung viral load and alleviated lung histopathologic changes of PR8 virus infected mice.

Three mice from each group were euthanized on day 4 post-inoculation and their lungs were extracted for lung index measurement and lung viral load titer. Compared with the untreated group, SJS at 1 g/kg/day significantly

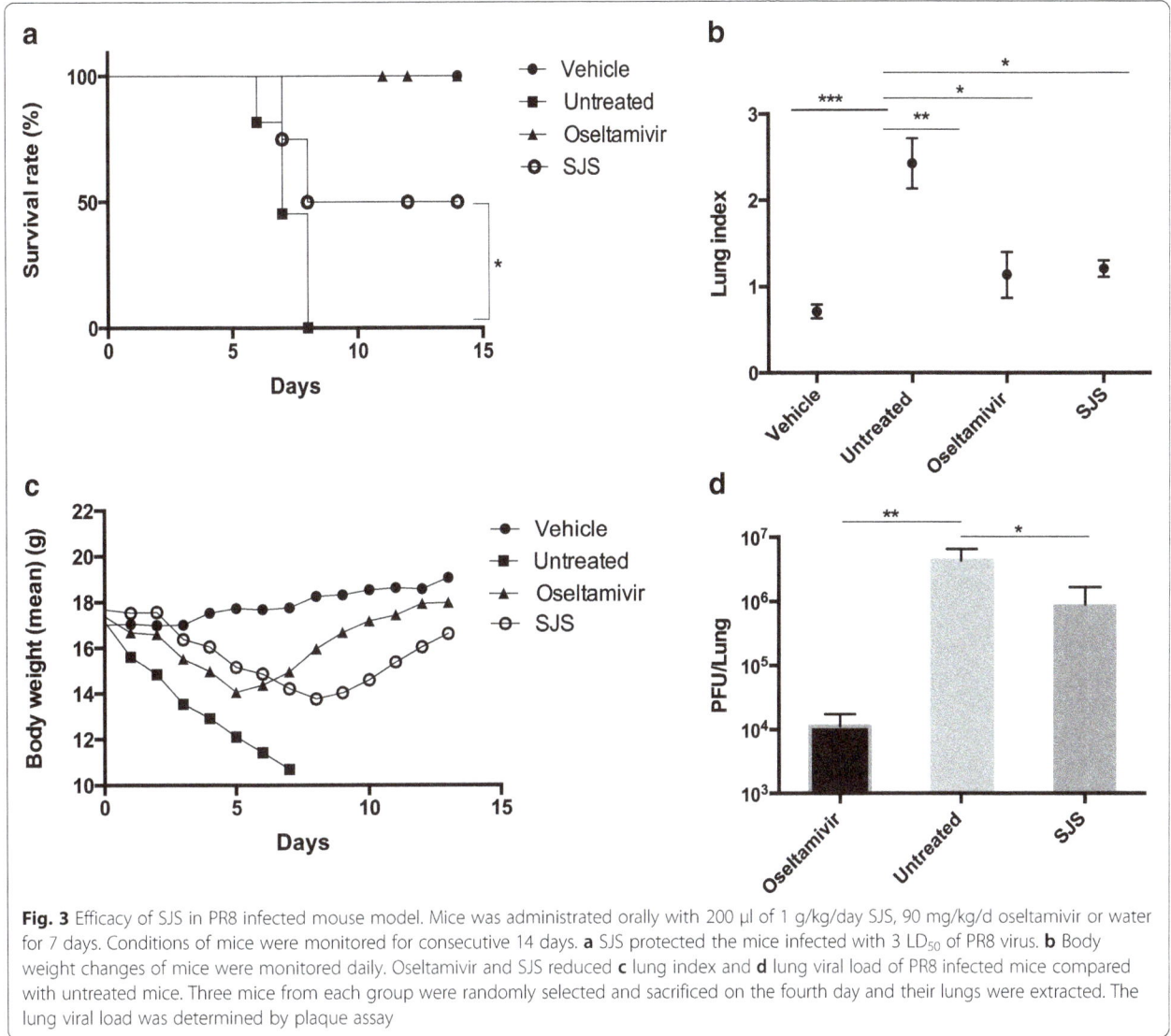

Fig. 3 Efficacy of SJS in PR8 infected mouse model. Mice was administrated orally with 200 μl of 1 g/kg/day SJS, 90 mg/kg/d oseltamivir or water for 7 days. Conditions of mice were monitored for consecutive 14 days. **a** SJS protected the mice infected with 3 LD_{50} of PR8 virus. **b** Body weight changes of mice were monitored daily. Oseltamivir and SJS reduced **c** lung index and **d** lung viral load of PR8 infected mice compared with untreated mice. Three mice from each group were randomly selected and sacrificed on the fourth day and their lungs were extracted. The lung viral load was determined by plaque assay

decreased the mice lung index (Fig. 3c) and inhibited the lung viral load (Fig. 3d).

Another three mice were also euthanized on the sixth day post-inoculation for observating the histopathologic changes. As shown in Fig. 4, untreated group showed pronounced lung inflammation, characterized by interstitial expansion, edema and inflammatory cell infiltration around small vessels. Inflammation cells could be observed in alveolar lumen. For SJS group, the histopathology was alleviated and mild lesions were observed. Less inflammatory cells were exuded and infiltrated around vessels and interstitial space. The results of lung index and

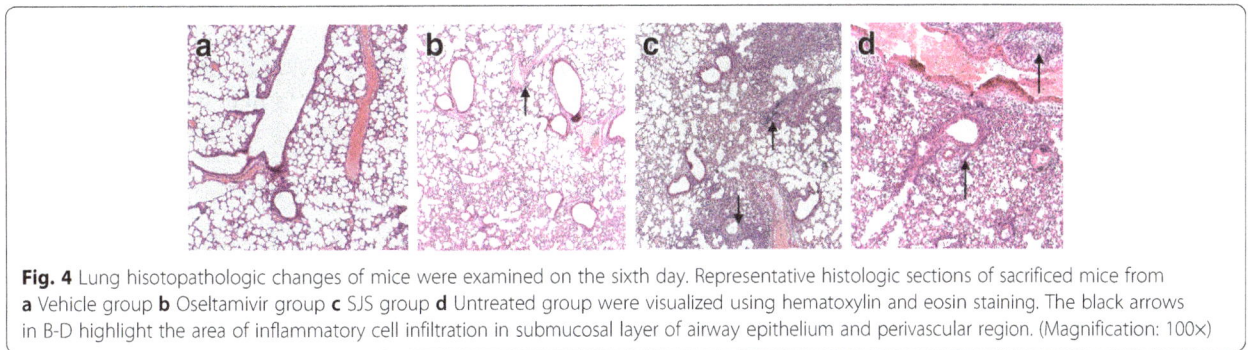

Fig. 4 Lung hisotopathologic changes of mice were examined on the sixth day. Representative histologic sections of sacrificed mice from **a** Vehicle group **b** Oseltamivir group **c** SJS group **d** Untreated group were visualized using hematoxylin and eosin staining. The black arrows in B-D highlight the area of inflammatory cell infiltration in submucosal layer of airway epithelium and perivascular region. (Magnification: 100×)

lung viral load following SJS treatment indicated that SJS treatment alleviated lung pathology and lesion of PR8 infected mice.

Effect of SJS on lung cytokine expression

To determine the inflammatory markers after SJS treatment, part of the lung homogenates collected on day 4 post-inoculation was used for Elisa assay on the level of cytokine TNF-α, IFN-α and IL-2 (Fig. 5). For the former two markers, their expression in infected group increased significantly compared with the vehicle group. Oseltamivir and SJS treatment both decreased the expression level of these two cytokines after PR8 infection, though IFN-α was only slightly reduced. Cytokine IL-2 in mice lung decreased after PR8 infection, oseltamivir and SJS displayed the same tendency that they increased the level of IL-2. In this Elisa analysis, SJS also showed better regulatory activity on TNF-α and IFN-α than oseltamivir group. These results showed that SJS could reduce the inflammatory responses in mice.

Discussion

SJS is a classical Chinese formulation for treating influenza virus infection. However, there has been no systematic study to substantiate the anti-influenza efficacy. The mechanism of SJS action also remained unclear.

We first found that SJS could inhibit flu A and B strains on MDCK cell line at less than 750 μg/ml, showing that SJS has a broad-spectrum inhibitory activity to influenza viruses. We also showed that SJS could protect mice from PR8 infection. Compared with the untreated group, SJS could significantly improve the survival rate and prolong the average survival day, also help the body weight of the mice to rebound. SJS treated mice not only had a lower lung viral load but also had reduced lung index and alleviated histopathology, suggesting that SJS might work on the virus directly and SJS could also decrease the lung injury induced by PR8 infection. Compared with oseltamivir, SJS is less effective in protecting

PR8 infected mice. However, considering that the formulation containing many phytochemicals, with each in a minute quantity, there is a high chance to have some potent fractions or phytochemicals in the extract.

Previous reports pointed out that over-expression of TNF-α and IFN-α induced by influenza virus is a cause of lung inflammation and can in turn result in tissue injury [20, 21]. In contrast, IL-2 decreases after infected by influenza virus and lower expression of IL-2 causes dysfunction of immune system [11]. In this study, the expression level of three cytokines (TNF-α, IFN-α, IL-2) after PR8 virus infection was examined. Our data showed SJS was beneficial to PR8 infected mice, as SJS could down-regulate TNF-α and up-regulate IL-2. The expression level of IFN-α under treatment of SJS also showed a down-regulatory trend, although there was no statistically significant difference with the untreated group. Meanwhile, compared with the treatment of oseltamivir, SJS showed a stronger regulation on the expression of these cytokines (Fig. 5). Thus, besides inhibiting virus replication directly through targeting on NA, SJS might also protect the mice through regulating the expression of cytokines. We are in the process of carrying out bioassay-guided fractionation to find the pure phytochemicals that inhibit NA and regulate the concerned cytokines.

As influenza infection is a common disease, there are many cold and flu herbal remedies in the market, such as Chinese patent drugs, traditional Chinese prescriptions, or even cooling herbal tea. However, their efficacy in treating influenza is not well investigated. Our research has provided an example on the evidence-based research on an anti-influenza formulation, which involves virus inhibitory studies in cell culture, animal model and mechanism elucidation. The work may be extended to other traditional or folk medicine, which will strengthen the confidence on their clinical uses and for downstream development of these formulations.

Conclusions

In this study, a Chinese prescription SJS was found to inhibit a number of influenza virus strains and act against influenza virus PR8 in mice. SJS exhibited anti-influenza activity through inhibiting NA activity and regulating cytokine expression. Our work has substantiated that SJS is an effective anti-influenza formulation, which may be further developed by the pharmaceutical industry.

Additional files

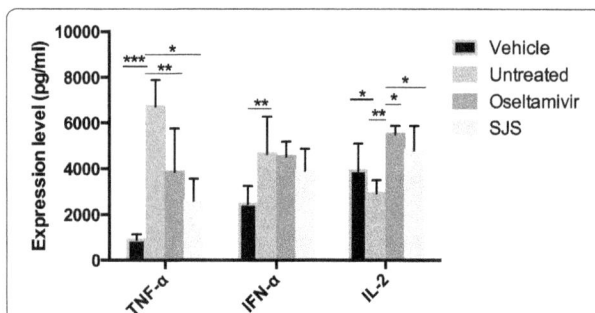

Fig. 5 Influence of SJS on cytokine expression in mouse lung infected with PR8 virus. The cytokine expression level of TNF-α, IFN-α and IL-2 was analyzed using Elisa. The experiments were carried out in triplicate and repeated three times for confirmation

Additional file 1: Method of High-performance liquid chromatography (HPLC) analysis of SJS. HPLC method was used to analyze the chemical profile of SJS. The HPLC condition is described in this additional file and the profile is shown in Additional file 2: Figure S1. By comparing with reference compounds, rhein, chrysophanol, emodin, aloe emodin and curcumin were found.

Additional file 2: Figure S1. HPLC analysis of SJS (a) HPLC profile of SJS (b) Some constituents were denoted by standard compounds.

Abbreviations
CPE: Cytopathic effect inhibition; DMEM: Dulbecco's Modified Eagle Medium; DMSO: Dimethyl sulfoxide; Elisa: Enzyme-linked immunosorbent assay; FBS: Fetal bovine serum; HA: Hemagglutinin; IC_{50}: 50% inhibitory concentration; IFN: Interferon; IL: Interleukin; LD_{50}: 50% lethal dose; MDCK: Madin-Darby canine kidney; MEM: Minimum essential medium; MOI: Multiplicity of infection; MTT: 3-(4,5-dimethylthiazol-2-yl)-2,5-diphenyltetrazolium bromide; NA: Neuraminidase; NP: Nucleoprotein; PA: Polymerase acidic protein; PB1: Polymerase basic protein 1; PB2: Polymerase basic protein 2; PBS: Phosphate buffered saline; Pfu: Plaque forming unit; PGG: Pentagalloylglucose; PR8: A/PR/8/34 (H1N1); RNP: Ribonucleoprotein; SI: Selective index; SJS: Sheng Jiang San; TC_{50}: 50% toxic concentration; TNF: Tumor necrosis factor; TPCK: Tolylsulfonyl phenylalanyl chloromethyl ketone; WSN: A/WSN/33 (H1N1)

Acknowledgements
The authors would like to extend their sincere appreciation to Dr. Zifeng Yang (Guangzhou Institute of Respiratory Disease, China) and Dr. Ervin Fodor (University of Oxford, UK) for providing viruses and plasmids respectively.

Funding
This work was supported in part by a Theme-based grant (Project No. T11-705/14 N) of the Research Grants Council of Hong Kong HKSAR and a grant from the National Natural Science Foundation of China (no. 31401662) and Science research project of the Guangdong Province (no. 2016A050503047).

Authors' contributions
TBZ, HHT, PCS co-conceived the study and designed the experiments. MJX, TBZ, XZ and HHT conducted the cell biology tests. MJX and HHT performed the animal experiments. CKW, KPM and PCS carried on the mechanisms investigation and data analysis. TBZ and PCS contributed to draft the manuscript. All authors read and approved the final manuscript.

Competing interests
The authors declare that they have no competing interests.

Author details
[1]School of Life Sciences, The Chinese University of Hong Kong, Shatin, N.T, Hong Kong, SAR 999077, People's Republic of China. [2]State Key Laboratory of Respiratory Disease, Guangdong Provincial Key Laboratory of Molecular Target & Clinical Pharmacology, School of Pharmaceutical Sciences and The Fifth Affiliated Hospital, Guangzhou Medical University, Guangzhou 510632, People's Republic of China. [3]Guangzhou Institutes of Biomedicine and Health, Chinese Academy of Science, Guangzhou 510632, People's Republic of China. [4]Department of Chemical Pathology, The Chinese University of Hong Kong, Prince of Wales Hospital, Shatin, N.T, Hong Kong, SAR 999077, People's Republic of China. [5]Institute of Chinese Medicine and State Key Laboratory of Phytochemistry and Plant Resources in West China, the Chinese University of Hong Kong, Shatin, N.T, Hong Kong, SAR 999077, People's Republic of China. [6]HKU-Pasteur Research Pole, School of Public Health, Li Ka Shing Faculty of Medicine, The University of Hong Kong, Pok Fu Lam, Hong Kong, SAR 999077, People's Republic of China. [7]Li Dak Sum Yip Yio Chin R & D Centre for Chinese Medicine, The Chinese University of Hong Kong, Shatin, N.T, Hong Kong, SAR 999077, P. R. China.

References
1. Regoes RR, Bonhoeffer S. Emergence of drug-resistant influenza virus: population dynamical considerations. Science. 2006;312(5772):389–91.
2. Klenk HD, Garten W, Matrosovich M. Molecular mechanisms of interspecies transmission and pathogenicity of influenza viruses: lessons from the 2009 pandemic. BioEssays. 2011;33(3):180–8.
3. Yang S, Chen Y, Cui D, Yao H, Lou J, Huo Z, Xie G, Yu F, Zheng S, Yang Y, et al. Avian-origin influenza a(H7N9) infection in influenza a(H7N9)-affected areas of China: a serological study. J Infect Dis. 2014;209(2):265–9.
4. Kamali A, Holodniy M. Influenza treatment and prophylaxis with neuraminidase inhibitors: a review. Infect Drug Resist. 2013;6:187–98.
5. Furuta Y, Takahashi K, Kuno-Maekawa M, Sangawa H, Uehara S, Kozaki K, Nomura N, Egawa H, Shiraki K. Mechanism of action of T-705 against influenza virus. Antimicrob Agents Chemother. 2005;49(3):981–6.
6. Vanderlinden E, Vrancken B, Van Houdt J, Rajwanshi VK, Gillemot S, Andrei G, Lemey P, Naesens L. Distinct effects of T-705 (Favipiravir) and ribavirin on influenza virus replication and viral RNA synthesis. Antimicrob Agents Chemother. 2016;60(11):6679–91.
7. Bai GR, Chittaganpitch M, Kanai Y, Li YG, Auwanit W, Ikuta K, Sawanpanyalert P. Amantadine- and oseltamivir-resistant variants of influenza a viruses in Thailand. Biochem Biophys Res Commun. 2009;390(3):897–901.
8. Newman DJ, Cragg GM. Natural products as sources of new drugs over the 30 years from 1981 to 2010. J Nat Prod. 2012;75(3):311–35.
9. Koh A. Wen Bing (warm diseases) and the 2009 H1N1 influenza. Australian journal of acupuncture and. Chin Med. 2010;5(2):23–9.
10. Liu Y, Ahmed S, Long C. Ethnobotanical survey of cooling herbal drinks from southern China. J Ethnobiol Ethnomed. 2013;9:82.
11. Wu QF, Zhu WR, Yan YL, Zhang XX, Jiang YQ, Zhang FL. Anti-H1N1 influenza effects and its possible mechanism of Huanglian Xiangru decoction. J Ethnopharmacol. 2016;185:282–8.
12. Peng XQ, Zhou HF, Zhang YY, Yang JH, Wan HT, He Y. Antiviral effects of Yinhuapinggan granule against influenza virus infection in the ICR mice model. J Nat Med. 2016;70(1):75–88.
13. Rong R, Li RR, Hou YB, Li J, Ding JX, Zhang CB, Yang Y. Mahuang-Xixin-Fuzi decoction reduces the infection of influenza a virus in kidney-Yang deficiency syndrome mice. J Ethnopharmacol. 2016;192:217–24.
14. Ding Y, Zeng L, Li R, Chen Q, Zhou B, Chen Q, Cheng PL, Yutao W, Zheng J, Yang Z, et al. The Chinese prescription lianhuaqingwen capsule exerts anti-influenza activity through the inhibition of viral propagation and impacts immune function. BMC Complement Altern Med. 2017;17(1):130.
15. Chen H, Jie C, Tang LP, Meng H, Li XB, Li YB, Chen LX, Yan C, Kurihara H, Li YF, et al. New insights into the effects and mechanism of a classic traditional Chinese medicinal formula on influenza prevention. Phytomedicine. 2017;27:52–62.
16. Kao RY, Yang D, Lau LS, Tsui WH, Hu L, Dai J, Chan MP, Chan CM, Wang P, Zheng BJ, et al. Identification of influenza a nucleoprotein as an antiviral target. Nat Biotechnol. 2010;28(6):600–5.
17. Gaush CR, Smith TF. Replication and plaque assay of influenza virus in an established line of canine kidney cells. Appl Microbiol. 1968;16(4):588–94.
18. Liu G, Xiong S, Xiang YF, Guo CW, Ge F, Yang CR, Zhang YJ, Wang YF, Kitazato K. Antiviral activity and possible mechanisms of action of pentagalloylglucose (PGG) against influenza a virus. Arch Virol. 2011;156(8):1359–69.
19. Bardsley-Elliot A, Noble S. Oseltamivir. Drugs. 1999;58(5):851–60. discussion 861-852
20. Vervelde L, Reemers SS, van Haarlem DA, Post J, Claassen E, Rebel JM, Jansen CA. Chicken dendritic cells are susceptible to highly pathogenic avian influenza viruses which induce strong cytokine responses. Dev Comp Immunol. 2013;39(3):198–206.
21. Loo YM, Gale M Jr. Influenza: fatal immunity and the 1918 virus. Nature. 2007;445(7125):267–8.

Comparative efficacy of Chinese herbal injections for treating chronic heart failure

Kai-Huan Wang, Jia-Rui Wu[*] , Dan Zhang, Xiao-Jiao Duan and Meng-Wei Ni

Abstract

Background: On account of deterioration of chronic heart failure (CHF) and extensive exploration of Chinese herbal injections (CHIs), we performed a network meta-analysis to investigate the efficacy of CHIs (Huangqi injection, Shenfu injection, Shengmai injection, Shenmai injection, Shenqi Fuzheng injection, Yiqifumai injection) on the basis of western medicine (WM) treatment in CHF.

Methods: Literature search was conducted in Embase, the Cochrane Library, Pubmed, Chinese Biological Medicine Database, China National Knowledge Infrastructure, Wanfang Database, Chinese Scientific Journal Database from inception to June 12nd 2017, and study selection was abided by a prior eligible criteria.

Results: Ultimately, a total of 113 randomized controlled trials (RCTs) were enrolled. The clinical data of the effective clinical rate, left ventricular ejection fraction, cardiac output and others outcomes was estimated by Stata software and Winbugs software. Risk of bias was assessed by Cochrane Collaboration's tools. Integrating the each outcome's results, a combination of Shengmai injection/Shenmai injection and WM obtain a first rank in most outcomes, particularly primary outcomes.

Conclusions: In conclusion, on the basis of WM, Shengmai injection or Shenmai injection may be a perforable treatment in CHF. In terms of insufficient of this study, more high quality RCTs needed to implement to support our conclusions.

Keywords: Network meta-analysis (NMA), Chronic heart failure (CHF), Chinese herbal injection (CHI)

Background

Chronic heart failure (CHF) refers to a pathologic condition that cardiac output is absolute or relative reduce and cannot meet the whole body tissue metabolism under the normal venous return, then result in decreasing the myocardial contractile force and ventricular compliance, ultimately dyspnea, edema, feeble and so on. It was estimated that five-year survival rate of CHF was lower as malignant tumor and CHF was a main reason of disability and death on a global scale [1–3]. Impaired cardiac function of CHF patients may lessen their ability of daily living and render them a heavy economic pressure [1, 4]. At present, the primary aims of alleviating CHF symptoms are to inhibit myocardial

remodeling, and perfect cardiac function [5]. Therefore, angiotensin-converting enzyme inhibitors (ACEIs), angiotensin II receptor blockers (ARBs), digoxin, and diuretics are become standard western medicine (WM) treatment in CHF [6], while it cannot obtain a desired effect own to poor compliance, lower heart rate of patients and others questions [5]. In consideration of its limitations, the application of Chinese herbal injections (CHIs) could be promoted. Currently, a combination between CHIs and WM treatment has already been a supportive measure in treatment of CHF in China. In accordance with traditional Chinese medicine (TCM) theories, CHF pertain to "heart impediment (xin bi)", "palpitation", "edema" and so forth, which caused by heart and then affect others organs. The clinical principle is to strengthen the body resistance to eliminate pathogenic factors [2]. Due to the relative low recognition of CHIs in CHF, this study selected six CHIs

* Correspondence: exogamy@163.com
Department of Clinical Pharmacology of Traditional Chinese Medicine,
School of Chinese Materia Medica, Beijing University of Chinese Medicine,
Beijing 100102, China

commonly used in CHF treatment, all of them were autho-rized by China Food and Drug Administration (CFDA), namely Huangqi injection (HQI), Shenfu injection (SFI), Shengmai injection (SI), Shenmai injection (SMI), Shenqi Fuzheng injection (SQFZI), Yiqifumai injection (YQFMI), to explore and rank their efficacy in CHF by the approach of network meta-analysis (NMA). Compared with conven-tional pairwise meta-analysis, NMA can sort the interven-tions via indirect comparison [7]. At the same time, the clinical trials compared those six CHIs head to head was lack. Thus, an attempt to conduct a NMA was necessarily. The goal of this study was to provide evidence-based hier-archies of the comparative efficacy and more insights for selection of CHF treatment.

Methods
The study was congrunt with The Prisma Extension Statement for Reporting of Systematic Reviews Incorpor-ating Network Meta-analyses of Health Care Interven-tions [8]. And the Prisma check list was displayed in Additional file 1.

Eligibility criteria and study selection
A study was considered eligible if it suited for these cri-teria: 1) randomized controlled trial (RCT); 2) patients enrolled were diagnosed as CHF according to "Guide-lines on the Diagnosis and Treatment of Heart Failure" conducted by The Chinese medical association cardio-vascular epidemiology branch in 2014 [9] or "Clinical Guideline of New Drugs for Traditional Chinese Medi-cine" released by CFDA in 2002 [10]. Both of them con-tained both western diagnostics, the latter included TCM diagnostics as well; 3) patients receive WM treat-ment (e.g. cardiotonic, diuretic, ACEIs, β-blocker and so forth), meanwhile patients needed relevant therapy if they had complications during therapeutic process. On the basis of it, the treatment group received one of the included CHIs, the control group received another or just adopted WM. Besides, the dosages of CHIs were re-ported; 4) RCTs tested the clinical effective rate. The clinical effective rate calculated by this formula: (number of remarkable recovery patients + number of basic recovery patients) / total number of patients * 100%. Cardiac function classification was conformed to the standard issued by New York Heart Association (NYHA) in the United States. Clinical symptoms disappeared and cardiac function improved 2 levels at least was deemed as the class of remarkable recovery, clinical symptoms relieved and cardiac function increase 1 level was classi-fied into the part of basic recovery, clinical symptoms and cardiac function was unaltered or worse belonged to deterioration. Besides, the incidence of left ventricular ejection fraction (LVEF), cardiac output (CO), stroke volume (SV), 6-min walk test (6MWT), brain natriuretic

peptide (BNP), left ventricular end-diastolic dimension (LVEDD), left ventricular end-systolic dimension (LVESD), adverse drug reactions/adverse drug events (ADRs/ADEs) were also evaluated. The clinical effective rate and LVEF were regarded as dominating outcomes of the study, because the clinical effective rate can inflect the efficacy directly and LVEF was a main indicator for CHF. And others were counted as secondary outcomes. A study was excluded when it met these following criteria: 1) the study without full text; 2) duplicated reports; 3) RCTs with incomplete or inaccurate data; 4) RCTs with wrong sequence generation method. For example, sequence gen-erated by odd or even date of birth, some rules based on date (or day) of admission and so forth; 5) patients received physiotherapy, acupuncture and moxibustion therapy, and Chinese materia medica preparation.

A comprehensive literatures searching was carried out in seven database including Embase, the Cochrane Library, Pubmed, Chinese Biological Medicine Database (CBM), China National Knowledge Infrastructure (CNKI), Wanfang Database, Chinese Scientific Journal Database (VIP) from their inception up to June 12nd 2017. In addition, there was no restriction on language. The method that incorporated the medical subject head-ings (MeSH) term and the free text was applied in searching process, and it would vary from different data-bases. Each searching item included three parts of terms that chronic heart failure, CHIs, and randomization. Detailed searching strategies were illustrated in Additional file 2.

After literatures duplicate checking, the rest literatures were firstly screened by titles and abstracts, reviews, irrele-vant literatures and animals' experiments reports were ex-cluded. Literatures passed the initial filtration were read full text in order to sort out the eligible RCTs. Two re-viewers undertook literature selection respectively, any di-vergences resolved by discussion or the third reviewer.

Data extraction and quality assessment
Information from the eligible RCTs was extracted based on a custom-made form. The data consisted of the fol-lowing items: 1) basic information of the eligibility: the first author, nationality, publication year, study desgin; 2) basic characteristics of patients: sample size, gender composition, average age, course of disease, primary dis-eases, cardiac function classification; 3) detail of RCTs' intervention; 4) outcomes results and RCTs' quality assessment.

The quality analysis was assessed with the Cochrane Collaboration's tools (version 5.1.0 the Nordic Chchrane Center, the Cochrane Collaboration, 2012 Copenhagen, Denmark) by two reviewers independently. The tool comprised following these 7 items: 1) the method of randomization; 2) the concealment of random allocation;

3) the blinding method for patients and clinicians; 4) the blinding method for assessor; 5) the integrality of outcomes data; 6) the condition of selective reporting; 7) others bias. Each item was rated as "high risk", "low risk" and "unclear". And any difference between two reviewers settled by discussion or the third reviewer.

It is not necessary for this meta-analysis to obtain an ethical approval, because this study was the procedure that just gathered the clinical data in each RCT without any leak of patients' information.

Statistical analysis

NMA was performed with Stata software (version 12, Stata Corporation, College Station, Texas, U.S.) and Winbugs (version 1.4, MRC Biostatistics Unit, Cambridge, UK) software by using Mantel-Haenszel random-effects model. In Winbugs software, the number of iteration was set as 50,000, the first 20,000 was used for annealing algorithm in order to eliminate the impact of initial value. For binary outcomes, the pooled results were calculated as odds ratios (ORs). For continuous outcomes, mean differences (MD) were used. Both types of outcomes were presented with their 95% credible intervals (95% CIs) as well. Besides, the network graph showed indirect comparative relationship between different interventions was described. The node area of each intervention on behalf of its number of patients, and the

thickness between different interventions represented the number of relative RCTs [11]. To rank various CHIs in treatment in CHF, the surface under the cumulative ranking curve (SUCRA) was utilized, which expressed each intervention's efficacy with percentages. A larger area of SCUAR indicated that corresponding intervention was more preferable in certain outcomes [12]. After that, the funnel plots were depicted to reflect publication bias. Due to non-close loops in this NMA, the assumption of consistency between direct and indirect evidence was not utilized.

Results

Literature selection

A total of 9968 literatures were identified in initial search (Fig. 1). After removing duplicates, there were 4852 remained. By screened titles and abstracts, 1491 literatures were excluded because they were irrelevant literatures, reviews and animals' experiments reports. 3361 literatures were eligible and then examined respectively, among which 3248 were further excluded, for the following reasons: 1) the RCT's intervention or diseases missed eligibility criteria ($n = 2694$); 2) the therapeutic effect standard missed eligibility criteria ($n = 256$);3) the RCT with wrong randomization ($n = 68$); 4) the RCT did not divide patients in two groups (n = 68); 5) case reports ($n = 40$); 6) the RCT without full-text ($n = 104$); 7)

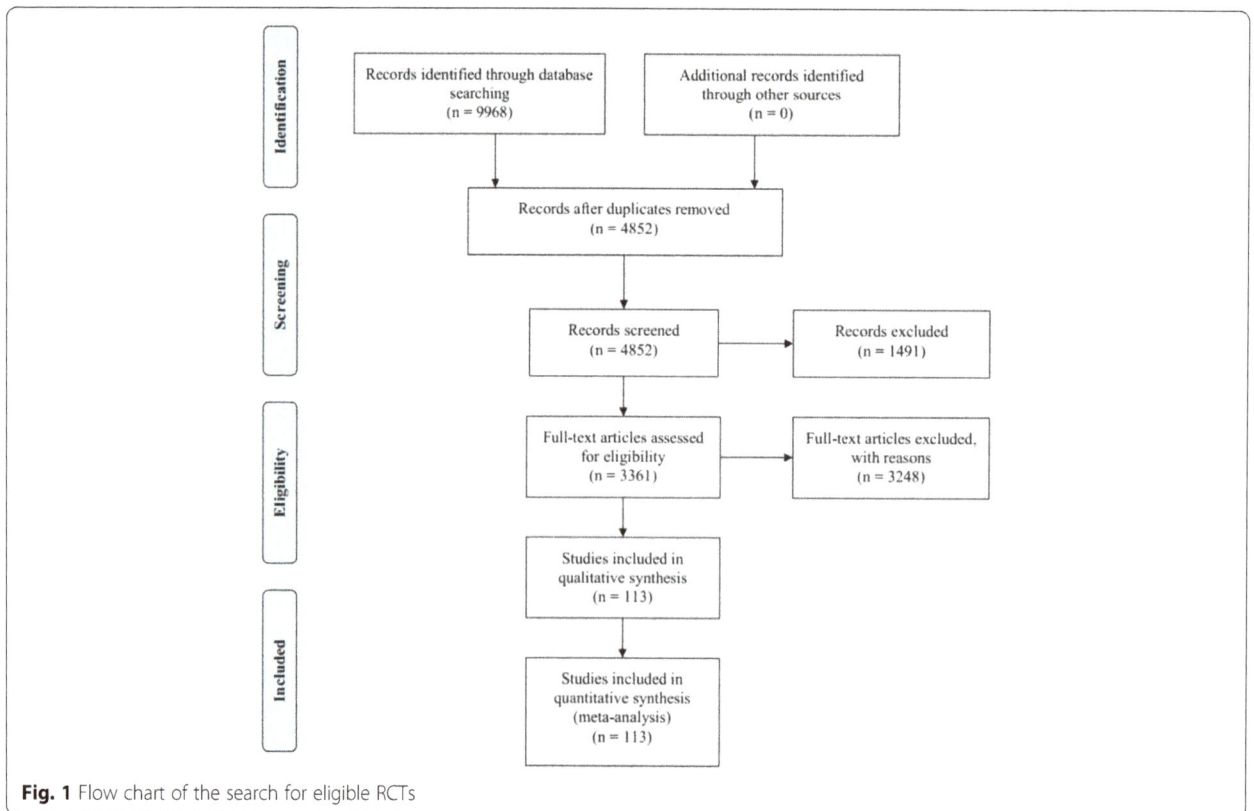

Fig. 1 Flow chart of the search for eligible RCTs

the RCT with duplicated data ($n = 18$). As results, 113 RCTs that evaluated CHIs combined with WM for CHF were eligible in the NMA, and all of then carried out in China between 2001 and 2017. Meanwhile, 6 types of CHIs were identified, including HQI (12 RCTs), SFI (39 RCTs), SI (31 RCTs), SMI (13 RCTs), SQFZI (12 RCTs) and YQFMI (6 RCTs).

Study characteristics and quality evaluation

One hundered thirteen [3, 13–124] RCTs with 9525 patients were accorded with the eligible criteria, among which 4852 patients in the treatment groups and 4673 patients in the control groups. Among patients, the male patients were about 55% of total, and majority of patients were middle aged and elderly people. The intervention of the control groups were WM treatment, for instance, ACEIs, β-blocker, cardiotonic, diuretic. In the meantime, the treatment groups received one of the identified CHIs on the basis of the control groups. HQI, SFI, SI, SMI was a kind of injection that clinicians

injected them with 5%–10% dextrose solution or 0.9% normal saline, the specific dosage were determined by clinicians. SQFZI was a kind of already made injection with menstruum. And YQFMI was a powder-injection, clinicians injected them with 5%–10% dextrose solution or 0.9% normal saline as well. All of identified CHIs were injected once a day via mainline. Characteristics of included RCTs can be found in Additional file 3. And the compared connections among each intervention for each outcome were displayed in Fig. 2.

For the eligible RCTs, 19 RCTs [15, 26, 32, 34, 37, 56, 57, 61, 64, 75, 81, 88, 96, 101, 103, 104, 107, 110, 118] used the random number table method or sortation randomization method to generate groups and 1 RCTs [88] utilized double blind method. Thus all of them were assessed as low risk. The rest RCTs were evaluated as high risk due to insufficient information. Besides, none of the included RCTs assessed had incomplete data, so the attrition bias was appraised as low risk. As for the part of reporting bias and others bias, the included RCTs

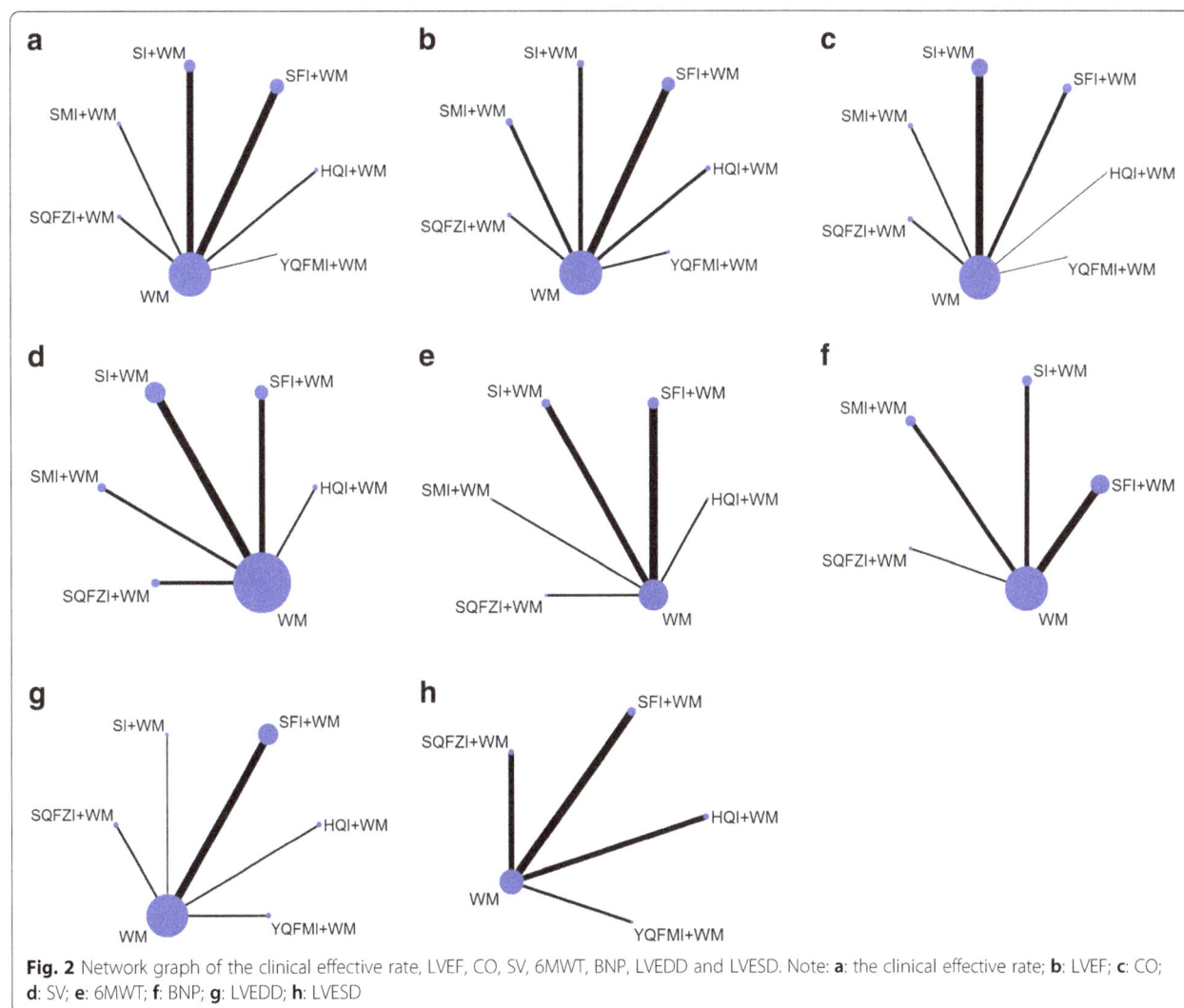

Fig. 2 Network graph of the clinical effective rate, LVEF, CO, SV, 6MWT, BNP, LVEDD and LVESD. Note: **a**: the clinical effective rate; **b**: LVEF; **c**: CO; **d**: SV; **e**: 6MWT; **f**: BNP; **g**: LVEDD; **h**: LVESD

did not provide relevant contents about selective report and mention any factors leading to high risk. Therefore these two items were evaluated as unclear risk. The graphical summary was depicted in Fig. 3.

Outcomes

The clinical effective rate

The clinical effective rate was deemed as the primary outcomes, as shown in the right upper part of Table 1 [3, 13–124], HQI + WM (OR = 0.28, 95% CIs: 0.19–0.41),SFI + WM (OR = 0.29, 95% CIs: 0.24–0.35), SI + WM (OR = 0.28, 95% CIs: 0.22–0.35), SMI + WM (OR = 0.25, 95% CIs: 0.17–0.36), SQFZI+WM (OR = 0.28, 95% CIs: 0.19–0.39), YQFMI+WM (OR = 0.42, 95% CIs: 0.25–0.70), these six interventions with 95% CIs between 0 and 1 possessed the obvious strengthen in increasing clinical effective rate.

In the Table 5 and Fig. 4, ranking analysis suggested that SMI + WM was the optimal combination, SI + WM was the second and the third was SQFZI+WM.

LVEF

As the other dominating outcomes, LVEF (%) was estimated in 57 RCTs [3, 13–15, 17, 19, 20, 23, 24, 32, 33, 36, 38, 39, 42, 45–49, 53, 55, 56, 58, 60, 61, 64, 65, 72, 75, 82, 84, 88, 91–93, 95–97, 99, 100–103, 105, 106, 109–111, 114, 116, 117, 119–123]. According to Table 1, if the 95% CIs was more than 0, the result was significant. Four of them were noticeably better than WM treatment for LVEF, as SFI + WM (MD = 4.05, 95% CIs: 1.00–7.59), SI + WM (MD = 8.61, 95% CIs: 4.22–10.99), SMI + WM (MD = 7.29, 95% CIs: 1.97–12.70), YQFMI+WM (MD = 7.26, 95% CIs: 0.42–13.64) were outstanding among them compared with WM.

Results of ranking analysis manifested that SI + WM was efficacious in LVEF. Another beneficial treatments were SMI + WM and YQFMI+WM (Table 5 and Fig. 4).

Co

CO (L/min) was tested in 22 RCTs [20, 30, 31, 34, 45, 61, 68, 73, 75, 76, 81–83, 87, 92, 97, 99, 102, 111, 112, 117, 119] involved seven interventions. Based on Table 2, only SI + WM (MD = 1.29, 95% CIs: 0.74–1.72) had excellent performance in improving CO.

The SUCRA mentioned above was also affirmed, SI + WM was the best choice, and the following two were SMI + WM, and SQFZI+WM (Table 5 and Fig. 4).

SV

SV (ml) was reported in 20 RCTs [20, 23, 30, 36, 38, 45, 61, 68, 73, 75, 81, 82, 87, 92, 97, 99, 102, 111, 112, 117] involved six interventions. In terms of Table 2, only SI + WM (MD = 9.35, 95% CIs: 3.75–14.90) was remarkable among them.

Base on its SUCRA, SI + WM was the optimum, SQFZI+WM was the second and SMI + WM was the third (Table 5 and Fig. 4).

6MWT

The potency of lengthening the distance of 6MWT (m) was assessed, and six interventions with 10 RCTs [24, 32, 39, 46, 51, 74, 85, 92, 106, 109] had data in contrast with WM, shown in Table 3. While the results showed no significant difference in most cases.

The ranking analysis indicated that SI + WM was the favorable intervention (Table 5).

BNP

In terms of BNP (pg/ml), five treatments with 21 RCTs [3, 33, 36, 38, 44, 46, 47, 53, 58, 64, 65, 69, 72, 88, 94–97, 104, 107, 109] were compared with WM in Table 3. SFI + WM vs SMI + WM (MD = 80.17, 95% CIs: 16.67–147.5), SFI + WM vs SQFZI+WM (MD = 110.00, 95% CIs: 35.08–186.40), SFI + WM vs WM (MD = 87.77, 95% CIs: 32.61–129.90) had statistically significance.

Based on ranking analysis, SQFZI+WM attained the first-rank (Table 5).

LVEDD & LVESD

The efficiency of decreasing LVEDD (mm) and LVESD (mm) was estimated as well. These two indexes were

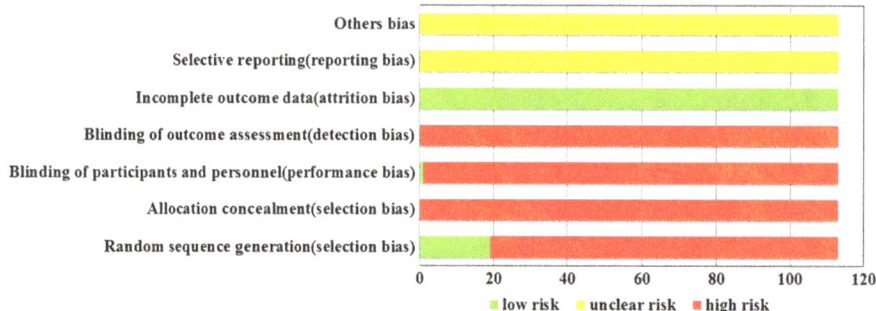

Fig. 3 Risk of bias graph

Table 1 Odds ratios/mean difference (95%CIs) of the clinical effective rate (right upper part) and LVEF (left lower part)

the clinical effective rate						
LVEF	**HQI + WM**	0.98(0.62,1.49)	1.03(0.62,1.59)	1.15(0.65,1.96)	1.00(0.60,1.76)	0.67(0.36,1.28)	0.28(0.19,0.41)
	0.13(−7.46,7.87)	**SFI + WM**	1.05(0.76,1.41)	1.17(0.79,1.83)	1.05(0.72,1.60)	0.69(0.42,1.21)	0.29(0.24,0.35)
	−4.31(−11.77,4.08)	− 4.50(−8.43,1.48)	**SI + WM**	1.12(0.73,1.75)	1.00(0.67,1.58)	0.66(0.39,1.16)	0.28(0.22,0.35)
	−3.08(−12.25,5.93)	−3.26(−9.21,3.26)	1.03(− 5.62,7.12)	**SMI + WM**	0.88(0.52,1.51)	0.59(0.31,1.10)	0.25(0.17,0.36)
	−2.60(−12.30,7.90)	− 2.69(− 10.87,5.50)	1.63(−6.79,9.48)	0.38(−8.25,9.34)	**SQFZI + WM**	0.66(0.36,1.23)	0.28(0.19,0.39)
	−3.11(−12.39,6.93)	− 3.17(− 10.26,4.48)	1.26(−6.88,8.28)	0.25(−8.18,8.53)	−0.50(− 10.09,9.22)	**YQFMI + WM**	0.42(0.25,0.70)
	4.27(− 2.61,11.46)	4.05(1.00,7.59)	8.61(4.22,10.99)	7.29(1.97,12.70)	6.81(−0.59,14.06)	7.26(0.42,13.64)	**WM**

Note: The result underlined meant it had statistical significant

tested in 22 RCTs [13, 19, 20, 28, 30, 33, 36, 38, 39, 45, 53, 55, 58, 61, 65, 72, 107, 109, 111, 119, 121, 122] and 8 RCTs [13, 20, 30, 55, 61, 107, 109, 119] respectively. According to Table 4, it appeared that there was no significant difference between each comparison.

The ranking analysis suggested that HQI + WM and SQFZI+WM was the optimum for these two indexes (Table 5).

ADRs/ADEs
Among 113 RCTs, a total of 36 [22, 23, 26, 30, 32, 33, 36, 39, 40, 43, 45, 48, 49, 51, 54, 64, 65, 67, 71–74, 77–81, 88, 93, 97–99, 103, 107, 108, 119, 120] RCTs (HQI (2 RCTs), SFI (13 RCTs), SI (13 RCTs), SMI (4 RCTs), SQFZI (2 RCTs), YQFMI (2 RCTs)) did not appear ADRs/ADEs during the trials. Another 72 RCTs (HQI (10 RCTs), SFI (25 RCTs), SI (17 RCTs), SMI (6 RCTs), SQFZI (10 RCTs),

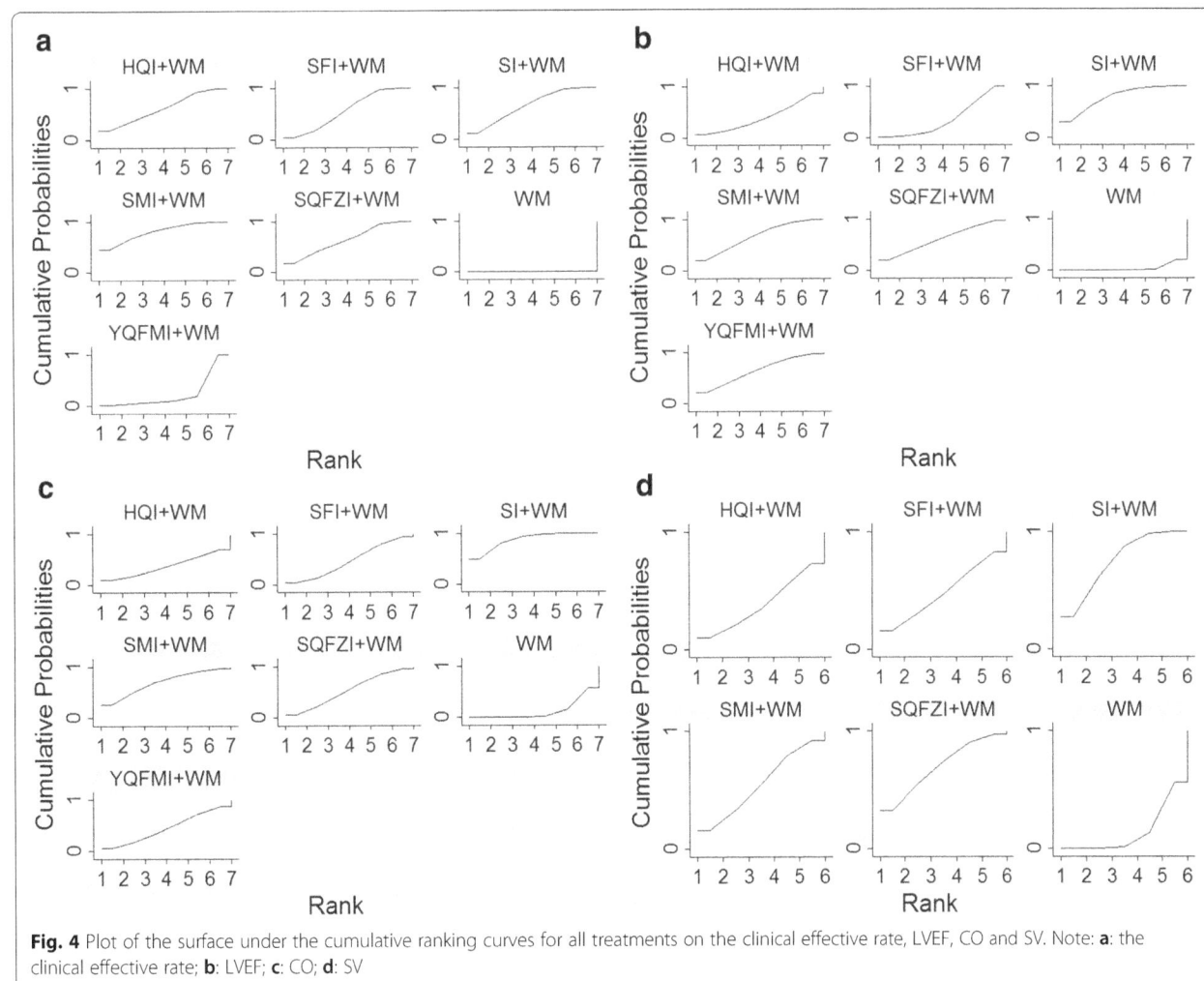

Fig. 4 Plot of the surface under the cumulative ranking curves for all treatments on the clinical effective rate, LVEF, CO and SV. Note: **a**: the clinical effective rate; **b**: LVEF; **c**: CO; **d**: SV

Table 2 Mean difference (95%CIs) of CO (right upper part) and SV (left lower part)

CO							
SV	HQI + WM	−0.22(−2.09,1.59)	−0.97(−2.61,0.80)	−0.64(−2.68,1.31)	−0.36(−2.21,1.53)	−0.20(−2.14,1.82)	0.32(−1.29,1.99)
	−1.92(−21.24,16.33)	SFI + WM	−0.73(−1.69,0.34)	−0.46(−1.89,1.03)	−0.12(−1.36,1.13)	0.03(−1.38,1.49)	0.55(−0.29,1.43)
	−6.07(−21.13,9.09)	−4.32(−17.07,9.69)	SI + WM	0.29(−1.02,1.51)	0.61(−0.46,1.58)	0.77(−0.54,1.98)	1.29(0.74,1.72)
	−3.05(−20.33,14.23)	−1.10(−17.34,15.64)	2.99(−8.76,14.46)	SMI + WM	0.32(−1.15,1.77)	0.46(−1.15,2.13)	0.99(−0.17,2.16)
	−5.74(−23.58,11.31)	−3.84(−20.16,12.65)	0.25(−11.63,12.08)	−2.51(−17.27,11.40)	SQFZI + WM	0.14(−1.31,1.65)	0.68(−0.21,1.57)
	—	—	—	—	—	YQFMI + WM	0.52(−0.64,1.68)
	3.28(−10.90,17.25)	5.12(−6.59,18.01)	9.35(3.75,14.90)	6.46(−3.94,16.34)	9.04(−1.36,19.54)	—	WM

Note: The result underlined meant it had statistical significant

YQFMI (4 RCTs)) did not mention the situation of ADRs/ADEs. In others RCTs, one of the SFI treatment group occurred 2 cases of mild elevation of blood pressure and 2 cases of slight dry cough, and the corresponding control group occurred 3 cases of slight dry cough and 2 cases of headache [37]. Besides, one of the SI treatment group occurred 2 cases of mild anaphylaxis. There were 3 RCTs with SMI treatment group appeared ADRs [96, 100, 104]. One RCT occurred 1 case of pruritus in the treatment group and 6 cases mild headache in the control group. Another occurred 3 cases of mild gum bleeding in the control group. Another occurred 2 cases of stomach upset in the treatment and control group respectively. All of the symptom were alleviated after corresponding treatment and did not influence the RCTs.

Funnel plot characteristics

A comparison-adjusted funnel plot for the clinical effective rate was displayed in Fig. 5. The funnel plot was general symmetrical in visual. Thus we concluded that the obvious publication bias did not exist.

Discussion

The impairment of CHF has been a global public health issue [125], with the utilization of a conjunction between CHIs and WM in its treatment, the efficacy of CHF has been promoted, meanwhile, more and more relevant RCTs and pairwise meta-analysis were carried out. But almost RCTs concerned about the efficacy between a kind of CHI plus WM and WM, many CHIs have not been compared head to head. Thus, researchers could merely figure out the efficacy of a CHI based on these RCTs via pairwise meta-analysis. While NMA can address this void, the efficacy of CHIs can be obtained at a time based on indirect comparison. By comparing with WM, the efficacy of CHIs for CHF and their rank can be demonstrated. we conducted a NMA in order to appraise the efficacy and safety of seven interventions: HQI + WM, SFI + WM, SI + WM, SMI + WM, SQFZI +WM, YQFMI+WM and WM.

This study made an extensive literature review and evaluation. The clinical data derived from 113 RCTs in the aspects of the clinical effective rate, LVEF, CO, SV, 6MWT, BNP, as well as the value of LVEDD and LVESD. CO, SV, LVEDD and LVESD was regarded as a supplement of cardiac condition, while the consequence of LVEDD and LVESD was no significant difference in most cases, these two outcomes' results were merely deemed as a reference. Besides, 6MWT was vital indicator of patients' recovery, and its importance was emphasized in the guide [9], though the amount of relevant RCTs in this study was small and its statistical power was low, we just treat it as a secondary outcome. In addition, the measurement of BNP was highlighted in guide as an exclusion for CHF [126]. Therefore, we viewed it as a secondary index as well. In terms of the

Table 3 Mean difference (95%CIs) of 6MWT (right upper part) and BNP (left lower part)

6MWT							
BNP	HQI + WM	−5.40(−71.99,70.70)	−29.10(−115.00,66.32)	16.53(−82.29,163.00)	7.97(−134.30,150.90)	—	17.38(−52.09,84.04)
	—	SFI + WM	−22.05(−91.18,37.25)	25.48(−84.97,155.60)	15.06(−137.40,161.20)	—	22.42(−9.55,53.97)
	—	54.65(−19.88,134.30)	SI + WM	50.83(−75.61,178.60)	36.18(−109.80,204.00)	—	45.03(−12.06,101,10)
	—	80.17(16.67,147.5)	24.53(−58.64,110.20)	SMI + WM	−16.56(−213.70,188.00)	—	−1.23(−133.50,100.10)
	—	110.00(35.08,186.40)	53.69(−41.32,151.3)	27.54(−44.17,108.30)	SQFZI + WM	—	—
	—	—	—	—	—	YQFMI + WM	7.12(−141.80,149.50)
	—	87.77(32.61,129.90)	34.25(−44.31,100.20)	8.33(−52.43,63.95)	−20.41(−87.19,35.51)	—	WM

Note: The result underlined meant it had statistical significant

Table 4 Mean difference (95%CIs) of LVEDD (right upper part) and LVESD (left lower part)

LVEDD							
LVESD	HQI + WM	−6.39(− 20.58,8.88)	−5.90(− 22.48,11.36)	—	− 7.40(− 21.99,8.39)	−5.02(− 20.71,10.80)	− 7.87(− 21.64,7.22)
	−1.36(− 17.43,15.51)	SFI + WM	0.32(−9.47,10.49)	—	−1.04(− 6.88,5.10)	1.08(− 8.40,10.10)	−1.49(− 5.58,2.45)
	—	—	SI + WM	—	−1.43(− 11.31,8.84)	0.68(− 12.36,13.41)	−1.88(− 10.71,7.12)
	—	—	—	SMI + WM	—	—	—
	−2.21(−17.01,13.77)	−0.72(− 10.35,8.84)	—	—	SQFZI + WM	2.22(−7.61,11.31)	− 0.37(−5.41,3.66)
	0.97(− 20.42,23.54)	2.30(− 15.51,17.43)	—	—	3.02(− 14.80,20.13)	YQFMI + WM	−2.68(−10.91,6.07)
	− 4.03(− 18.02,10.96)	−2.57(− 10.73,5.24)	—	—	− 1.82(− 7.68,3.52)	−4.80(− 21.19,12.13)	WM

primary outcomes, SI + WM and SMI + WM exhibited superior performance. What more, these two interventions did a noteworthy effect on CO and SV. And SI + WM also obtained a first-rank with respect to 6MWT. Overall, on the basis of receiving WM, CHF patients received SI or SMI may be more efficacious. Both of them were approved by CFDA on the market of CHF. SI was derived from Shengmai San which has been widely used for cardiovascular diseases since 1186 in China [127]. It was mainly made from the extractive of *Panax ginseng, Radix Ophiopogonis* and *Schisandra chinensis,* and had a function as replenishing qi-yin deficiency. Pharmacological researches have confirmed that SI had features in perfecting cardiac function and alleviating heart failure, enhancing myocardial contractility and cardiac pumping [128]. Under the guideline of TCM, SI was employed in CHF treatment routinely with its preferable curative effect, and several pairwise meta-analysis manifested that a conjunctive between SI and WM owned a superior capability on increasing the effective rate and LVEF [128–130]. As for SMI, it stemmed from Shenmai Yin which was prescribed by Simiao Sun in the Tang Dynasty [131], and its ingredients did not contain *Schisandra chinensis* compared with SI, but it also had a superior capacity in nourishing yin and benefiting qi. Upon pharmacological researches, the effect of SMI on promoting myocardial contractility and antiarrhythmic action has been verified [132]. Besides, several pairwise meta-analysis demonstrated that SMI plus WM exhibited a better performance in improving the effective rate, LVEF, CO, SV and decreasing BNP than WM [133–135].

Apart from efficacy, the safety of interventions was the other crucial element that must be considered in clinical trials. In this study, the occurrence rate of ADRs/ADEs was small, but about 64% of the research did not report the ADRs/ADEs. Hence, we could not draw a certain conclusion on it. As suggested in previous study, anaphylaxis was the main ADRs/ADEs of CHIs, and it would appear within 30 min at first time [136–139]. Hence, it is crucial for clinicians to monitor the ADRs/ADEs after using CHIs. Meanwhile, it is necessary to reported exactly if ADRs/ADEs occurred [136].

Upon the design and contents, three merits enhanced the creditable of this study. Firstly, this study made a comprehensive literature search and a contrast for six CHIs which have been already adopted in CHF treatment. Besides, this study expressed the efficacy of CHIs objectively due to the relevant large number of eligible RCTs. Furthermore, a strict eligibility criterion was formulated before implementing NMA. The consistency of the intervention and the curative standard lowered the clinical heterogeneity. What's more, it was significant that the outcomes demonstrated cardiac condition in multiaspect. According to corresponding conclusions, this study provided several clinical suggestions for treatment in CHF.

Table 5 Ranking probability for all treatments on the clinical effective rate, LVEF, CO, SV, 6MWT, BNP, LVEDD and LVESD

Treatment	Outcomes							
	the clinical effective rate	LVEF	CO	SV	6MWT	BNP	LVEDD	LVESD
HQI + WM	0.615	0.391	0.370	0.384	0.507	—	0.795	0.583
SFI + WM	0.559	0.359	0.462	0.481	0.596	0.020	0.503	0.533
SI + WM	0.649	0.783	0.872	0.747	0.776	0.392	0.499	—
SMI + WM	0.806	0.670	0.695	0.550	0.378	0.575	—	—
SQFZI+WM	0.635	0.613	0.530	0.697	0.460	0.849	0.361	0.501
YQFMI+WM	0.236	0.650	0.449	—	—	—	0.563	0.619
WM	0.00	0.034	0.122	0.141	0.284	0.664	0.279	0.263

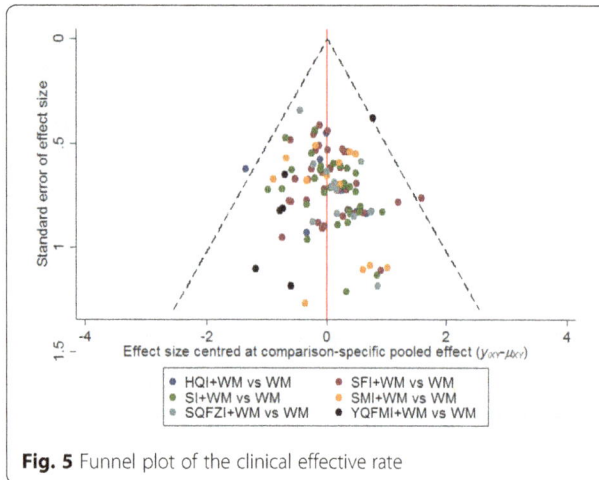

Fig. 5 Funnel plot of the clinical effective rate

Abbreviations
6MWT: 6-min walk test; 95% CIs: 95% credible intervals; ACEIs: Angiotensin-converting enzyme inhibitors; ADRs/ADEs: Dverse drug reactions/adverse drug events; ARBs: Angiotensin II receptor blockers; BNP: brain Natriuretic peptide; CBM: Chinese Biological Medicine Database; CFDA: China Food and Drug Administration; CHF: Chronic heart failure; CHIs: Chinese herbal injections; CNKI: China National Knowledge Infrastructure; CO: Cardiac output; HQI: Huangqi injection; LVEDD: Left ventricular end-diastolic dimension; LVEF: Left ventricular ejection fraction; LVESD: Left ventricular end-systolic dimension; MD: Mean differences; MeSH: Medical subject headings; NMA: Network meta-analysis; NYHA: New York Heart Association; ORs: Odds ratios; RCTs: Randomized controlled trials; SFI: Shenfu injection; SI: Shengmai injection; SMI: Shenmai injection; SQFZI: Shenqi Fuzheng injection; SUCRA: Surface under the cumulative ranking curve; SV: Stroke volume; TCM: Traditional Chinese medicine; VIP: Chinese Scientific Journal Database; WM: Western medicine; YQFMI: Yiqifumai injection

Funding
National Natural Science Foundation of China (No. 81473547; No.81673829).

Authors' contributions
Conception and design of the network meta-analysis: JRW, KHW. Performance of the network meta-analysis: KHW. Quality assessment of the network meta-analysis: MWN, KHW, JRW. Analysis of study data: DZ, XJD. Writing of the paper: KHW, DZ. All authors read and approved the final version of the manuscript.

Competing interests
The authors declare no competing interests in any aspects.

Limitation

Nevertheless, there was still insufficient in this study. Frist, the enrolled patients in RCTs were merely Chinese, which may lead to a bias on whether non-Chinese use eligible CHIs effectively or not. Although CHIs was mostly adopted in China, clinicians also can not only recruit Chinese. Next, just ten of included RCTs reported 6MWT in this study. While it is 6MWT, and readmission rate that associate with CHF patients closely and influence patients' survival quality. Thus, these aspects should be paid more emphasis when RCTs are designed. In addition, the methodological quality was general, and most included RCTs did not mention the details of randomization and allocation concealment, which may generate an overestimate for eligible CHIs. It should be note that clinicians utilize low risk randomization and concealment method as possible. Based on the limitations, the RCTs conducted in the future should be perfected in relevant areas.

Conclusion

To sum up, this study found that a combination between SI/SMI and WM exerted a positive effect on improving efficacy of CHF. However, the strength of evidence needed be promoted by more high quality RCTs. Moreover, safety of SI and SMI should be cautious monitoring in trials.

Additional files

Additional file 1: PRISMA checklist for network meta-analysis. This file contained items about PRISMA checklist for network meta-analysis and corresponding pages of this study.

Additional file 2: Search strategy. This file contained the search strategy of traditional Chinese medicine injections and English database. (DOC 39 kb)

Additional file 3: Characteristics of included randomized controlled trials. This file contained the information about included randomized controlled trials.

References

1. Wang E-W, Jia X-S, Ruan C-W, et al. miR-487b mitigates chronic heart failure through inhibition of the IL-33/ST2 signaling pathway. Oncotarget. 2017;8: 51688–702.
2. Zhao Z-Q, Mao J-Y, Wang X-L, et al. Application and evaluation of Chinese medicine in treatment of chronic heart failure. Chin J Integ Med. 2013;33:1701.
3. Wu D-H. Effects of the shenfu injection on the level of serum cerebral sodium peptide in patients with chronic heart failure. Zhejiang J Integ Tradit Chin West Med. 2013;23:837–8.
4. Vetrovsky T, Siranec M, Parenica J, et al. Effect of a 6-month pedometer-based walking intervention on functional capacity in patients with chronic heart failure with reduced (HFrEF) and with preserved (HFpEF) ejection fraction: study protocol for two multicenter randomized controlled trials. J Transl Med. 2017;15:153.
5. Wang Y-Z, Zhuang Y, Gu Y, Chen Q-Q, Wang Z-X. Progress in the evolution of chronic heart failure syndrome. Guiding J Tradit Chin Med Pharmacol. 2016;22:62–8.
6. Sane R, Aklujkar A, Patil A, et al. Effect of heart failure reversal treatment as add-on therapy in patients with chronic heart failure: a randomized open-label study. Indian Heart J. 2017;69:299.
7. Leucht S, Cipriani A, Spineli L, et al. Comparative efficacy and tolerability of 15 antipsychotic drugs in schizophrenia: a multiple-treatments meta-analysis. Lancet. 2013;382:951–62.
8. Hutton B, Salanti G, Caldwell DM, et al. The PRISMA extension statement for reporting of systematic reviews incorporating network meta-analyses of health care interventions: checklist and explanations. Ann Intern Med. 2015; 162:777–84.
9. Cardiology Branch of the Chinese Medical Association. Guidelines for the diagnosis and treatment of heart failure in China 2014. Chin J Cardiol. 2014; 42:98–122.
10. Zheng Y-Y. Clinical guideline of new drugs for traditional Chinese medicine. Beijing: Chin Med Sci and Tech Press; 2013. p. 77–85.
11. Zhang D, Wu J-R, Liu S, Zhang X-M, Zhang B. Network meta-analysis of Chinese herbal injections combined with the chemotherapy for the treatment of pancreatic cancer. Med. 2017;96:e7005.

12. Chang L, Guo R. Comparison of the efficacy among multiple chemotherapeutic interventions combined with radiation therapy for patients with cervix cancer after surgery: a network meta-analysis. Oncotarget. 2017;8:49515–33.

13. Xing G-P, Nie X-M. Effects of astragalus injection on hemodynamics in patients with congestive heart failure. Med ind inf. 2006;3:67–9.

14. Gu X, Shang S-Z, Guo R. 68 cases of congestive heart failure assisted by astragalus injection. Her Med. 2003;22:556–7.

15. Zhang Z-B. Clinical observation of astragalus injection combined with conventional western medicine for senile patients of chronic congestive heart failure. J New Chin Med. 2017;49:25–8.

16. Luo X-C. Clinical observation of 30 cases of congestive heart failure treated by huangqi injection. J Emerg Syndromes Tradit Chin Med. 2003;12:35.

17. Feng L-Y, Hao W. Clinical observation of 34 cases of congestive heart failure treated with astragalus injection. Chin J Integr Med Cardio/ Cerebrovasc Dis. 2008;6:1362–3.

18. Gao J-H. Clinical observation of astragalus injection for treating congestive heart failure. Acad J Guangdong Coll Pharm. 2005;21:610–1.

19. Yan F-Y, Lin H-Z. 80 cases of chronic congestive heart failure treated with astragalus injection. Jiangxi J Tradit Chin Med. 2009;40:27–8.

20. Lin Y, Huang C-L, Zhu C-L. Clinical study on astragalus injection in treating chronic congestive heart failure. Chin Pharm. 2009;18:22–3.

21. Zhang C-M, Duan Q-F, Bian X-J. Clinical observation of astragalus injection in the treatment of chronic heart failure. Med Front. 2013;17:19–20.

22. Yuan G-P. Evaluation of clinical efficacy of astragalus injection for treatment of chronic heart failure. Chin J Clin Pharmacol Ther. 2003;8:710–1.

23. Wang X-X. Treatment of chronic heart failure by astragalus injection. Chin Foreign Health Abstr. 2015;14:53–4.

24. Jia B-Q, Xu L. Effect of astragalus injection on chronic heart failure. Chin J Clin Res. 2013;26:654–6.

25. Wang X-G. Effects of shenfu injection on chronic heart failure induced by different etiology and the effect of b-type natriuretic peptide. Speci health. 2014;4:598.

26. Wang H, Hu Y-H, Song Q-Q, Qiu Z-L, Bo R-Q. The impact of shenfu injection on the immune function in patients with chronic heart failure and heart kidney yang deficiency syndrome. Chin J Integr Med Cardio/ Cerebrovasc Dis. 2016;14:1441–6.

27. Zhou K, Lin S-Y, Yang WM. Effects of injection on NT-proBNP in heart failure patients with coronary heart disease. J Emerg Syndromes Tradit Chin Med. 2013;22:1625–6.

28. Xu L-L, Guan C-Y, Wang C-Y, Chen J, Zhang L-L. Effects of shenfu injection on the nt-probnp and life quality of chronic heart failure patients. J Emerg Syndromes Tradit Chin Med. 2015;24:918–20.

29. Cui Y, et al. Effect of shenfu injection on cardiac function and blood index in patients with chronic heart failure. Hebei med. 2016;22:1623–5.

30. Wu H-Q. Study about efficacy of shenfu injection on cardiac function and bone marrow stem cell mobilization in cardiac failure. Guang'anmen hospital. 2008;

31. Chen G-Q, Wu H-Q, Chen G-L, Dong L-M, Wang Z-M. Effect of shenfu injection on the serum NT-proBNP level of patients with heart failure. J Emerg Syndromes Tradit Chin Med. 2014;24:134–5.

32. Ren Q, Wang Q, Lin P. Clinical observation of the effect of shenfu injection on chronic heart failure. Zhejiang J Integr Tradit Chin West Med. 2015;25:350–2.

33. Cheng G, et al. Observation of clinical efficacy of shenfu injection in patients with congestive heart failure. Shaanxi Med J. 2014;43:482–4.

34. Li L-N. Observation of clinical efficacy of shenfu injection in treating congestive heart failure. J Emerg Syndr Tradit Chin Med. 2016;25:2375–7.

35. Mao X-Z. Clinical effect of shenfu injection on patients with chronic heart failure. J Baotou Med Coll. 2016;32:92–3.

36. Wu H-J, Duan H-W. Clinical study of shenfu injection for heart failure of coronary heart disease. Chin J Integr Med Cardio/ Cerebrovasc Dis. 2009;7:505–7.

37. Li C-Y. Observation of the effect of shenfu injection on chronic heart failure in elderly patients. Academic Conference of Gansu Province Medical Association; 2012.

38. Lv H-Y. Effects of shenfu injection on treatment of chronic heart failure and its effect on plasma BNP. Liaoning J Tradit Chin Med. 2014;41:726–7.

39. Yang Z-Y, Dong J-Y, Miao L-H. Clinical observation of shenfu injection in elderly patients with chronic heart failure. J Emerg Syndr Tradit Chin Med. 2010;19:2058–9.

40. Cao Z-Q. Observation of efficacy of shenfu injection in treating congestive heart failure in elderly patients. Chin Foreign Med Treat. 2014;30:118–9.

41. Bao G-H, Yu L-H. 30 cases of chronic congestive heart failure were treated with shenfu injection. Chin Med Mod Dis Educ China. 2011;9:27.

42. Zhang A-P, Song G-P, Cai J-S. Clinical observation of 40 cases of chronic congestive heart failure treated with shenfu injection. J Emerg Syndromes Tradit Chin Med. 2011;20:1140–1.

43. Liu Y. Clinical observation of 40 cases of chronic congestive heart failure treated with shenfu injection. J Emerg Syndromes Tradit Chin Med. 2008;16:51–2.

44. Ma L-P. Clinical study on 98 cases of chronic congestive heart failure treated with shenfu injection. World Health Dig. 2013;9:117.

45. Yao J, Lu X-R. Clinical observation on the treatment of chronic congestive heart failure with shenfu injection. J Med Theory Pract. 2010;23:287–8.

46. Ran X, Chen L, Wu W. Clinical observation of shenfu injection for chronic congestive heart failure. J New Chin Med. 2012;44:15–7.

47. Ding L. Observation of the effect of shenfu injection on chronic heart failure. Clin J Tradit Chin Med. 2013;25:482–3.

48. Zhu G-Y. Clinical observation of shenfu injection in the treatment of chronic heart failure. Hubei University of Traditional Chinese Medicine. 2013;

49. Qiu Q. Clinical observation of shenfu injection in treating chronic heart failure. Hunan J Tradit Chin Med. 2013;29:33–5.

50. Wang C-L. Clinical observation of 100 cases of chronic heart failure treated with shenfu injection. J Emerg Syndromes Tradit Chin Med. 2012;29:958–9.

51. Liu D-H, Chen G-Y, Chen W-X. Clinical observation of the curative effect of shenfu injection on chronic heart failure. The fourth Traditional Chinese Medicine continued education peak conference. 2011;

52. Qiu W-W. Clinical observation of the effectiveness of shenfu injection on chronic heart failure. J Emerg Syndromes Tradit Chin Med. 2010;19:420–1.

53. Qin Y, Zhou Q, Chen Y, Li J-P, Lv X-F. Clinical observation on the treatment of chronic heart failure with shenfu injection. J Emerg Syndromes Tradit Chin Med. 2015;24:161–2.

54. Fan T-B, Yang Z-X. Clinical observation on the treatment of chronic heart failure with shenfu injection. J Emerg Syndromes Tradit Chin Med. 2012;21:1851–2.

55. Fu R. Clinical observation on the treatment of chronic heart failure with shenfu injection. J Chin Tradit Chin Med Inf. 2011;3:245–6.

56. Jin Z-C, Jin Z-X, Han L. Study on clinical efficacy of shenfu injection in the treatment of chronic heart failure. Pharmacol Clin Chin Mater Med. 2015;31:159–61.

57. Gao F. Effect of shenfu injection on inflammatory cytokines in patients with chronic heart failure. J Emerg Syndromes Tradit Chin Med. 2012;21:1646–7.

58. Wang J, Zhang J, Ran G-Y. Clinical effect of shenfu injection on chronic heart failure and its impact on serum hs-CRP and IL-6. J Hubei Univ Chin Med. 2015;17:10–2.

59. Jiang L-X, Luo P. 96 cases of heart failure in treatment with shenfu injection. Shaanxi J Tradit Chin Med. 2011;32:1285–6.

60. Zhang Z-F, Lv H-G. Observation on the curative effect of shenfu injection on chronic heart failure in elderly patients. People's Mil Surg. 2009;52:360–1.

61. Liu D-Q, Zheng Z-M, Zhang K. Treatment of chronic congestive heart failure with shenfu injection. Jiangxi J Med Pharm. 2005;40:529–30.

62. Yu H-B, et al. Changes of nitric oxide synthase, adrenal medulla lignin, interleukin-10 in heart failure patients and the intervention effect of shenfu injection. Chin J Gerontol. 2014;34:7085–6.

63. Wang Y-X. Clinical observation on the short-term treatment of chronic congestive heart failure in elderly patients with shengmai injection. Chin Tradit Pat Med. 2010;32:713–4.

64. Wang G-T, He Y-Q, Yang P. Effects of shengmai injection on cardiac function and plasma brain natriuretic peptide in patients with congestive heart failure. Chin J Integr Med. 2010;30:551–3.

65. Zhou J. Clinical effect of shengmai injection on plasma BNP in patients with congestive heart failure. J Emerg Syndromes Tradit Chin Med. 2009;18:732–3.

66. Pan J-J. Therapeutic effect of shengmai injection on chronic heart failure. China Contemp Med. 2014;20:70–1.

67. Wang Z-Y, Hu X-Y, Liu F-Z. Clinical observation of shengmai injection for congestive heart failure. Lishizhen Med Mater Med Res. 2004;15:353.

68. Zhao Q-F, Dai J, Bai X-L. Clinical efficacy of shengmai injection as adjuvant therapy for elderly patients with chronic congestive heart failure: an analysis of 31 cases. Hunan J Tradit Chin Med. 2015;31:23–5.

69. Wu C-Z, Hu M. Clinical observation of 36 cases of chronic congestive heart failure in elderly patients. Yunnan J Tradit Chin Med Mater Med. 2011;32:30.

70. Yang Z-Z, Zhang Z. Clinical observation of 43 cases of chronic congestive heart failure assisted by shengmai injection. Chin Med Her. 2010;7:80–1.

71. Cheng F-Y. Clinial treatment of 45 cases of chronic congestive heart failure with shengmai injection. Chin J Integr Med Cardio/ Cerebrovasc Dis. 2007;5:1239–40.
72. Ni Y-M. 43 cases of chronic heart failure in treatment with shengmai injection. Her Med. 2012;31:171–2.
73. Xu J. 50 cases of chronic heart failure in treatment with shengmai injection. J M Udanjiang M Ed Coll. 2004;25:32–3.
74. Wen Y. Shengmai injection combined with conventional drug in the treatment of chronic heart failure for 20 cases. Chin Med Mod Dis Educ China. 2016;14:139–41.
75. Wen Y. Efficacy of shengmai injection in treatment of 64 cases with chronic heart failure. J Chengdu Univ Tradit Chin Med. 2013;36:76–8.
76. Kong LG, Zhu KW. Clinical observation of 30 cases of congestive heart failure in treatment of congestive heart failure. J Clin Emerg Call. 2004;5:26–7.
77. Tang E-W, Zeng Y-R. Observation of 33 cases of congestive heart failure treated by shengmai injection. Youjiang Med J. 2011;29:10–1.
78. Li W-D, Zhang T-S. Therapeutic effect of shengmai injection on congestive heart failure. Chin Commun Doct. 2002;18:35.
79. Chen Z-G. Therapeutic effect of shengmai injection on chronic heart failure in elderly patients. For All Health. 2016;10:28.
80. Luo X-Y. Therapeutic effect of shengmai injection on chronic heart failure in elderly patients. Med Inf. 2014;27:271.
81. Zhai Y-M. Clinical research of pulse-activating injection on 30 cases of chronic congestive heart failure. J Henan Univ Chin Med. 2009;24:59–61.
82. He D-Y, Wang P, Liu Q. Clinial treatment of 20 cases of chronic heart failure with shengmai injection. Henan Tradi Chin Med. 2006;26:71–2.
83. Chen K-H, Xu Z-Q, Liu QS. Analysis of 36 cases of chronic heart failure treated by shengmai injection. Zhejiang J Integr Tradit Chin West Med. 2008;18:155–6.
84. Wu X. Clinical observation of 52 cases of chronic heart failure treated by shengmai injection. For All Health. 2013;7:56.
85. Lu F. Clinical observation of 68 cases of chronic heart failure treated by shengmai injection. J Emerg Syndromes Tradit Chin Med. 2012;21:1695.
86. Liu S-H. Clinical observation of 120 cases of chronic heart failure treated by shengmai injection. National academic seminar on Wang qingren thought. 2008;
87. Zou X, Shi S-Q, Han Y. Clinical observation of the treatment of chronic heart failure by shengmai injection. Clin J Tradit Chin Med. 2011;23:777–8.
88. Kong W-W. Study on shengmai injeetion in patients with chronic heart failure of type qi and yin deficiency. Guangdong University Traditional Chinese Medicine; 2010.
89. Ni L-M, Ding C-Y. Curative effect observation on the treatment of congestive heart failure. Zhejiang J Tradit Chin Med. 2007;42:668.
90. Wang R-L, Zhou X-Y, Tian X-Z. 80 cases of chronic heart failure in treated with shengmai injection. Med Inf. 2007;20:326–7.
91. Li S-G. Clinical study on effects of shengmai injection with chronic heart failure treatment by monitoring the level of plasma NT-probnp. Fujian College of Traditional Chinese Medicine. 2009;
92. Zhang Y-T. Clinical effect of Chinese and western medicine on 103 cases of chronic congestive heart failure. Xinjiang J Tradit Chin Med. 2015;33:42–3.
93. Shi G-R. Treatment of chronic heart failure by Chinese and western medicine. Liaoning University of Traditional Chinese Medicine. 2009;
94. Pan Q-H, Chu S-X, Zheng Z-X, Jiang L-Q, Chen J-S. Effect of shenmai injection on the efficacy and plasma BNP of chronic congestive heart failure. Zhejiang J Tradit Chin Med. 2014;49:422.
95. Huang S-E, Huang Q, Yao Q, Pei D-A. Influence of shenmai injection on chronic contractive heart failure patients' heart function and BNP. J Zhejiang Univ Tradit Chin Med. 2011;35:718–9.
96. Hou X-L, Hong J-K, Xiao X-Y, Chen S-X. Effect of shenmai injection on cardiac function and brain natriuretic peptide in patients with chronic heart failure. Mod J Integ Tradit Chin West Med. 2014;23:2904–5.
97. Wang J-L, Zhou W-J, Shi G-P. Clinical observation of 51 cases of senile heart failure assisted by shenmai injection. Suzhou Univ J Med Sci. 2010;30:1289–90.
98. Liu XR. Clinical study of combined western medicine with shenmai injection to treat chronic heart failure. World Health Dig Med Period. 2011;8:103.
99. Qu F. Clinical observation of shenmai injection to treat congestive heart failure. J Emerg Syndromes Tradit Chin Med. 2006;15:1102.
100. Wu QG. Effect of shenmai injection on chronic congestive heart failure. Mod J Integr Tradit Chin West Med. 2011;20:3961–2.
101. Tian J-H, Zhang R-H. Clinical efficacy of shenmai injection in chronic heart failure. Chin Med Mod Dis Educ China. 2010;8:98–9.
102. Cui H-S. Analysis of 42 cases of chronic heart failure treated by shenmai injection. Neimonggu J Tradit Chin Med. 2008;27:65–6.
103. Hu C-L. Effective observation on shenmai injection for chronic heart failure of 132 cases. Med J West China. 2011;23:2162–3.
104. Ye J-F. Effect of shenmai injection on the treatment of chronic heart failure and its effect on plasma cerebral natriuretic peptide. Mod Pract Med. 2015;27:201–2.
105. Wang J. Therapeutic effective observation on 22 cases of congestive heart-failure treated with combined Chinese traditional and western therapy. Hunan J T Radit Chin Med. 2002;18:7–8.
106. Guo H-J, Tao Q-X, Li S-L. Chinese and western medicine combined treatment of 58 cases of chronic heart failure. Jilin J Tradit Chin Med. 2012;32:681–3.
107. Wu Y. Effect of shenqi fuzheng injection on the left ventricle of the heart and BNP on patients with chronic heart failure. Pract J Cardiac Cereb Pneum Vasc Dis. 2014;22:45–6.
108. Su H-M. Observation of the quality of chronic ischemic slow heart failure in the injection of shenqi fuzheng injection. Chin Commun Doct. 2009;11:163–4.
109. Wang L-W. Observation of shenqi fuzheng injection on cardiac function, BNP and myocardial troponin in patients with chronic congestive heart failure. Mod J Integ Tradit Chin West Med. 2014;23:1766–8.
110. Wang L, Ye B-H, Wang D-X, Li BT. Effects of shenqi fuzheng injection on plasma n terminal pro-brain natriuretic peptide in patients with chronic heart failure. Pract J Cardiac Cereb Pneum Vasc Dis. 2011;19:1774–5.
111. Liu P, Xu X-Y, Li N. Effect of shenqi fuzheng injection on peripheral blood ANGII, ET-1 levels and clinical curative effect in patients with congestive heart failure. Chin J Biochem Pharm. 2015;35:81–3.
112. Liang S-X. Observation of 43 cases of chronic congestive heart failure with elderly patients in treating with shenqi fuzheng injection. J New Chin Med. 2009;47:74–5.
113. Chen F-J, Chen L-C. Clinical curative effect and safety of shenqi fuzheng injection in the treatment of elderly patients with chronic heart failure. Chin J Biochem Pharm. 2017;37:137–9.
114. Yang S-J. Observation of curative effect of shenqi fuzheng injection on chronic congestive heart failure. World Latest Med Inf. 2015;15:166–7.
115. He F-T. Observation of curative effect of shenqi fuzheng injection on congestive heart failure. J Emerg Syndromes Tradit Chin Med. 2003;12:399–40.
116. Yun M-L. Clinic observation of 55 cases with chronic heart failure treated by shenqi fuzheng injection. Nat Sci J Hainan Univ. 2006;24:371–3.
117. Wu Z-G, Feng F-J, Xie W-B. Clinical effect of shenqi fuzheng injection on the treatment of chronic heart failure. Res Integrated Tradit West Med. 2015;7:236–7.
118. Mao H-Y. Clinical observation of chinese and western medicine in treating chronic congestive heart failure. J Pract Tradit Chin Med. 2014;30:120–1.
119. Wang H-P, Wu Z-G. Clinical observation of digoxin tablet combined with yiqifumai in treatment of chronic heart failure. Drugs & Clin. 2014;29:532–5.
120. Zhao Y-B. Clinical observation on treating chronic heart failure by yiqifumai injection. Mod Med J China. 2015;17:72–3.
121. Xue L-X, Wang H-L, Lei X, Feng L. Effects of yiqifumai injection on cardiac function and plasma BNP in chronic heart failure. Chin J Integr Med Cardio/ Cerebrovasc Dis. 2014;12:279–80.
122. Ren H. Clinical observation on treating chronic heart failure by yiqifumai injection (freeze-dried) combined with trimetazidine. The World Clin Med. 2016;10:4–5.
123. Yang C-L, Liu Z-H. Clinical study on the treatment of chronic heart failure in elderly patients with coronary heart disease by yiqifumai injection (freeze-dried). Pract Geriatr. 2014;28:607–8.
124. Zhao X-F, Liu J-Y, Zhang M-L. Clinical efficacy of injection therapy for chronic heart failure with yiqifumai injection (freeze-dried). Shanxi Med J. 2015;44:1533–5.
125. Punchik B, et al. Can home care for homebound patients with chronic heart failure reduce hospitalizations and costs? PLoS One. 2017;12:e0182148.
126. Cui W. Highlights of european society of cardiology guidelines for the diagnosis and treatment of acute and chronic heart failure 2012. Chin J Cardiovasc Med. 2012;16:324–6.
127. Chen C-Y, Lu L-Y, Chen P, et al. Shengmai injection, a traditional Chinese patent medicine, for intradialytic hypotension: a systematic review and meta-analysis. Evid Based Complement Alternat Med. 2013;2013:1-14.
128. Chen J, Luo M-X, Zheng Q, Zhou Y-C. Effect of shengmai injection on patients with chronic heart failure: a meta-analysis. Chin J Inf Tradit Chin Med. 2011;18:25–9.
129. Hu Z-Z, Tang L-M, Lin Y. Meta-analysis of the efficacy of shengmai injection in treating congestive heart failure. Zhejiang J Integr Tradit Chin West Med. 2016;26:32–7.

130. Yuan Y, Mao J-Y, Tang E, Hou Y-Z, Wang X-L. Treatment of chronic heart failure with western drugs combining shengmai injection: a systematic review on randomized controlled trials. Chin J Evid Based Cardiovasc Med. 2014;6:519–24.
131. Shi L, Xie Y, Liao X, Luo Y. Shenmai injection as an adjuvant treatment for chronic cor pulmonale heart failure: a systematic review and meta-analysis of randomized controlled trials. BMC Complement Altern Med. 2015;15:1.
132. Duan Y-P, Meng C-L, Li P. Pharmacological action and clinical application of shenmai injection. Chin Med Abstr. 2007;23:698–700.
133. Chen H-D, Xie Y-M, Wang L-X, Wu J-B. Systematic review of efficacy and safety of shenmai injection for chronic heart failure. China J Chin Mater Med. 2014;39:3650–62.
134. Hou Y-Z, Mao J-Y, Wang X-L, Liu C-X, Zhang C. Shenmai injection in heart failure patients: a systematic review and meta-analysis. Chin J Evid Base Med. 2010;10:939–45.
135. Duan P. Systematic review of efficacy and safety of shenmai injection in treatment of heart failure. J Taishan Med Coll. 2014;35:1063–4.
136. Yan W-L, Tong X-T, Yang S-Q. The causes and countermeasures of adverse reactions of traditional Chinese medicine injection. Mod Tradit Chin Med. 2016;36:56–8.
137. Liu J-G, Liu Y-L, Zhang H-M, Li Y-L. Exploration on the adverse reactions of chinese herbal injection and the preventive measures. World J Integr Tradit West Med. 2017;12:81–4.
138. Hao C, Liu F-Q. Progress on cause of adverse reaction of traditional Chinese medicine. J Pharm Res. 2017;36:369–72.
139. Zhang X-X. A review on adverse reaction from TCM injection. Clin J Chin Med. 2017;9:141–2.

4

Using the Chinese herb *Scutellaria barbata* against extensively drug-resistant *Acinetobacter baumannii* infections: in vitro and in vivo studies

Chin-Chuan Tsai[1†], Chi-Shiuan Lin[1†], Chun-Ru Hsu[2], Chiu-Ming Chang[1], I-Wei Chang[3], Li-Wei Lin[1], Chih-Hsin Hung[4*] and Jiun-Ling Wang[5*] (ORCID)

Abstract

Background: No animal model studies have been conducted in which the efficacy of herbal compounds has been tested against multidrug-resistant *Acinetobacter baumannii* infections. Very few antibiotics are available for the treatment of pulmonary infections caused by extensively drug-resistant *Acinetobacter baumannii* (XDRAB). To find alternative treatments, traditional Chinese herbs were screened for their antimicrobial potential.

Methods: The present study screened 30 herbs that are traditionally used in Taiwan and that are commonly prescribed for heat clearing and detoxification. The herbs with antibacterial activities were analysed by disc diffusion assays, time-kill assays and a murine lung infection model.

Results: Of the 30 herbs tested, only *Scutellaria barbata* demonstrated 100% in vitro activity against XDRAB. Furthermore, we compared the antibacterial effect of the *S. barbata* extract with that of colistin, and the *S. barbata* extract showed better antibacterial effect. In the XDRAB pneumonia murine model, we compared the antimicrobial effects of the orally administered *S. barbata* extract (200 mg/kg, every 24 h), the intratracheally administered colistin (75,000 U/kg, every 12 h), and the control group. The bacterial load in the lungs of the treatment group that received the oral *S. barbata* extract showed a significant decrease in comparison to that in the lungs of the control group. In addition, histopathological examinations also revealed better resolution of perivascular, peribronchial, and alveolar inflammation in the oral *S. barbata* extract-treated group.

Conclusions: Our in vitro and in vivo data from the animal model support the use of *S. barbata* as an alternate drug to treat XDRAB pulmonary infections. However, detailed animal studies and clinical trials are necessary to establish the clinical utility of *S. barbata* in treating XDRAB pulmonary infections.

Keywords: Multidrug-resistant *Acinetobacter baumannii*, *Scutellaria barbata*, Disc diffusion method, Time-kill curve, Animal model

Background

Since 2000, multidrug-resistant *Acinetobacter baumannii* (MDRAB) strains have rapidly emerged, and their prevalence has increased worldwide, including in Taiwan. Currently, MDRAB is one of the most important pathogens associated with nosocomial pneumonia in hospitals, and it can lead to further complications, such as bacteraemia and sepsis. There are a limited number of effective antibiotics to treat MDRAB infections, including colistin and tigecycline [1–3]. However, the efficacy of colistin is limited by its nephrotoxicity and by the development of colistin-resistant MDRAB strains [4, 5]. Moreover, several retrospective studies on the effectiveness of tigecycline against MDRAB infections have suggested that the clinical efficacy of tigecycline-based therapy is still controversial. The development of breakthrough bacteraemia and the

* Correspondence: chhung@isu.edu.tw; jiunlingwang@gmail.com
†Equal contributors
[4]Department of Chemical Engineering, and Institute of Biotechnology, I-Shou University, Kaoshiung, Taiwan
[5]Department of Internal Medicine, National Cheng Kung University Hospital and College of Medicine,National Cheng Kung University, No. 138, Sheng Li Road, Tainan 70403, Taiwan
Full list of author information is available at the end of the article

emergence of drug resistance during the course of therapy limit the efficacy of tigecycline therapy for MDRAB when used as the single therapeutic agent [3, 6].

A study conducted by Savoia on the potential antimicrobial activity of plant-derived substances suggested that naturally bioactive plant compounds can be a source of new drugs in the future [7]. Some of the active compounds extracted from herbs have shown potential activity against *A. baumannii* and other gram-negative bacteria. Many plant-based natural compounds that show considerable antimicrobial activity against *Escherichia coli* or *Pseudomonas aeruginosa* have not been tested against *A. baumannii* [8]. Several medicinal plants extracts such as those from *Calotropis procera*, *Aegle marmelos*, *Actinidia deliciosa* and *Punica granatum* peel or nanomaterial-based therapies have been found to have antimicrobial activity against MDRAB [9–12]. After screening sixty herbal extracts, Miyasaki et al. reported that approximately 30% of the screened herbs displayed potential in vitro antimicrobial activity against MDRAB. The six most active compounds identified from the herbal extracts were ellagic acid from *Rosa rugosa*, norwogonin from *Scutellaria baicalensis,* and chebulagic acid, chebulinic acid, corilagin, and terchebulin from *Terminalia chebula* [13, 14]. However, further attempts to develop potent antimicrobials from plants were not successfully undertaken by pharmaceutical or biotechnology firms. One reason is that antibacterial compounds act more effectively in combination but show much lower efficacy when used in their isolated and purified forms [8].

In this context, searching for effective natural antimicrobial agents from Chinese herbs that have been used for centuries seems to be an alternative solution. Several heat-clearing and detoxifying Chinese herbs have been reported to have anti-inflammatory and antimicrobial effects through different mechanisms of action and on multiple targets [15]. In this study, we screened the commonly used heat-clearing Chinese herbs for activity against MDRAB by in vitro methods. Due to difficulty in conducting randomized controlled clinical trials for MDRAB infection, animal models (using the compounds that showed in vitro efficacy) are usually employed to evaluate the efficacy of test compounds in the treatment of MDRAB infection. There are several reports available in which animal models of *A. baumannii* pneumonia have been used to assess the efficacy of inhaled colistin against MDRAB pneumonia [16, 17], but no animal model studies have been conducted in which the efficacy of herbal compounds against MDRAB infection has been tested. In this study, we evaluated the antimicrobial effect of Chinese herbs against MDRAB infection in a mouse model.

Methods
In vitro studies
Microorganisms
Thirty-four clinical strains of *A. baumannii* were collected from five medical centres in Taiwan. All the isolates were subjected to MIC testing for various drugs using the CLSI (Clinical and Laboratory Standards Institute) guidelines [18]. Extensively drug-resistant *A. baumannii* (XDRAB) strains were defined as the bacterial isolates resistant to all authorized antibiotics except for tigecycline and polymyxin. There were seventeen XDRAB strains among the isolates.

Genomic DNA was extracted using a standard protocol. The genomic DNA of all 34 strains was digested with *Apa*I and separated by PFGE. Different DNA patterns were seen after PFGE, which indicated that all 34 strains were different genotypes (data not shown).

Screening of antimicrobial activity
To evaluate the antimicrobial potential of Chinese herbs against XDRAB, we obtained 30 Chinese herbs from a traditional herb store in Kaohsiung City in Taiwan. These herbs are the most commonly prescribed Chinese herbs for heat clearing and detoxification in the Taiwan National Health Insurance Database (Table 1). All herbs included in this study are considered important species for heat clearing and detoxification in traditional Chinese medicine and classical prescription in Taiwan. They have traditionally been used for respiratory-, digestive- and urinary tract infection-related ailments, such as cough and diarrhoea. Modern pharmacological reports have also demonstrated their antimicrobial, anti-inflammatory and analgesic effects, as well as their antitumour effects. Water extracts of these Chinese herbs were prepared using the following procedure: (a) 100 g of the raw herb was ground to a fine powder, (b) the powder was mixed with 1000 mL of distilled water, (c) the water mixture was boiled for 60 min, and (d) the extract was decanted and concentrated in a vacuum evaporator and then frozen to dry before use.

We screened 30 clinical isolates of *A. baumannii* for antimicrobial activity by the disc diffusion method on Muller-Hinton agar plates [19]. Each disc contained 20 μL of the herb extract (128 g/L) that was placed on MHA agar inoculated with 5×10^5 cfu/mL of XDRAB. The zone of inhibition was determined after incubation at 37 °C for 16–18 h.

Determination of MICs and MBCs
The broth microdilution method was used to determine the MIC (minimum inhibitory concentration) and MBC (minimal bactericidal concentration) [18]. An inoculum containing 5×10^5 cfu/mL of XDRAB in the exponential growth phase was used. The microtiter plates were inoculated with the bacterial suspension and the diluted antimicrobials. After incubating the plates at 37 °C for 16–18 h,

Table 1 The 30 traditional Chinese herbal extracts (128 g/L) and the zone of inhibition (mm)

Isolates	Ab019	Ab14	Ab15	Ab16	Ab19	Ab23	Ab26	Ab29	Ab35	Ab39	Ab40	Ab54	TVG55	KM5	Ab21	TVG68	Ab002	Ab010	Ab011	Ab015	Ab021	KM16	KM18	TSG2	TSG4	TSG5	TSG6	TVG52	TVG57	TVG58	TZ1
Scutellaria baicalensis (Huang Qin)	–	11	–	12	–	–	–	–	–	–	–	–	–	–	–	–	–	–	–	–	–	–	–	–	–	–	–	–	–	–	–
Houttuynia cordata (Yu Xing Cao)	–	–	–	–	–	–	–	–	–	–	–	–	–	–	–	–	11	–	–	–	–	–	–	–	–	–	–	–	–	–	–
Taraxacum mongolicum (Pu Gong Ying)	–	–	–	10	–	–	–	–	–	–	–	–	–	–	–	–	–	–	–	–	–	–	–	–	–	–	–	–	–	–	–
Scrophularia ningpoensis (Xuan Shen)	–	11	–	–	–	–	–	–	–	–	–	–	–	–	–	–	–	–	–	–	–	–	–	–	–	–	–	–	–	–	–
Anemarrhena asphodeloides (Zhi Mu)	–	12	–	10	–	–	–	–	–	–	–	–	–	–	–	–	–	–	–	–	–	–	–	–	–	–	–	–	–	–	–
Forsythia suspensa (Lian Qiao)	–	12	–	12	–	–	–	–	–	–	–	–	–	–	–	–	–	–	–	–	–	–	–	–	–	–	–	–	–	–	–
Rehmannia glutinosa (Sheng Di Huang)	–	12	–	–	–	–	–	–	–	–	–	–	–	–	–	–	–	–	–	–	–	–	–	–	–	–	–	–	–	–	–
Belamcanda chinensis (She Gan)	–	14	–	–	14	–	–	–	–	–	–	–	–	–	–	–	–	–	–	–	–	–	–	–	–	–	–	–	–	–	–
Paeonia suffruticosa (Mu Dan Pi)	–	14	–	–	–	–	–	–	–	–	–	–	–	–	–	–	–	–	–	–	–	–	–	–	–	–	–	–	–	–	–
Phellodendron amurense (Huang Bo)	–	–	–	–	–	–	–	–	–	–	–	–	–	–	–	–	–	–	–	–	–	–	–	–	–	–	–	–	–	–	–
Coptis chinensis (Huang Lian)	–	–	–	–	–	–	–	–	–	–	–	–	–	–	–	–	–	11	–	–	–	–	–	–	–	–	–	–	–	–	–
Gardenia jasminoides (Zhi Zi)	–	–	–	–	–	–	–	–	–	–	–	–	–	–	–	–	–	–	–	–	–	–	–	–	–	–	–	–	–	–	–
Isatis indigotica (Ban lan Gen)	–	–	–	–	–	–	–	–	–	–	–	–	–	–	–	–	–	–	–	–	–	–	–	–	–	–	–	–	–	–	–
Smilax glabra (Tu Fu Ling)	–	–	–	–	–	–	–	–	–	–	–	–	–	–	–	–	–	–	–	–	–	–	–	–	–	–	–	–	–	–	–
Gypsum fibrosum (Shi Gao)	–	–	–	–	–	–	–	–	–	–	–	–	–	–	–	–	–	–	–	–	–	–	–	–	–	–	–	–	–	–	–
Prunella vulgaris (Xia Ku Cao)	–	–	–	–	–	–	–	–	–	–	–	–	–	–	–	–	–	–	–	–	–	–	–	–	–	–	–	–	–	–	–
Cassia obtusifolia (Jue Ming Zi)	–	–	–	–	–	–	–	–	–	–	–	–	–	–	–	–	–	–	–	–	–	–	–	–	–	–	–	–	–	–	–

Table 1 The 30 traditional Chinese herbal extracts (128 g/L) and the zone of inhibition (mm) (*Continued*)

Isolates	Ab019	Ab14	Ab15	Ab16	Ab19	Ab23	Ab26	Ab29	Ab35	Ab39	Ab40	Ab54	TVG55	KM5	Ab21	TVG68	Ab002	Ab010	Ab011	Ab015	Ab021	KM16	KM18	TSG2	TSG4	TSG5	TSG6	TVG52	TVG57	TVG58	TZ1
Dictamnus dasycarpus (Bai Xian Pi)	–	–	–	–	–	–	–	–	–	–	–	–	–	–	–	–	–	–	–	–	–	–	–	–	–	–	–	–	–	–	–
Lycium chinense (Di Gu Pi)	–	–	–	–	–	–	–	–	–	–	–	–	–	–	–	–	–	–	–	–	11	–	–	–	–	–	–	–	–	–	–
Torenia concolor (Dao Di Wu Gong)	–	–	–	–	–	–	–	–	–	–	–	–	–	–	–	–	–	–	–	–	–	–	–	–	–	–	–	–	–	–	–
Lonicera japonica (Jin Yin Hua)	–	–	–	–	–	–	–	–	–	–	–	–	–	–	–	–	–	–	–	–	–	–	–	–	–	–	–	–	–	–	–
Hedyotis diffusa (Bai Huan She She Cao)	–	–	–	–	–	–	–	–	–	–	–	–	–	–	–	–	–	–	–	–	–	–	–	–	–	–	–	–	–	–	–
Sophora tokiensis (Shan Dou Gen)	–	–	–	–	–	–	–	–	–	–	–	–	–	–	–	–	–	–	–	–	–	–	–	–	–	–	–	–	–	–	–
Isatis indigotica (Da Qing Ye)	–	–	–	–	–	–	–	–	–	–	–	–	–	–	–	–	–	–	–	–	–	–	–	–	–	–	–	–	–	–	–
Polygonum cuspidatum (Hu Zhang)	–	–	–	–	–	–	–	–	–	–	–	–	–	–	–	–	–	–	–	–	–	–	–	–	–	–	–	–	–	–	–
Patrinia scabiosaefolia (Bai Jiang Cao)	–	–	–	–	–	–	–	–	–	–	–	–	–	–	–	–	–	–	–	–	–	–	–	–	–	–	–	–	–	–	–
Haliotis diversicolor (Shi Jue Ming)	–	–	–	–	–	–	–	–	–	–	–	–	–	–	–	–	–	–	–	–	–	–	–	–	–	–	–	–	–	–	–
Gentiana scabra (Long Dan)	–	–	–	–	–	–	–	–	–	–	–	–	–	–	–	–	–	–	–	–	–	–	–	–	–	–	–	–	–	–	–
Sophora flavescens (Ku Shen)	–	–	–	–	–	–	–	–	–	–	–	–	–	–	–	–	–	–	–	–	–	–	–	–	–	–	–	–	–	–	–
Scutellaria barbata (Ban Zhi Lian)	14	15	18	16	17	17	16	14	18	14	15	16	18	14	17	15	16	16	17	14	16	18	16	18	15	17	17	16	17	16	15

the growth of the organism in each well was visually detected. The MIC was defined as the lowest concentration of the antimicrobial agent that completely inhibited the growth of the organism in the microdilution wells as detected by unaided eyes. The MBC was defined as the lowest concentration of the antibacterial agent that resulted in ≥99.9% reduction of the initial bacterial inoculum [18] (Table 2).

Time-kill curve

Initial inoculums of 5×10^5 cfu/mL XDRAB isolates were prepared. Two sets containing the herb extract of the Chinese herb and colistin at concentrations equal to (1×), twice (2×) and four (4×) times the MIC were employed for each strain. Bacterial growth was measured after 0, 1, 2, 4, 8 and 24 h of incubation by plating on BHI agar and incubating at 37 °C for 16–18 h.

Plant identification and authentication method

Since only the *Scutellaria barbata* extract showed 100% antimicrobial activity in the in vitro experiments, we sent the herbal extract for authentication by a non-profit organization, the Brion Research Institute of Taiwan. Authentication of Scutellaria barbata was performed according to Doc No. BR3-TE01 Authentication SOP by Non-profit organization Brion Research Institute of Taiwan, New Taipei City, Taiwan. Paraffin method was modified from Taiwan Herbal Pharmacopeia [20]. In brief, raw materials were cutting into smashed powder (about 1 cm). After dehydration with mixture of t-Butanol and alcohol (TBA-series), t-Butanol is generally replaced with a pure wax (called infiltration of paraffin) and then the sample was embedded with paraffin. Sectioning with selected thickness, deparaffinization and staining were carried out and sample was observed under an inverted microscope. Identification of tissue mark meets description of Herba of Scutellaria barbata D. Don of Labiatae family [21].

The authentication of *Scutellaria barbata* was performed according to Doc No. BR3-TE01 Authentication Standard Operation Procedure (SOP). We used the paraffin method for the identification of the leaf. The smashed powder of the raw materials was processed with chloral hydrate or water and observed under an inverted microscope.

Animal model
Mice

According to reference material and our experience, 8–12-week-old mice were ideal for this experiment. Younger mice would be too fragile to withstand such a challenge. Inbred female BALB/c mice, 8 to 12 weeks of age, were purchased from the National Experimental Animal Center (Taipei, Taiwan). The mice were kept in animal cages with a 12 h light/dark cycle, with ad libitum access to food and

Table 2 MIC and MBC values of colistin and *S. barbata* extract against various *A. baumannii* strains

Strain	Colistin		*S. barbata* extract	
	MIC/MBC (µg/mL)		MIC/MBC (mg/mL)	
Ab019	4	8	6.4	6.4
Ab14	8	8	6.4	6.4
Ab15	4	4	6.4	6.4
Ab16	8	16	6.4	6.4
Ab19	4	4	6.4	6.4
Ab23	4	8	6.4	12.8
Ab26	4	8	6.4	6.4
Ab29	4	4	6.4	6.4
Ab35	8	16	6.4	6.4
Ab39	8	16	6.4	6.4
Ab40	8	8	6.4	6.4
Ab54	4	4	6.4	6.4
TVG55	4	8	6.4	12.8
KM5	4	8	6.4	6.4
Ab21	8	8	6.4	6.4
TVG68	4	4	6.4	6.4
Ab002	8	8	6.4	6.4
Ab010	4	4	6.4	6.4
Ab011	4	4	6.4	6.4
Ab015	4	4	12.8	12.8
Ab021	4	16	12.8	12.8
KM16	4	8	6.4	12.8
KM18	4	8	6.4	6.4
TSG2	8	8	6.4	6.4
TSG4	4	4	6.4	6.4
TSG5	8	16	6.4	6.4
TSG6	8	16	6.4	6.4
TVG52	4	8	6.4	6.4
TVG57	2	2	6.4	6.4
TVG58	4	8	6.4	6.4
TZ1	16	16	12.8	12.8

water. All animal experiments were approved by the Animal Use Protocol IACUC of I-Shou University (IACUC-ISU-102032). Tribromoethanol, an injectable anaesthetic agent used in mice, was used in our animal model. Tribromoethanol is prepared by the mixing 2,2,2-tribromoethyl alcohol with tert-amyl alcohol (SIGMA). The material is mixed by swirling prior to administration and given by IP injection at a dose of 250 mg/Kg. This amounts to 0.5 ml of the above solution to a 25 g mouse. Tribromoethanol is effective and simple to use; it provides rapid induction and deep surgical anaesthesia in mice followed by faster postoperative recovery and low morbidity and mortality [22, 23].

In the end time point of animal experiments, all animals were sacrificed by cervical dislocation with anaesthesia. Post induction of anaesthesia (tribromoethanol, 250 mg/Kg, IP injection), the thumb and index finger are placed on either side of the neck at the base of the skull or, alternatively, a rod is pressed at the base of the skull with the animal lying on a table surface. With the other hand, the bases of the tail or hind limbs are firmly and steadily pulled to cause separation of the cervical vertebrae and spinal cord from the skull.

Experimental design

Since only the *Scutellaria barbata* extract showed 100% antimicrobial activity in the in vitro experiments, it was used in the animal studies. The mouse model of *A. baumannii*-associated pneumonia was generated as described previously, with minor modifications [24]. Briefly, anaesthetized mice were suspended vertically and given an intratracheal (i.t.) inoculation of aliquots containing the bacterial suspension (the inoculum dose was 1×10^9 cfu in 50 µL of phosphate-buffered saline (PBS)). After an incubation period of 4 h, all the infected mice were randomly divided into three groups as follows: (1) the control group (without treatment); (2) the colistin treatment group (i.t. administration of colistin at 75000 U/kg every 12 h); and (3) the Sb treatment group (oral administration of *S. barbata* extract at 200 mg/kg every 24 h) [25]. The dose of Sb that we used in this study (200 mg/kg) is the same as the dose used for cancer treatment.

Pulmonary bacterial loads and histopathological studies

Mice were sacrificed at 72 h post treatment. Homogenized lung samples were examined for pulmonary bacterial loads after 72 h of treatment (*n* = 5 per group). Serial tenfold dilutions of the lung homogenates were prepared in saline, and 0.1 mL of each dilution was spread on LB agar plates. The results were expressed as cfu per homogenized lung. For the histopathological studies, the lungs were fixed immediately in 10% neutral buffered formalin and processed by

standard paraffin embedding methods. Sections 4 µm thick were cut, stained with haematoxylin-eosin (HE) or Gram stained, and examined under the light microscope (*n* = 4).

Statistical analysis

Data are presented as the mean ± standard deviation for each group. Differences in quantitative measurements were assessed by Student's t-test or one-way or two-way analysis of variance (ANOVA). Differences were considered statistically significant at $P < 0.05$.

Results

Screening of antimicrobial activity

Among the 30 Chinese herbs screened by the disc diffusion method, only the extract of *Scutellaria barbata* showed 100% antimicrobial activity against the 30 clinical isolates of *A. baumannii*, including the XDRAB strains with different pulsotypes (Table 1 and Fig. 1). The mean diameters of the zones of inhibition ranged from 14 to 18 mm. The MIC and MBC values are shown in Table 1. We also tested five active compounds of *Scutellaria barbata*, including apigenin, baicalin, hispidulin, luteolin, naringenin, wogonin and protocatechuic acid. The data show no antibacterial effect of any single compound at the highest concentration (1280 µg/ml), but we found synergistic effects of several formulas, including hispidulin (640 µg/ml) + protocatechuic acid (640 µg/ml), luteolin (640 µg/ml) + naringenin (640 µg/ml) and pigenin (320 µg/ml) + hispidulin (320 µg/ml) + protocatechuic acid (320 µg/ml) (data not shown).

Time-kill curve

The time-kill curve for the *S. barbata* extract showed better bactericidal activity than that of colistin against two selected strains of *A. baumannii*, TSG2 and Ab011. The XDRAB growth was persistent even after 8 h at 1× the MIC concentration of colistin. However, under similar conditions, the *S. barbata* extract could successfully kill the bacteria. Bactericidal activity (≥ 3 $\log_{10}$ cfu/mL)

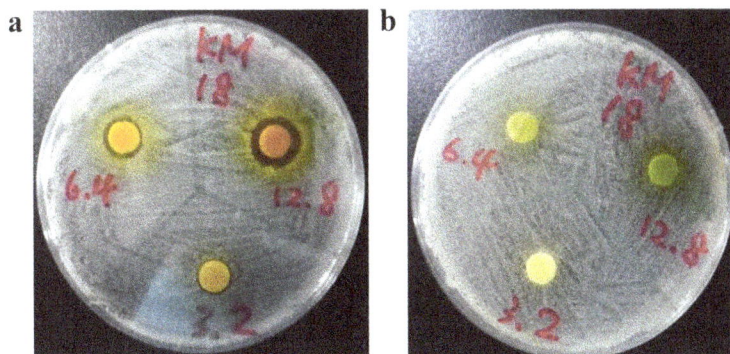

Fig. 1 The antibacterial effect of *S. barbata* extract (**a**) and *L. japonica* extract (**b**) assayed at concentrations of 3.2 mg/mL, 6.4 mg/mL and 12.8 mg/mL against *A. baumannii* strain KM18

was achieved within 2 to 4 h against two *A. baumannii* isolates treated with the *S. barbata* extract at 1×, 2× and 4× times the MIC concentration (Fig. 2).

Plant identification

The herbal extract was authenticated as the dried herb of *Scutellaria barbata* D. Don of the Lamiaceae family by the non-profit organization the Brion Research Institute of Taiwan. Briefly, the powder was yellowish-green (Fig. 3-a). The epidermal cells of the leaf walls were slightly curved, and the stoma (Fig. 3-b) were of the diacytic type, with 2–7 subsidiary cells. The glandular scales (Fig. 3-c) were 4- to 8-celled, subrounded or elliptical, and 24–47 μm in diameter. The glandular hairs (Fig. 3-d) consisted of a few-celled head and a single-celled stalk. The non-glandular hairs (Fig. 3-e) consisted of 1–4 cells, with very long apical cells and a fine, warty protuberance on the surface. Bordered-

pitted vessels (Fig. 3-f) and spiral vessels (Fig. 3-g) were visible. The fibres (Fig. 3-h) were often in bundles 8–36 μm in diameter that were usually broken, and they had relatively thick walls.

Histopathological studies of pneumonia

Compared with the lungs of uninfected mice (Fig. 4a), the infected lungs revealed acute inflammation, with the infiltration of numerous polymorphonuclear cells and consolidation, which was consistent with pneumonia. The accumulation of invasive gram-negative diplococci was also observed (Fig. 4b). In the colistin treatment group, lung consolidation and infiltration of polymorphonuclear cells were noted (Fig. 4c). However, this inflammatory status abated after Sb extract treatment, indicating the therapeutic efficacy of oral Sb extract against *A. baumannii* infections (Fig. 4d).

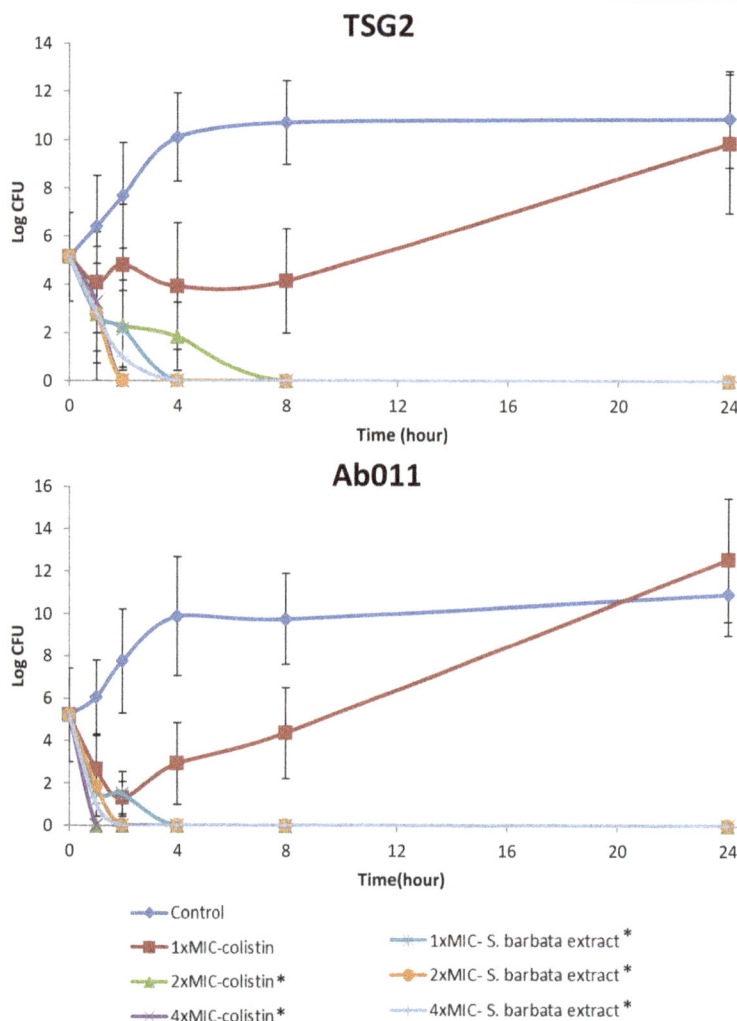

Fig. 2 Time-killing curves of colistin and *S. barbata* extract assayed on two selected strains of *A. baumannii* TSG2 and Ab011. "*" Significantly lower bacterial load compared to the control group at 24 h ($P < 0.05$). $n = 3$ per group

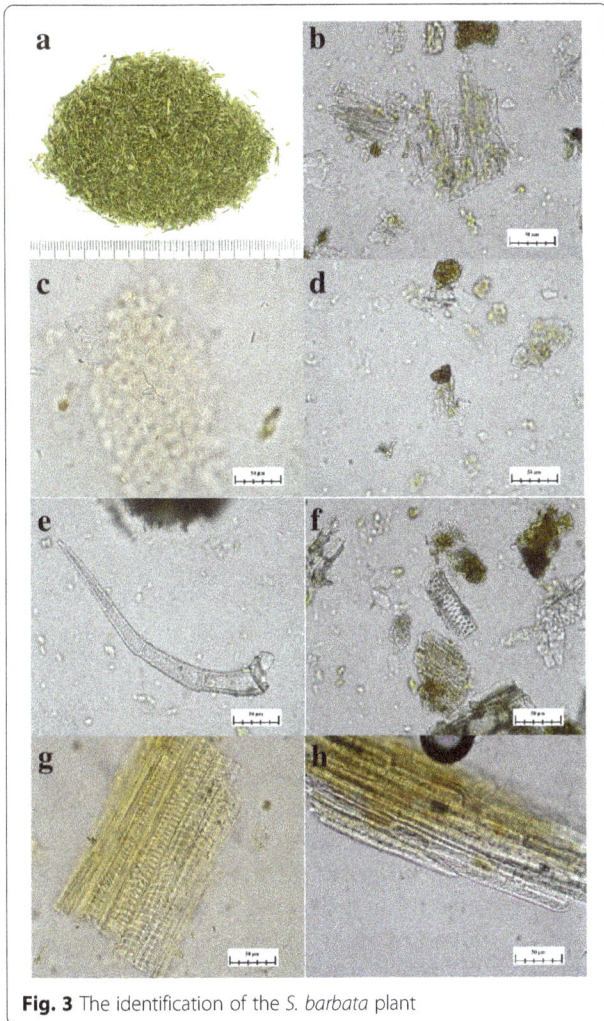

Fig. 3 The identification of the *S. barbata* plant

Pulmonary bacterial clearance

In the murine model, we compared the efficacy of oral *S. barbata* extract (Sb treatment group) with inhaled colistin (colistin treatment group). All the mice survived until day 3. After sacrificing the mice, the lungs of the mice were examined. It was observed that the bacterial load decreased significantly in the Sb treatment group ($P < 0.05$), whereas a decrease in the bacterial load was not seen in the colistin treatment group or the control group (Fig. 5).

Discussion

Previous studies have shown that many heat-clearing and detoxifying Chinese herbs have antimicrobial effects [15]. Miyasaki et al. found that plant herbal extracts contain flavones, tannins, and phenolic compounds that are active against MDRAB strains. In their study, they also found that among all the screened herbs, *Scutellaria baicalensis* demonstrated the lowest MIC value against MDRAB [13, 14]. *Scutellaria* species (Lamiaceae) have widely been used in traditional medical systems in China, India, Korea, Japan,

European countries, and North America because of their potential antimicrobial activity [26, 27]. In our study, we screened the commonly used heat-clearing and detoxifying Chinese herbs used in Taiwan against MDRAB strains and found that *S. barbata* showed the best antimicrobial activity against MDRAB. The time-kill curve for the *S. barbata* extract against XDRAB showed marked bactericidal activity compared to colistin under similar conditions. Furthermore, in the murine XDRAB pneumonia model, the *S. barbata* extract-treated group showed a decrease in the bacterial load and inflammation in the lungs when compared to the intratracheal colistin-treated group.

S. barbata is a perennial herb prevalent in Korea and southern China [28, 29]. Its English common name is barbed skullcap, and its Chinese name is Ban Zhi Lian. *S. barbata* has been used along with other herbs in traditional Chinese and Korean medicine to treat bacterial infections (including carbuncles, cellulitis, and pneumonia), hepatitis, and tumours [30]. Six phenolic compounds, namely, p-coumaric acid, scutellarin, apigenin 5-O-β-glucopyranoside, luteolin, apigenin and 4′-hydroxywogonin, were obtained from *S. barbata* during the phytochemical analyses [31]. Recent studies in many animal models and small clinical trials have demonstrated the antitumour activity of *S. barbata*. The safety and efficacy of an aqueous extract of the aerial parts of *S. barbata* (Bezielle: BZL101) for breast cancer treatment have also been analysed in the Phase I clinical trial undertaken by Bionovo [32–34]. *S. barbata* and *Hedyotis diffusa* are the most commonly prescribed Chinese herbs for breast cancer and post-surgery colon cancer, as reported by Taiwanese nationwide surveys [35, 36]. In addition to anticancer properties, *S. barbata* has been reported to have anti-inflammatory, anticomplementary, antioxidant and antimicrobial properties [36]. A previous study showed that the antimicrobial effect of *S. barbata* is broad spectrum, possessing antibacterial activity against many bacterial strains, including *Escherichia coli*, *Staphylococcus aureus*, *Pseudomonas aeruginosa* and *Salmonella typhimurium*. It was also reported that the antibacterial effect of *S. barbata* is mediated via ROS generation, intracellular protein leakage, and the rupture of bacterial cell membranes [17]. The antimicrobial effect of the essential oil derived from *S. barbata* (50% ethanolic extract) against methicillin-resistant *Staphylococcus aureus* (MRSA) has also been studied. Both of these studies showed that *S. barbata* has better activity against gram-positive cocci than against gram-negative bacteria [37, 38]. Apigenin and luteolin were isolated from the plant as active constituents against MRSA [37]. There are neither in vitro data nor animal model studies available on the utility of *S. barbata* in the treatment of *Acinetobacter* infection, although several animal models of cancer have been reported [39, 40]. A company in

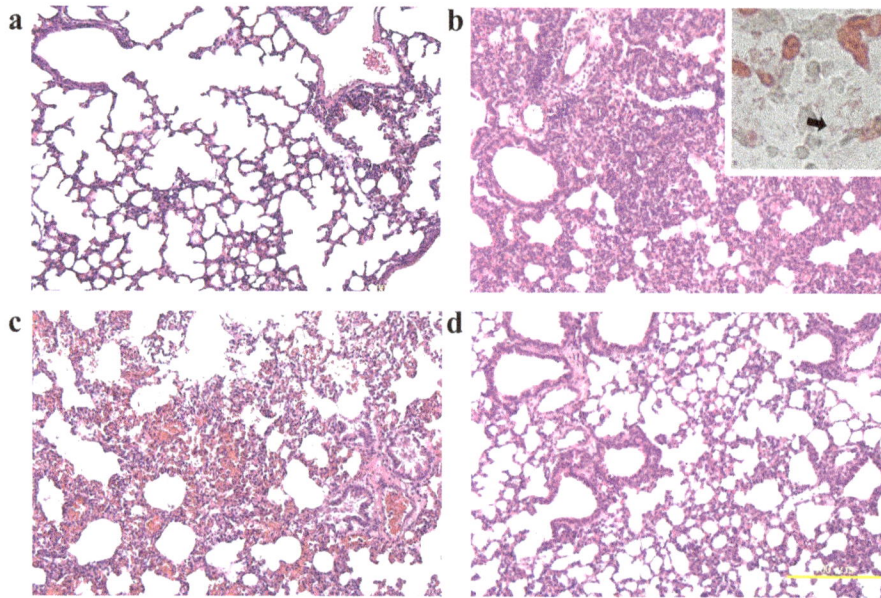

Fig. 4 Pathological pulmonary findings after intratracheal inoculation of KM18. Uninfected mice (a, H&E, × 100), control group mice (b, H&E, × 100) and diplococci (arrowhead) in an alveolar sac with Gram staining (right upper panel of b, × 1000), colistin treatment group mice (c, H&E, × 100) and Sb extract treatment group mice (d, H&E, × 100)

China used a combination of lobelia extract (50%) and *S. barbata* extract (50%) and showed that it has 90% efficiency in treating pneumonia caused by mixed a bacterial and viral infection in pigs and in treating mastitis in cows. In addition, they reported that *S. barbata* extract alone has a comparatively lower efficacy (70%) [41]. Another study in China also showed that *S. barbata* can inhibit the expression of the quorum sensing gene

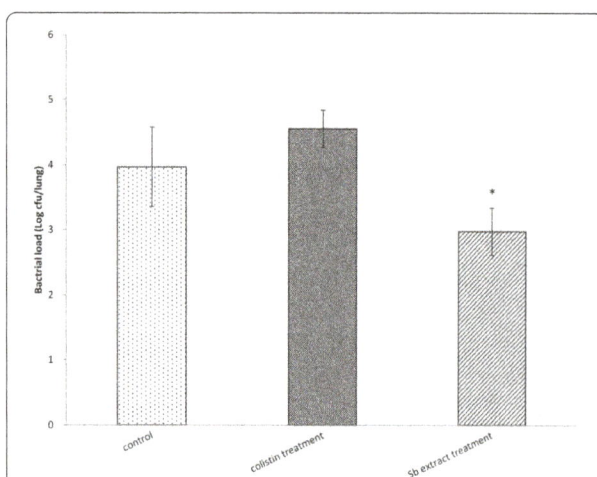

Fig. 5 Bacterial load in the lungs of the infected mice without therapy (control group) and infected mice treated with colistin or *S. barbata* (Sb) extract after inoculation with 3.97 ± 0.61, 4.56 ± 0.28 and 2.97 ± 0.36 log CFU/lung (Data are expressed as the mean ± SD of five mice for each group). "*" Significantly lower bacterial load in the *S. barbata* (Sb) extract treatment group compared to the control group ($P < 0.05$)

involved in *Pseudomonas* infections [42]. In this study, we found that among the commonly used heat-clearing and detoxifying Chinese herbs, *S. barbata* displayed the maximum potency against XDRAB. This finding was further validated by animal model studies. Furthermore, an active component study showed that while no single compound was active against XDRAB, combinations of two or more active compounds displayed considerable antimicrobial activity against XDRAB (data not shown). An explanation for this observation could be that the antibacterially active compounds act effectively in combination but show very low efficacy when used alone [8].

The limitations of this study are as follows: (1) Our in vitro tests showed good activity of *S. barbata* extract against XDRAB; however, the outcome of the tested bacterial isolates cannot conclude that *S. barbata* would also be active against other worldwide clinical isolates. The inclusion of more clinical isolates of *A. baumannii* may improve the generalizability of the study. (2) The animal model study was preliminary, and the ideal dosage needs to be optimized. The dose we used in this study (200 mg/kg) was similar to the dose used in human clinical trials and in the animal model studies of cancer. (3) Inhaled colistin might produce a local effect in the control group. Further animal model studies comparing intravenous and inhaled colistin need to be conducted. (4) In conventional use, the water decoction of the herbs can be administered orally to treat infection or used externally on skin wounds. In this study, we wanted to identify herbs with the potential to treat

XDRAB infections in clinical settings. In our future study, we will apply another extraction method (polar and non-polar) to determine the active compounds and antibacterial mechanisms.

Conclusion

S. barbata could be an alternative therapy in the treatment of infection caused by the superbug *Acinetobacter baumannii*. Further human clinical trials are necessary to determine whether it can be used for the treatment of XDRAB pulmonary infection.

Acknowledgements
We are grateful to the members of the medicine laboratory for their excellent work. And we thanks American Journal Experts for English Editing.

Funding
This work was supported by research grants from the Taiwan Ministry of Science and Technology MOST 103–2314-B-214-001 and E-DA Hospital EDAHP105009, EDAHP104050 and EDAHP103016.

Authors' contributions
This study was designed by CSL, JLW and TCC. CSL, CRH and CCH performed all the experiments, and JLW drafted the manuscript. CSL, LWL and CMC performed the plant extractions. IWC performed the pathological experiments. TCC and CHH critically reviewed the manuscript. All authors reviewed the manuscript and read and approved the final version.

Competing interests
The authors declare that they have no competing interests.

Author details
[1]School of Chinese Medicine for Post-Baccalaureates, Chinese Medicine Department, I-Shou University and E-DA Hospital, Kaoshiung, Taiwan. [2]Department of Medical Research, E-DA Hospital and School of Medicine, I-Shou University, Kaoshiung, Taiwan. [3]Department of Pathology, Taipei Medical University Hospital and , School of Medicine, College of Medicine, Taipei Medical University , Taipei, Taiwan. [4]Department of Chemical Engineering, and Institute of Biotechnology, I-Shou University, Kaoshiung, Taiwan. [5]Department of Internal Medicine, National Cheng Kung University Hospital and College of Medicine,National Cheng Kung University, No. 138, Sheng Li Road, Tainan 70403, Taiwan.

Reference
1. Peleg AY, Seifert H, Paterson DL. Acinetobacter baumannii: emergence of a successful pathogen. Clin Microbiol Rev. 2008;21(3):538–82.
2. Karageorgopoulos DE, Falagas ME. Current control and treatment of multidrug-resistant Acinetobacter baumannii infections. Lancet Infect Dis. 2008;8(12):751–62.
3. Garnacho-Montero J, Amaya-Villar R. Multiresistant Acinetobacter baumannii infections: epidemiology and management. Curr Opin Infect Dis. 2010;23(4):332–9.
4. Yahav D, Farbman L, Leibovici L, Paul M. Colistin: new lessons on an old antibiotic. Clin Microbiol Infect. 2012;18(1):18–29.
5. Justo JA, Bosso JA. Adverse reactions associated with systemic polymyxin therapy. Pharmacotherapy. 2015;35(1):28–33.
6. Ni W, Han Y, Zhao J, Wei C, Cui J, Wang R, Liu Y. Tigecycline treatment experience against multidrug-resistant Acinetobacter baumannii infections: a systematic review and meta-analysis. Int J Antimicrob Agents. 2016;47(2):107–16.
7. Savoia D. Plant-derived antimicrobial compounds: alternatives to antibiotics. Future Microbiol. 2012;7(8):979–90.
8. Miyasaki Y, Nichols WS, Morgan MA, Kwan JA, Van Benschoten MM, Kittell PE, Hardy WD. Screening of herbal extracts against multi-drug resistant Acinetobacter baumannii. Phytotherapy research: PTR. 2010;24(8):1202–6.
9. Tiwari M, Roy R, Tiwari V. Screening of herbal-based bioactive extract against Carbapenem-resistant strain of Acinetobacter baumannii. Microbial drug resistance (Larchmont, NY). 2016;22(5):364–71.
10. Tiwari V, Tiwari M, Solanki V. Polyvinylpyrrolidone-capped silver nanoparticle inhibits infection of Carbapenem-resistant strain of Acinetobacter baumannii in the human pulmonary epithelial cell. Front Immunol. 2017;8:973.
11. Khan I, Rahman H, Abd El-Salam NM, Tawab A, Hussain A, Khan TA, Khan UA, Qasim M, Adnan M, Azizullah A, et al. Punica granatum peel extracts: HPLC fractionation and LC MS analysis to quest compounds having activity against multidrug resistant bacteria. BMC Complement Altern Med. 2017;17(1):247.
12. Tiwari V, Tiwari D, Patel V, Tiwari M. Effect of secondary metabolite of Actinidia deliciosa on the biofilm and extra-cellular matrix components of Acinetobacter baumannii. Microb Pathog. 2017;110:345–51.
13. Miyasaki Y, Rabenstein JD, Rhea J, Crouch ML, Mocek UM, Kittell PE, Morgan MA, Nichols WS, Van Benschoten MM, Hardy WD, et al. Isolation and characterization of antimicrobial compounds in plant extracts against multidrug-resistant Acinetobacter baumannii. PLoS One. 2013;8(4):e61594.
14. Tiwari V, Roy R, Tiwari M. Antimicrobial active herbal compounds against Acinetobacter baumannii and other pathogens. Front Microbiol. 2015;6:618.
15. Muluye RA, Bian Y, Alemu PN. Anti-inflammatory and antimicrobial effects of heat-clearing Chinese herbs: a current review. Journal of traditional and complementary medicine. 2014;4(2):93–8.
16. Chiang SR, Chuang YC, Tang HJ, Chen CC, Chen CH, Lee NY, Chou CH, Ko WC. Intratracheal colistin sulfate for BALB/c mice with early pneumonia caused by carbapenem-resistant Acinetobacter baumannii. Crit Care Med. 2009;37(9):2590–5.
17. Lu C-X, Tang Q-L, Kang A-R. Phytochemical analysis, antibacterial activity and mode of action of the Methanolic extract of Scutellaria barbata against various clinically important bacterial pathogens. Int J Pharmacol. 2016;12(2):116–25.
18. Methods for dilution antimicrobial susceptibility tests for bacteria that grow aerobically approved standard—ninth edition M07-A9. Wayne: Clinical and Laboratory Standards Institute; 2012.
19. Performance standards for antimicrobial disk susceptibility tests; approved standard—eleventh edition M02-A11. Wayne: Clinical and Laboratory Standards Institute; 2012.
20. Microscopic identification. In: Taiwan Herbal Pharmacopeia. 2.: Ministry of Health and Welfare. Taiwan; 2013: 50–53.
21. Chinese Pharmacopoeia Commission. Labiatae family. In: Pharmacopoeia of the People's Republic of China. Beijiung: China Medical Science Press. 2015;117–118.
22. Papaioannou VE, Fox JG. Efficacy of tribromoethanol anesthesia in mice. Lab Anim Sci. 1993;43(2):189–92.
23. Weiss M, Zimmermann F. Tribromoethanol (Avertin) as an anaesthetic in mice. Lab Anim. 1999;33(2):192–3.
24. Joly-Guillou ML, Wolff M, Pocidalo JJ, Walker F, Carbon C. Use of a new mouse model of Acinetobacter baumannii pneumonia to evaluate the postantibiotic effect of imipenem. Antimicrob Agents Chemother. 1997;41(2):345–51.
25. Xu H, Yu J, Sun Y, Xu X, Li L, Xue M, Du G. Scutellaria barbata D. Don extract synergizes the antitumor effects of low dose 5-fluorouracil through induction of apoptosis and metabolism. Phytomedicine: international journal of phytotherapy and phytopharmacology. 2013;20(10):897–903.
26. Tan BK, Vanitha J. Immunomodulatory and antimicrobial effects of some traditional chinese medicinal herbs: a review. Curr Med Chem. 2004;11(11):1423–30.
27. Skullcap: Potential Medicinal Crop [https://www.hort.purdue.edu/newcrop/ncnu02/v5-580.html].
28. Hyman P, Abedon ST. Bacteriophage host range and bacterial resistance. Adv Appl Microbiol. 2010;70:217–48.
29. Scutellaria barbata D. Don. [http://www.koreantk.com/ktkp2014/medicine/medicine-view.view?medCd=M0006293&tempLang=en].
30. Integrative Medicine, About Herbs, Botanicals & other products, search about herbs, Scutellaria barbata [https://www.mskcc.org/cancer-care/integrative-medicine/herbs/scutellaria-barbata#msk_professional].
31. Yao H, Li S, Hu J, Chen Y, Huang L, Lin J, Li G, Lin X. Chromatographic fingerprint and quantitative analysis of seven bioactive compounds of Scutellaria barbata. Planta Med. 2011;77(4):388–93.
32. Rugo H, Shtivelman E, Perez A, Vogel C, Franco S, Tan Chiu E, Melisko M, Tagliaferri M, Cohen I, Shoemaker M, et al. Phase I trial and antitumor effects of BZL101 for patients with advanced breast cancer. Breast Cancer Res Treat. 2007;105(1):17–28.

33. Perez AT, Arun B, Tripathy D, Tagliaferri MA, Shaw HS, Kimmick GG, Cohen I, Shtivelman E, Caygill KA, Grady D, et al. A phase 1B dose escalation trial of Scutellaria barbata (BZL101) for patients with metastatic breast cancer. Breast Cancer Res Treat. 2010;120(1):111–8.

34. Tao G, Balunas MJ. Current therapeutic role and medicinal potential of Scutellaria barbata in traditional Chinese medicine and western research. J Ethnopharmacol. 2016;182:170–80.

35. Yeh YC, Chen HY, Yang SH, Lin YH, Chiu JH, Lin YH, Chen JL. Hedyotis diffusa combined with Scutellaria barbata are the Core treatment of Chinese herbal medicine used for breast cancer patients: a population-based study. Evidence-based complementary and alternative medicine: eCAM. 2014;2014:202378.

36. Chao TH, Fu PK, Chang CH, Chang SN, Chiahung Mao F, Lin CH. Prescription patterns of Chinese herbal products for post-surgery colon cancer patients in Taiwan. J Ethnopharmacol. 2014;155(1):702–8.

37. Sato Y, Suzaki S, Nishikawa T, Kihara M, Shibata H, Higuti T. Phytochemical flavones isolated from Scutellaria barbata and antibacterial activity against methicillin-resistant Staphylococcus aureus. J Ethnopharmacol. 2000;72(3):483–8.

38. Yu J, Lei J, Yu H, Cai X, Zou G. Chemical composition and antimicrobial activity of the essential oil of Scutellaria barbata. Phytochemistry. 2004;65(7):881–4.

39. Dai ZJ, Lu WF, Gao J, Kang HF, Ma YG, Zhang SQ, Diao Y, Lin S, Wang XJ, Wu WY. Anti-angiogenic effect of the total flavonoids in Scutellaria barbata D. Don. *BMC complementary and alternative medicine*. 2013;13:150.

40. Dai ZJ, Wu WY, Kang HF, Ma XB, Zhang SQ, Min WL, Kang WF, Ma XB, Zhang SQ, Min WL, et al. Protective effects of Scutellaria barbata against rat liver tumorigenesis. Asian Pacific journal of cancer prevention: APJCP. 2013; 14(1):261–5.

41. Chen L. 'Shuanglian' injection and preparation process thereof. Chinese patent (CN101167800A). 2008.

42. Xiao J, Shen L, Zhao L, Wu Y, Duan K, Guo Q. Inhibition of the quorum sensing system in Pseudomonas aeruginosa PAO1 by Sculellaria barbata. Zhongguo Kang Sheng Su Za Zhi. 2004;12:885–90.

5

Comparative efficacy of Chinese herbal injections for treating acute cerebral infarction: a network meta-analysis of randomized controlled trials

Shi Liu, Jia-Rui Wu*⬧, Dan Zhang, Kai-Huan Wang, Bing Zhang, Xiao-Meng Zhang, Di Tan, Xiao-Jiao Duan, Ying-Ying Cui and Xin-Kui Liu

Abstract

Background: Chinese herbal injections (CHIs) are prepared by extracting and purifying effective substances from herbs (or decoction pieces) using modern scientific techniques and methods. CHIs combined with aspirin + anticoagulants + dehydrant + neuroprotectant (AADN) are believed to be effective for the treatment of acute cerebral infarction (ACI). However, no randomized controlled trial (RCT) has been performed to directly compare the efficacies of different regimens of CHIs. Therefore, we performed a systematic review and network meta-analysis (NMA) to compare the efficacies of different regimens of CHIs for ACI.

Methods: We conducted an overall and systematic retrieval from literature databases of RCTs focused on the use of CHIs to treat ACI up to June 2016. We used the Cochrane Handbook version 5.1.0 and CONSORT statement to assess the risk of bias. The data were analyzed using STATA 13.0 and WinBUGS 1.4.3 software.

Results: Overall, 64 studies with 6225 participants involving 15 CHIs were included in the NMA. In terms of the markedly effective rate, Danhong (DH) + AADN had the highest likelihood of being the best treatment. In terms of the improvement of neurological impairment, Shuxuening (SXN) + AADN had the highest likelihood of being the best treatment. Considering two outcomes, injections of SXN, Yinxingdamo (YXDM), DH, Shuxuetong (SXT), HongHuaHuangSeSu (HHHSS), DengZhanXiXin (DZXX) and Shenxiong glucose (SX) plus AADN were the optimum treatment regimens for ACI, especially SXN + AADN and YXDM + AADN.

Conclusions: Based on the NMA, SXN, YXDM, DH, SXT, HHHSS, DZXX and SX plus AADN showed the highest probability of being the best treatment regimens. Due to the limitations of the present study, our findings should be verified by well-designed RCTs.

Keywords: Network meta-analysis, Acute cerebral infarction, Chinese herbal injection

Background

Acute cerebral infarction (ACI) is one of the most common cerebral vascular diseases, also referred to as ischemic stroke, which is result from ischemia, hypoxia and cerebral blood circulation [1–3]. ACI has the characteristics of high disability and recurrence [4–6]. Besides, it is a major disease leading to serious damage of central nervous system or death [4, 7]. It was estimated that ACI cause 6.2 million mortalities annually worldwide [8]. In traditional Chinese medicine (TCM) theories, ACI refers to "apoplexy", majorly due to blood stasis syndrome [3]. Therefore, promoting blood flow is of primary importance. It has been proven that TCM is an effective complementary intervention for stroke, especially in the treatment of ischemic stroke [9–13].

Currently, therapies for ACI include thrombolytics, antithrombotics, anticoagulants, and neuroprotectants [14]; this was the Grade-I recommendation in the guidance of diagnosis and treatment of acute ischemic stroke in China 2010, which fully considered the national

* Correspondence: exogamy@163.com
Department of Clinical Chinese Pharmacy, School of Chinese Materia Medica, Beijing University of Chinese Medicine, Beijing 100102, China

conditions and clinical experience. Among them, thrombolytic has a short therapeutic time window. Thus, many patients easily miss the effective time window of thrombolysis. ACI patients who are not eligible for thrombolysis therapy should be given oral aspirin, which was approved by the US Food and Drug Administration (FDA), at a dose ranging from 150 to 300 mg/d as soon as possible (level of evidence: A) [15, 16]. And patients with brain edema could use a mannitol intravenous drip. Although more high-quality clinical trials are needed to further demonstrate the efficacy and safety of neuroprotective agents, a number of RCTs have suggested that edaravone and cerebroprotein hydrolysate improve functional outcomes and the safety of patients with ACI [17–20]. Additionally, the therapeutic principle of invigorating blood circulation for removing blood stasis of TCM holds a significant position for ACI. Chinese herbal injections (CHIs) have the characteristics of rapid efficacy and high bioavailability [21–23].Presently, 37 injections are often used in the treatment of cerebral infarction, such as Xueshuantong injection, Shuxuening injection, Mailuoning injection, and Danshenchuanxiongqin injection [24–27]. Clinical data [28–32] from systematic reviews of RCTs have demonstrated the beneficial effects of CHIs for inhibiting platelet aggregation, improving blood microcirculation and nerve function, enhancing the tolerance of ischemic tissue to hypoxia, and protecting against ischemic reperfusion injury.

Hence, this study systematically evaluated the clinical effectiveness of CHIs combined with an aspirin + anticoagulants + dehydrant + neuroprotectant (AADN) regimen in ACI patients that conformed to the standardized treatment of ischemic cerebrovascular disease: integration, individualization and sequencing. However, there is no direct head-to-head evidence revealing the best CHIs for ACI treatment. Determining the superiority of a treatment based on a pairwise comparison meta-analysis is difficult. A network meta-analysis (NMA), which is an extension of a traditional meta-analysis, synthesizes the available evidence to enable simultaneous comparisons of different treatment options that lack direct head-to-head evaluations [33–35]. Therefore, the present study performed a NMA to compare the clinical efficacy of 37 CHIs combined with the AADN regimen to reveal the best CHIs for ACI, aiming to provide more sights for selection of ACI.

Methods
Eligibility criteria
Studies meeting the following criteria were included: (1) Clinical randomized controlled trials (RCTs) using CHIs + AADN to treat ACI regardless of blinding. (2) Cerebrovascular disease was diagnosed according to the standards revised by the Fourth National Conference on Cerebrovascular Disease by the Chinese Medical Association in 1995 [36]. The acute phase of ACI generally refers to 2 weeks after the onset of disease. Thus, this NMA enrolled patients with the course of disease within 2 weeks. No cerebral hemorrhage was detected using cranial computed tomography (CT) or magnetic resonance imaging (MRI). There were no limits on age, gender, race or disease severity. (3) Eligible comparisons were CHIs + AADN regimens versus the AADN regimen alone and CHIs + AADN regimens versus other CHIs + AADN regimens. There was no limitation on the dosages or treatment courses. (4) Outcome measures included the markedly effective rate, improvement of neurological impairment, activities of daily living function, and death from all causes within the treatment and during the entire follow-up period. The following formula was used: the markedly effective rate (%) = (number of recovered patients + number of patients with significant progress) / total number × 100%. The efficacy criteria were predominantly based on the reduction of the neurological deficit score and could be divided into four grades: recovery, significant progress, progress, and no change or deterioration. Recovery, significant progress, progress, and no change or deterioration were determined when the neurological deficit score decreased from 91% to 100%, between 46% and 90%, between 18% and 45%, and < 17%, respectively. The improvement of neurological impairment is expressed as the mean ± standard deviation.

The following studies were excluded: (1) studies that did not refer to the acute phase; (2) studies that did not meet the curative effect valuation standard; (3) studies involving patients who had a severe cognitive disorder, hemorrhagic tendency, or serious complications, such as atrial fibrillation, severe heart failure, severe liver and kidney diseases, undergoing surgery, acupuncture or other physical therapy; (4) data that were incorrect, incomplete or unavailable; (5) reviews or meta-analyses, experimental research, retrospective studies, case reports, and conference abstracts.

Data sources and search strategy
A systematic literature search was performed using the following databases from inception to June 2016: PubMed, Cochrane Library, Embase, China National Knowledge Infrastructure Database (CNKI), Wanfang Database, and Chinese Biomedical Literature Database (CBM). The medical subject headings (MeSH) and free text words were used. No language or other restrictions were imposed. Furthermore, we hand searched the reference lists of all retrieved studies. The specific Chinese and English search terms for each CHIs are shown in Additional file 1: Table S1 and the detailed search strategy is shown in Additional file 2.

Literature selection and data extraction

Two reviewers independently read the titles and abstracts of the literature to exclude literature that was obviously not relevant as well as reviews and pharmacological experiments. We retrieved the full text of the articles to determine whether they were eligible.

The data of interest from each included RCT were collected using a standard data abstraction form created in Microsoft Excel 2013 (Microsoft Corp, Redmond, WA, USA). The main components of the extracted data were as follows: (1) General information: author names and publication data; (2) Patient information: median age, number of patients, gender, and acute phase; (3) Intervention: names, dosages, and treatment; (4) Outcomes: the markedly effective rate, improvement of neurological deficit score, adverse drug reactions/adverse drug events (ADRs/ADEs), activities of daily living function, and death from all causes within the treatment and during the entire follow-up period.

Quality assessment

The methodological quality of each included study was evaluated using the Cochrane Risk of Bias tool [37] and the CONSORT statement [38]. The items included randomization, blinding, dropout, eligibility criteria for participants, adverse events, and statistical methods. The judgments for each entry involved were divided into 3 grades: "high", "unclear", and "low". A quality assessment was performed by two independent reviews, and disagreements were resolved by consensus.

Statistical analysis

We performed a pairwise meta-analysis using STATA 13.0 software (Stata Corporation, College Station, TX, USA). The pooled odds ratios (ORs) were calculated for dichotomous data and standardized mean differences (SMDs) were calculated for continuous variables, both with 95% confidence interval (95% CI). The Chi-squared test was used to evaluate the heterogeneity between studies, and I^2 was used to show the extent of heterogeneity. When P was ≥ 0.1 and I^2 was $\leq 50\%$, no statistical heterogeneity was suggested and the Mantel-Haenszel fixed-effects model was used for the meta-analysis. When $P < 0.1$ and I^2 was $> 50\%$, we explored the sources of heterogeneity using a subgroup analysis and meta-regression. When there was no clinical heterogeneity, the Mantel-Haenszel random-effects model was used to perform the meta-analysis [37].

A Bayesian NMA was conducted using WinBUGS 1.4.3 software (MRC Biostatistics Unit, Cambridge, UK). The random-effects model with vague priors for multi-arm trials was used [39]. The model parameters were estimated using a Markov chain Monte Carlo method called Gibbs sampling. Convergence was found to be adequate after running 1000 samples. These samples were discarded as "burn-in," and posterior summaries were based on 100,000 subsequent simulations. The results are reported as the OR and SMD with 95% CI. To evaluate the inconsistency between direct and indirect effect estimates for the same comparison, we evaluated each closed loop in the network. In a closed loop, we employed the inconsistency factor (IF) to evaluate heterogeneity among the included studies. If the 95% CIs of the IF values were truncated at zero, it indicated that the 2 sources were in agreement [39]. To rank the treatments, we used the surface under the cumulative ranking probabilities (SUCRA); a SUCRA value of 100% is assigned to the best treatment and 0% for the worst treatment [39]. A comparison-adjusted funnel plot was used to assess the presence of small-study effect [40]. Egger's test was used to assess the symmetry of the funnel plot [41].

To account for both the markedly effective rate and neurological deficits, we used multivariate methods to determine the dependency between outcomes. Clustering methods and 2-dimensional plots were used to produce clusters of treatments [42]. Using the clusterank command, clustered ranking plots can be obtained using the STATA program. The markedly effective rate and neurological deficits became the data variable containing the SUCRA scores for all treatments in this network. The different colors correspond to the estimated clusters and were utilized for grouping the treatments according to their similarity for both outcomes.

Results

Literature search and characteristics of the included studies

Figure 1 shows the PRISMA flow diagram. A total of 13,764 articles were identified from electronic databases. After the exclusion of duplications, reviews, and obviously irrelevant studies by reading titles and abstracts, 3493 papers were downloaded for additional review. A total of 3429 RCTs were excluded for the following reasons: non-RCTs, non-acute phase, not meeting intervention and the curative effect valuation standard, incorrect data, no treatment time, and no outcomes of interest. Hence, 64 studies and 15 CHIs were included in the NMA. All studies were published in Chinese from 2006 to 2015.

Characteristics of the included studies

The 64 RCTs [28, 43–105] included 6225 participants, with sample sizes varying from 26 to 300 participants. All RCTs were conducted among Chinese populations in China. All participants were evaluated using cranial CT or NMRI. The rang of participants was approximately 35 to 87 years. There were more male patients (59.4%) than females. This study included 16

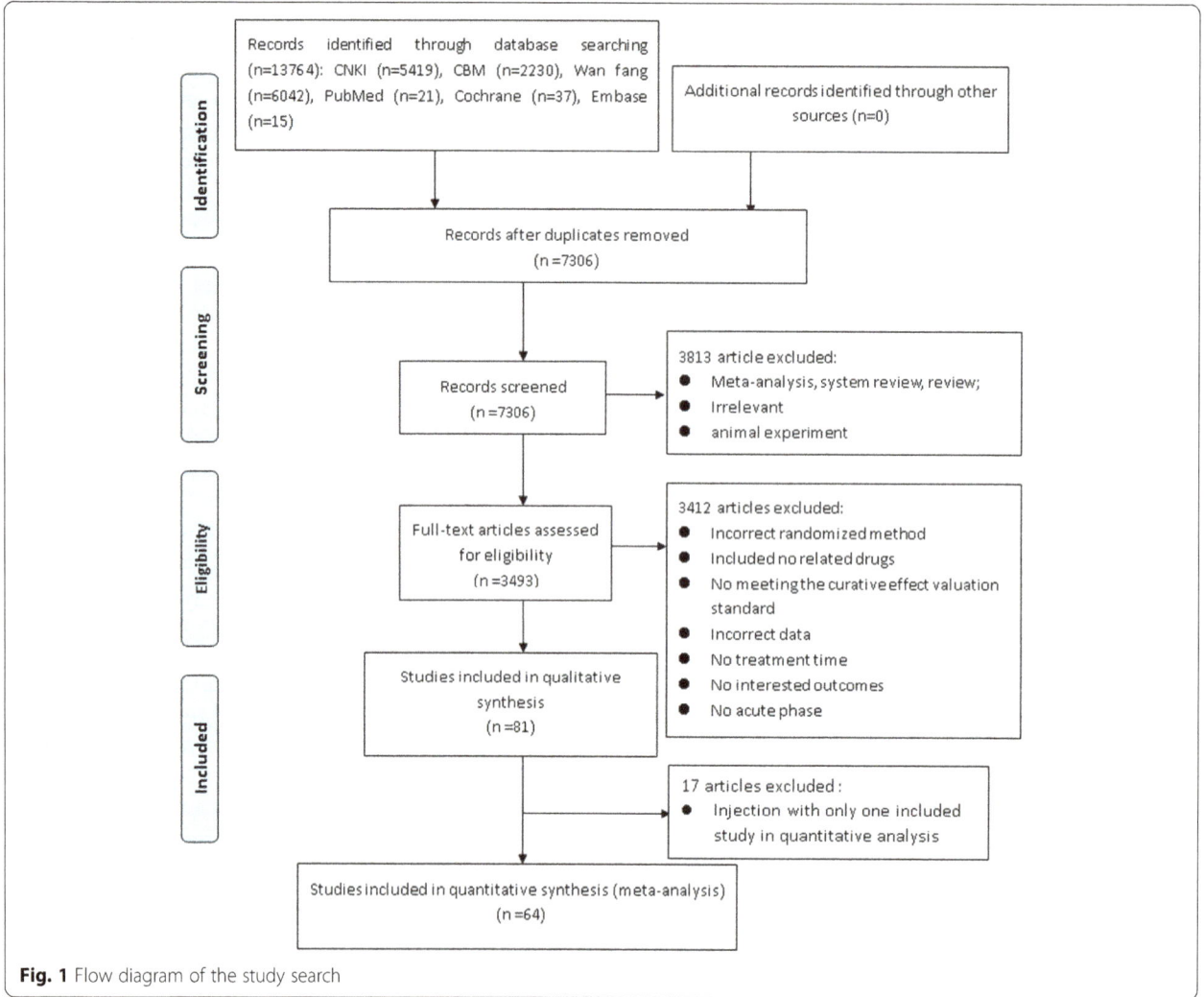

Fig. 1 Flow diagram of the study search

treatments for ACI: AADN, Shuxuening injection(SXN) + AADN, Shuxuetong injection (SXT) + AADN, Shenxiong injection (SX) + AADN, Mailuoning injection (MLN) + AADN, Honghuahuangsesu injection (HHHSS) + AADN, Fufangdanshen injection (FFDS) + AADN, Dengzhanhuasu injection (DZHS) + AADN, Dengzhanxixin injection (DZXX) + AADN, Danshenchuanxiongqin injection (DSCXQ) + AADN, Danshen injection (DS) + AADN, Danhong injection (DH) + AADN, Yinxingdamo injection (YXDM) + AADN, Ligustrazine injection (LI) + AADN, Xuesaitong injection (XST2) + AADN, and Xueshuantong injection (XST1) + AADN; to concisely express the results of this research, we used the abbreviations of the TCM injections to replace the treatments. The treatment abbreviations are shown in Table 1. The acute phase was no more than 30 days, with 62.5% of the cases having an acute phase of less than 72 h. The duration of treatment for both the experimental and control groups was no more than 30 days. Figure 2 shows

a network graph comparing fifteen CHIs. There were 120 pairwise comparisons including 40 direct comparisons. Table 2 provides a summary of the included studies. Additional file 3 showed the more details of included CHIs.

Quality of the included studies

We used the Cochrane Handbook version 5.1.0 and CONSORT statement to conduct a quality evaluation of the included studies. All studies mentioned the use of random distribution, while ten studies [44, 64, 68, 73, 75, 82, 95–97, 101] described a satisfactory method of randomization including random number tables or the envelope method. Two studies [60, 85] reported information about blinding. All studies provided information on patients who were lost to follow-up or dropped out. All studies reported the eligibility criteria for participants and statistical methods. Approximately 74.6% of the studies provided

Table 1 Treatment abbreviations

Full name	Abbreviations
Aspirin + Anticoagulants + Dehydrant + Neuroprotectant	AADN
Ligustrazine injection	LI
Xueshuantong injection	XST1
Xuesaitong injection	XST2
Shuxuening injection	SXN
Dengzhanxixin injection	DZXX
Dengzhanhuasu injection	DZHS
Shuxuetong injection	SXT
Danhong injection	DH
Fufangdanshen injection	FFDS
Yinxingdamo injection	YXDM
Mailuoning injection	MLN
Honghuahuangsesu injection	HHHSS
Shenxiong glucose injection	SX
Danshen Chuanxiongqin injection	DSCXQ
Danshen injection	DS

information about adverse events. Details on risk of bias are shown in Additional file 4: Figure S1.

Pairwise meta-analysis

Pairwise meta-analysis of the markedly effective rate

Fifty-nine RCTs reported markedly effective rates; in these RCTs, 5864 patients were involved and 34 regimens were included. Table 3 summarizes the results of the pairwise meta-analysis regarding the markedly effective rates. There was no significant heterogeneity in the pooled analysis of all included studies ($P > 0.1$; $I^2 < 50\%$); the results of the heterogeneity test are shown in Table 2. The direct

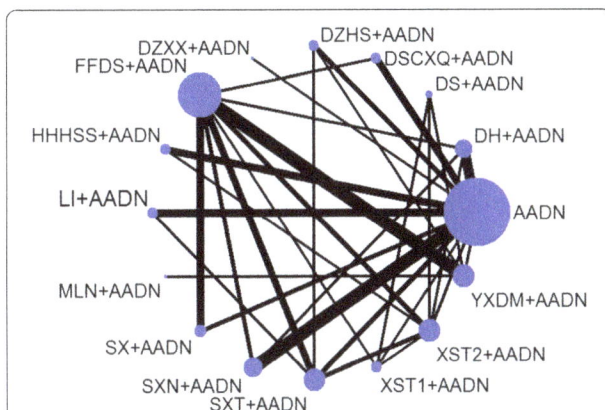

Fig. 2 Network of the included comparisons. Note: Nodes are proportional to the number of patients included in the corresponding treatments, and edges are weighted according to the number of studies included in the respective comparisons

comparison showed that DH and SXN were more beneficial in improving the markedly effective rate than AADN (AADN versus DH: $OR = 0.61$, 95% $CI = 0.45–0.84$; versus SXN: $OR = 0.57$, 95% $CI = 0.44–0.73$). SX and XST2 were more beneficial than FFDS (FFDS versus SX: $OR = 0.61$, 95% $CI = 0.38–0.98$; versus XST2: $OR = 0.54$, 95% $CI = 0.34–0.86$). Other treatment comparisons failed to reach statistical significance (the 95% CI included 1). The detailed results are shown in Fig. 3.

Pairwise meta-analysis of the improvement of neurological impairment

Forty-one RCTs reported an improvement of neurological impairment; in these RCTs, 3828 patients were involved and 29 regimens were included. When P was ≥0.1 and I^2 was ≤50%, the Mantel-Haenszel fixed-effects model was used for the meta-analysis and vice versa. The results of the heterogeneity test are shown in Table 4. Table 4 summarizes the results of the pairwise meta-analysis regarding the improvement of neurological impairment. The direct comparison showed that DH, DZHS, HHHSS, SX, SXT, XST2, LI, YXDM, and SXN were more effective than AADN alone in the reduction of the neurological impairment score (AADN versus DH: $SMD = 0.54$, 95% $CI = 0.33–0.75$; versus DZHS: $SMD = 1.01$, 95% $CI = 0.04–1.98$; versus HHHSS: $SMD = 0.64$, 95% $CI = 0.44–0.84$; versus SX: $SMD = 0.77$, 95% $CI = 0.43–1.11$; versus SXT: $SMD = 0.79$, 95% $CI = 0.44–1.14$; versus XST2: $SMD = 0.53$, 95% $CI = 0.01–1.04$; versus LI: $SMD = 0.83$, 95% $CI = 0.51–1.16$; versus YXDM: $SMD = 1.03$, 95% $CI = 0.56–1.50$; versus SXN: $SMD = 0.41$, 95% $CI = 0.15–0.66$). DH was more effective than FFDS ($SMD = -1.01$, 95% $CI = -1.40$ to -0.62) and XST2 ($SMD = -0.61$, 95% $CI = -1.02$ to -0.20). DSCXQ was more effective than FFDS ($SMD = -0.82$, 95% $CI = -1.27$ to -0.37). YXDM and SXT were more effective than DZHS (DZHS versus YXDM: $SMD = 0.75$, 95% $CI = 0.24–1.26$; versus SXT: $SMD = 0.84$, 95% $CI = 0.35–1.33$). SX, XST1, XST2, and SXN were more effective than FFDS (FFDS versus SX: $SMD = 0.79$, 95% $CI = 0.45–1.13$; versus XST1: $SMD = 1.15$, 95% $CI = 0.58–1.71$; versus XST2: $SMD = 0.95$, 95% $CI = 0.49–1.41$; versus SXN: $SMD = 2.41$, 95% $CI = 1.85–2.97$). SXT was more effective than LI ($SMD = -0.79$, 95% $CI = -1.19$ to -0.39). YXDM was more effective than LI (LI versus YXDM: $SMD = 0.96$, 95% $CI = 0.51–1.42$). MLN was more effective than YXDM (YXDM versus MLN: $SMD = 0.51$, 95% $CI = 0.06–0.95$). Other treatment comparisons failed to reach statistical significance (the 95% CI included 0). The detailed results are shown in Fig. 4.

Pairwise meta-analysis of the death

Most studies did not report any deaths during the treatment period or during follow up after the treatment

Table 2 Characteristics of the studies included in this meta-analysis

Study	Acute phase	Sex (M/F)	Age	Experimental group			Control group			Course	Outcomes	ADRs/ ADEs
				N	T1	Dosage	N	T2	Dosage			
Yu YC 2014	72 h	38/30	62.5 (44–76)	34	XST1	500 mg	34	AADN	–	14d	(1)	None
Yu YM 2009	72 h	71/45	62.5 (40–72)	58	DH	20 ml	58	FFDS	20 ml	15d	(1)(2)	Unclear
Yu Y 2015	72 h	35/21	54.3 (38–71)	28	XST1	500 mg	28	FFDS	20 ml	14d	(1)(2)	6
Zhang ZJ 2008	74 h	41/30	64.3	35	SX	100 ml	36	FFDS	20 ml	14d	(1)	None
Zheng XD 2007	72 h	39/21	66.4	30	YXDM	20 mL	30	FFDS	30 ml	14d	(1)	None
Zhou SJ 2011	1 M	46/34	62 (42–75)	40	SX	100 ml	40	AADN	–	14d	(1)(2)	None
Zhou SF 2009	48 h	52/42	65.6 (62–86)	48	SX	200 ml	46	FFDS	20 mL	21d	(1)(2)	10
Zhou SH 2013	72 h	50/40	62	45	SXN	20 ml	45	AADN	–	14d	(1)(4)	None
Xu XY 2011	12 h	40/20	55.9 (45–73)	30	YXDM	20 ml	30	DS	20 ml	21d	(1)(2)(3)	Unclear
Xie S 2011	24 h	42/30	61.4 (53–78)	36	SXT	6 ml	36	FFDS	20 ml	14d	(1)	None
Xie YG 2010	48 h	39/31	61.6 (50–76)	35	SXT	6 ml	35	DZHS	50 mg	14d	(1)(2)	None
Xu LL 2011	72 h	48/34	63.0 (55–81)	42	LI	120 mg	42	AADN	–	14d	(1)(2)	Unclear
Xu XQ 2012	72 h	64/44	57.9	54	YXDM	20 ml	54	FFDS	20 ml	14d	(1)(2)	1
Yang HJ 2007	24 h	50/34	53.6 (39–75)	48	DSCXQ	10 ml	36	FFDS	10 ml	30d	(1)(2)	1
Yang YF 2012	48 h	–	68	112	DH	30 ml	101	AADN	–	21d	(1)(2)	Unclear
Yao QY 2010	72 h	64/40	70.8 (54–82)	56	SXT	6 ml	48	LI	12 ml	14d	(1)(2)	2
Yao J 2010	72 h	37/27	60.5 (49–76)	32	YXDM	20 ml	32	DZHS	50 mg	14d	(1)(2)	None
Xie RP 2010	72 h	52/28	42–80	40	SXN	20 ml	40	FFDS	20 mL	15d	(1)	None
Tan SY 2016	72 h	49/37	39–82	43	DH	30 ml	43	AADN	–	14d	(1)(2)	None
Wang WP 2015	72 h	49/41	68.2 (60–78)	45	SXN	20 mL	45	FFDS	20 mL	14d	(1)(2)	Unclear
Ren HM 2009	72 h	38/26	40–78	32	SX	100 ml	32	AADN	–	14d	(1)(2)	None
Sun HJ 2013	72 h	42/36	60.9 (40–70)	39	LI	120 mg	39	AADN	–	14d	(1)(2)	Unclear
Tang JP 2013	72 h	47/45	51.8 (43–73)	46	HHHSS	100 mg	46	AADN	–	14d	(1)(2)	None
Tang FY 2009	72 h	39/33	64.0 (50–78)	36	DZHS	50 mg	36	AADN	–	14d	(1)(2)	None
Tang XJ 2013	72 h	45/33	58	39	YXDM	20 mg	39	AADN	–	14d	(1)(2)	None
Wang L 2010	48 h	26/22	65.6 (62–86)	40	SX	200 mL	40	FFDS	20 mL	21d	(1)(2)	Unclear
Wang YL 2013	168 h	33/23	32–88	28	SXT	6 ml	28	DZHS	40 ml	14d	(2)	Unclear
Lan Y 2015	72 h	41/39	54–72	40	DSCXQ	10 ml	40	AADN	–	14d	(1)(2)	3
Li M 2014	24 h	63/17	48–76	40	DH	30 ml	40	AADN	–	14d	(2)	Unclear
Liu YP 2010	72 h	45/35	51–71	40	DH	40 ml	40	AADN	–	15d	(1)	1
Ma J 2010	24 h	29/31	59.1 (50–68)	30	DZHS	20 mg	30	AADN	–	14d	(1)(2)	Unclear
Ma J 2015	72 h	49/41	65.5 (45–79)	45	DH	20 ml	45	AADN	–	28d	(1)(4)	Unclear
Chen H 2015	24 h	74/60	59.4 (46–87)	67	SXT	6 ml	67	AADN	–	14d	(1)(2)	5
Luan T 2014	48 h	52/43	57.5	50	XST2	0.4 g	45	DS	20 ml	15d	(1)(4)	7
Huang ML 2012	72 h	158/142	62.6 (42–71)	150	XST1	500 mg	150	DS	25 ml	14d	(1)	1
Li X 2015	72 h	129/71	62.9	100	HHHSS	0.1 g	100	AADN	–	14d	(1)(2)	Unclear
Ma ZL 2011	72 h	74/46	62.8 (45–84)	60	HHHSS	0.1 g	60	AADN	–	14d	(1)(2)	None
Zhang Y 2012	48 h	52/28	57.5 (35–80)	40	DSCXQ	100 mg	40	AADN	–	14d	(1)(2)	1
Liu M 2014	48 h	79/57	60.2 (40–76)	68	DSCXQ	10 mL	68	AADN	–	14d	(1)(2)	2
Chen YC 2011	72 h	44/24	57.9	34	YXDM	20 ml	34	FFDS	20 ml	14d	(1)(2)	1
Yang RF 2013	48 h	52/48	60.8 (30–83)	50	SXT	6 g	50	AADN	–	14d	(1)	Unclear
Lin YF 2008	72 h	39/21	66.5	30	YXDM	20 ml	30	FFDS	20 ml	14d	(1)(3)	None
Peng T 2006	48 h	51/48	68	49	SXT	7 ml	50	FFDS	20 ml	14d	(1)(3)	1

Table 2 Characteristics of the studies included in this meta-analysis *(Continued)*

Study	Acute phase	Sex (M/F)	Age	Experimental group			Control group			Course	Outcomes	ADRs/ ADEs
				N	T1	Dosage	N	T2	Dosage			
Li XH 2011	168 h	–	63.5(40–78)	120	SXN	20 ml	120	AADN	–	14d	(1)(2)	Unclear
Liu L 2015	6-72 h	74/46	61.4 (39–76)	60	DH	20 ml	60	SXN	20 ml	14d	(1)	None
Zhang YH 2010	6-72 h	62/34	58.9 (39–81)	48	DH	30 ml	48	XST2	400 mg	14d	(1)(2)	5
Fan J 2006	72 h	56/32	64 (41–82)	44	YXDM	20 ml	44	FFDS	20 ml	14d	(2)	Unclear
Liu HY 2014	96 h	67/57	61.9 (38–83)	64	XST2	0.4 g	60	FFDS	30 ml	15d	(1)	None
Li FQ 2010	72 h	74/46	64	60	YXDM	30 ml	60	FFDS	40 ml	15d	(1)	Unclear
Lian CL 2013	360 h	49/43	62 (43–77)	46	LI	120 mg	46	AADN	–	30d	(1)	None
Chen S 2006	72 h	81/53	67.9	70	XST2	800 mg	64	XST1	10 ml	14d	(1)(2)	None
Cao LZ 2012	72 h	71/9	59.3	40	XST2	500 mg	40	FFDS	1.0 g	14d	(1)(2)	Unclear
Liu Y 2009	72 h	79/43	65.1 (43–73)	62	SXT	6 ml	60	XST2	8 ml	14d	(1)	1
Luo XD 2011	72 h	35/25	61.8	30	XST2	0.4 g	30	AADN	–	14d	(1)(2)	3
Liao MJ 2014	6-72 h	43/17	62.5 (36–80)	30	HHHSS	100 ml	30	XST2	400 mg	14d	(1)	Unclear
Shi JL 2010	72 h	51/33	62	42	YXDM	20 ml	42	LI	200 mg	30d	(2)	Unclear
Ni H 2010	24 h	61/55	62.7 (54–74)	59	SXN	20 ml	57	AADN	–	14d	(1)	Unclear
Li CP 2007	8-72 h	106/54	63.8 (42–85)	80	SXN	10-20 ml	80	AADN	–	14d	(1)	Unclear
Zhou ZP 2011	24 h	48/33	62.2	42	DZXX	30 ml	39	AADN	–	15d	(1)	Unclear
Chen C 2015	72 h	37/31	67.5	34	SXT	6 ml	34	XST2	400 mg	14d	(1)(2)	14
Chen JY 2012	72 h	73/35	67 (40–76)	54	SXT	6 ml	54	FFDS	20 ml	14d	(1)(2)	Unclear
Luo QY 2007	72 h	54/36	63.6 (37–81)	45	SXN	6 ml	45	AADN	20 ml	14d	(1)	None
Chen J 2007	72 h	45/35	61	40	YXDM	20 ml	40	MLN	20 ml	15d	(1)(2)(3)	Unclear
Zhang XL 2005	6d	37/13	35–80	26	MLN	20 ml	24	FFDS	20 m l	21d	(2)	None

M male, *F* female, *AVG* average, *E* experimental group, *C* control group, *W* week, *D* day, *AADN* aspirin + anticoagulants + dehydrant + neuroprotectant, *DH* Danhong injection + AADN, *DS* Danshen injection + AADN, *DSCXQ* Danshenchuangxiongqin injection + AADN, *DZHS* Dengzhanhuasu injection + AADN, *DZXX* Dengzhanxixin injection + AADN, *FFDS* Fufangdanshen injection + AADN, *HHHSS* Honghuahuangsesu injection + AADN, *SX* Shenxiong glucose injection + AADN, *SXT* Shuxuetong injection + AADN, *XST1* Xueshuantong injection + AADN, *XST2* Xuesetong injection + AADN, *LI* Ligustrazine injection + AADN, *YXDM* Yinxingdamo injection + AADN, *SXN* Shuxuening injection + AADN, *MLN* Mailuoning injection + AADN, *ADRs* adverse drug reactions, *ADEs* adverse drug events; (1): markedly effective rate; (2): neurological impairment; (3): death; (4): activities of daily living function; N: sample size; T1: therapy of experiment; T2: Therapy of control; N:Number of studies; –: No report

ended in all trials. Four studies [50, 81, 82, 102] reported no death during the treatment period. This result may mean that CHIs plus AADN is an effective approach in the treatment of ACI or short follow-up time.

Pairwise meta-analysis of the activities of daily living function

Three studies [46, 67, 71] assessed the activities of daily living function using the Barthel Index. Due to the limited quantity of the included studies, the Mantel-Haenszel random-effects model was used. There was a significant difference between the treatment group and the control group (SX versus AADN: $SMD = 0.83$, *95% CI* = 0.41–1.25; DSCXQ versus AADN: $SMD = 0.73$, *95% CI* = 0.28–1.18; DH versus AADN: $SMD = 1.69$, *95% CI* = 1.21–2.17).

Results of the Bayesian network meta-analysis

In the original analysis, most studies did not mention the activities of daily living function or death from all causes within the treatment period or during the entire follow-up period. Therefore, the present study did not compare death or the activities of daily living function among different treatments; we only performed a NMA to compare the markedly effective rate and the improvement of neurological impairment among the different regimens of CHIs for ACI.

Bayesian network meta-analysis of the markedly effective rate

According to the network of comparisons (Table 3), DH, DSCXQ, DZXX, HHHSS, SX, SXT, XST2, YXDM, and SXN improved the markedly effective rate more significantly than AADN alone (DH: $OR = 3.89$, *95% CI* = 2.26–6.26; DSCXQ: $OR = 2.14$, *95% CI* = 1.02–3.99; DZXX: $OR = 5.36$, *95% CI* = 1.06–16.68; HHHSS: $OR = 3.34$, *95% CI* = 1.66–6.14; SX: $OR = 2.90$, *95% CI* = 1.36–5.46; SXT: $OR = 3.27$, *95% CI* = 1.86–5.35; XST2: $OR = 2.24$, *95% CI* = 1.23–3.77; YXDM: $OR = 2.99$, *95% CI* = 1.53–5.34; SXN: $OR = 3.3$, *95% CI* = 2–5.14). Moreover, DZXX,

Table 3 A summary of the meta-analysis for the markedly effective rate

The upper-right corner is the Meta-analysis results. The bottom-left corner is the network Meta-analysis results. Values are odds ratios (OR) with 95% credibility intervals (95% CI) of the row-defining treatment compared with the column-defining treatment. Significant effects are printed in **bold**. A dash (–) indicates no comparison available.

	AADN	DH	DS	DSCXQ	DZHS	DZXX	FFDS	HHHSS	SX	SXT	XST1	XST2	LI	YXDM	SXN	MLN
AADN	AADN	**0.61(0.45,0.84)** P=0.96 i²=0%	0.75(0.48,1.16) P=0.97 I²=0%	0.72(0.42,1.23) P=0.82 I²=0%	0.56(0.26,1.17)		0.74(0.54,1.01) P=0.91 I²=0%	0.67(0.40,1.14) P=0.92 I²=0%	0.90(0.61,1.32) P=0.71 I²=0%	0.93(0.46,1.90)	0.72(0.33,1.59)	0.81(0.54,1.21) P=0.79 I²=0%	0.61(0.30,1.26)	**0.57(0.44,0.73)** P=0.19 I²=35.4%		–
DH	3.89(2.26,6.26)	DH	–	–	–	–	–	–	1.73(0.89,3.34)	–	–	–	–	1.22(0.69,2.16)	–	–
DS	0.8(0.29,1.8)	0.22(0.07,0.52)	DS	–	–	–	–	–	0.79(0.53,1.19)	0.75(0.41,1.36)	–	–	0.64(0.28,1.47)	–	–	–
DSCXQ	**2.14(1.02,3.99)**	0.59(0.23,1.23)	3.3(0.91,8.58)	DSCXQ	–	–	–	–	–	–	–	–	–	–	–	–
DZHS	2.22(0.95,4.47)	0.61(0.22,1.35)	3.38(0.92,8.96)	1.16(0.37,2.82)	DZHS	–	–	–	0.70(0.32,1.48)	–	–	–	0.75(0.33,1.72)	–	–	–
DZXX	**5.36(1.06,16.68)**	1.47(0.26,4.87)	**8.32(1.12,30.55)**	2.82(0.44,9.73)	2.82(0.42,9.88)	DZXX	–	–	–	–	–	–	–	–	–	–
FFDS	0.94(0.57,1.46)	0.25(0.13,0.44)	1.41(0.51,3.11)	0.48(0.19,1.01)	0.49(0.21,0.96)	**0.29(0.05,0.93)**	FFDS	**0.61(0.38,0.98)** P=0.89 I²=0%	**0.54(0.34,0.86)** P=0.70 I²=0%	0.76(0.33,1.76)			0.75(0.53,1.06) P=0.98 I²=0%	0.81(0.50,1.31) P=0.65 I²=0%		
HHHSS	**3.34(1.66,6.14)**	0.91(0.37,1.91)	**5.14(1.48,13.28)**	1.75(0.56,4.22)	1.75(0.62,4)	1.02(0.16,3.51)	**3.76(1.61,7.65)**	HHHSS	0.65(0.37,1.15)	1.38(0.86,2.22) P=0.86 I²=0%	1.47(0.79,2.78)		0.79(0.31,1.68)			
SX	**2.9(1.36,5.46)**	0.79(0.32,1.65)	**4.43(1.29,11.37)**	1.52(0.53,3.47)	1.51(0.49,3.6)	0.89(0.14,3.03)	**3.18(1.56,5.83)**	0.97(0.34,2.21)	SX	0.65(0.37,1.15)		0.79(0.37,1.15)		0.96(0.45,1.82)		0.91(0.11,3.45)
SXT	**3.27(1.86,5.35)**	0.89(0.42,1.66)	**4.96(1.68,11.54)**	1.71(0.68,3.58)	1.68(0.67,3.51)	1(0.17,3.27)	**3.6(2.03,5.97)**	1.09(0.44,2.23)	1.25(0.52,2.55)	SXT						
XST1	1.27(0.53,26)	0.34(0.13,0.76)	1.78(0.7,3.81)	0.66(0.21,1.62)	0.66(0.2,1.63)	0.39(0.06,1.38)	1.39(0.59,2.84)	0.42(0.14,1)	0.49(0.16,1.16)	0.41(0.16,0.87)	XST1	0.65(0.37,1.15)				
XST2	**2.24(1.23,3.77)**	0.61(0.29,1.12)	**3.31(1.25,7.23)**	1.17(0.46,2.51)	1.16(0.43,2.56)	0.68(0.12,2.28)	**2.47(1.36,4.14)**	0.74(0.31,1.5)	0.86(0.35,1.77)	0.71(0.38,1.25)	1.99(0.85,3.94)	XST2	0.79(0.31,1.68)		1.21(0.54,2.33)	0.45(0.08,1.44)
LI	1.64(0.78,3.09)	0.45(0.18,0.96)	2.54(0.7,6.6)	0.86(0.29,2.01)	0.86(0.27,2.06)	0.5(0.08,1.73)	1.85(0.76,3.8)	0.55(0.19,1.25)	0.64(0.22,1.48)	0.53(0.22,1.07)	1.52(0.47,3.66)	0.79(0.31,1.68)	LI	YXDM		0.45(0.08,1.44)
YXDM	**2.99(1.53,5.34)**	0.81(0.36,1.6)	**4.43(1.57,10.1)**	1.52(0.59,3.24)	1.56(0.59,3.4)	0.91(0.15,3.1)	**3.24(1.85,5.34)**	1(0.37,2.17)	1.14(0.46,2.36)	0.96(0.45,1.82)	**2.69(1.01,5.84)**	1.41(0.65,2.69)	2.05(0.74,4.58)	YXDM		1.32(0.67,2.61)
SXN	**3.3(2,5.14)**	0.9(0.46,1.59)	**5.09(1.64,12.18)**	1.73(0.64,3.79)	1.73(0.71,3.61)	1.01(0.18,3.3)	**3.69(1.97,6.31)**	1.1(0.45,2.25)	1.28(0.53,2.61)	1.08(0.52,1.98)	**3.04(1.12,6.65)**	1.59(0.75,2.97)	2.27(0.91,4.75)	1.21(0.54,2.33)	SXN	–
MLN	1.33(0.2,4.65)	0.36(0.05,1.3)	1.98(0.24,7.46)	0.69(0.09,2.61)	0.68(0.09,2.47)	0.41(0.03,1.84)	1.45(0.23,4.95)	0.44(0.06,1.65)	0.51(0.07,1.86)	0.43(0.06,1.52)	1.2(0.15,4.48)	0.63(0.09,2.24)	0.91(0.11,3.45)	0.45(0.08,1.44)	0.42(0.06,1.51)	MLN

The upper right corner is the Meta-analysis results. The bottom left corner is the network Meta-analysis results. Results are the odds ratios (OR) and related 95% credibility interval (95% CI) in the row-defining treatment compared with the column-defining treatment. OR higher than 1 favor the row-defining treatment, and vice versa. Significant effects are printed in bold. AADN aspirin + anticoagulants + dehydrant + neuroprotectant, DH Danhong injection + AADN, DS Danshen injection + AADN, DSCXQ Danshenchuangxiongqin injection + AADN, DZHS Dengzhanhuasu injection + AADN, DZXX Dengzhanxixin injection + AADN, FFDS Fufangdanshen injection + AADN, HHHSS Honghuahuangsesu injection + AADN, SX Shenxiong glucose injection + AADN, SXT Shuxuetong injection + AADN, XST1 Xueshuantong injection + AADN, XST2 Xuesetong injection + AADN, LI Ligustrazine injection + AADN, YXDM Yinxingdamo injection + AADN, SXN Shuxuening injection + AADN, MLN Mailuoning injection + AAD

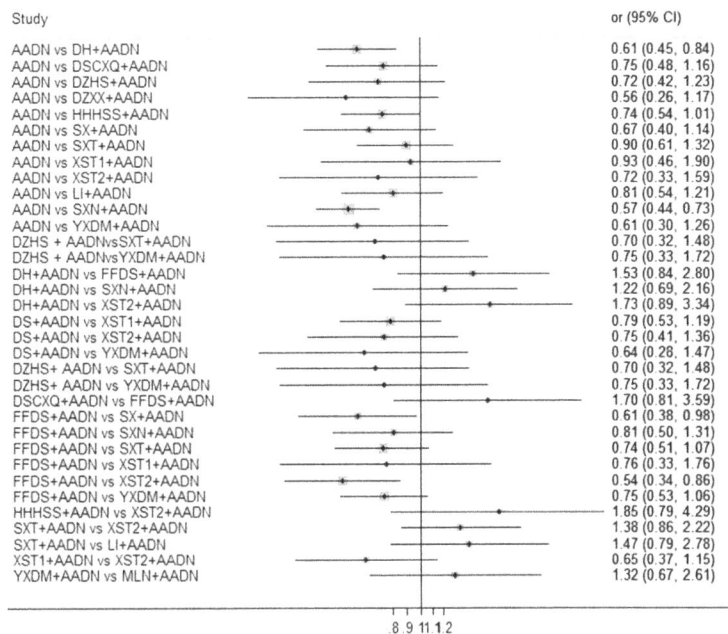

Study	or (95% CI)
AADN vs DH+AADN	0.61 (0.45, 0.84)
AADN vs DSCXQ+AADN	0.75 (0.48, 1.16)
AADN vs DZHS+AADN	0.72 (0.42, 1.23)
AADN vs DZXX+AADN	0.56 (0.26, 1.17)
AADN vs HHHSS+AADN	0.74 (0.54, 1.01)
AADN vs SX+AADN	0.67 (0.40, 1.14)
AADN vs SXT+AADN	0.90 (0.61, 1.32)
AADN vs XST1+AADN	0.93 (0.46, 1.90)
AADN vs XST2+AADN	0.72 (0.33, 1.59)
AADN vs LI+AADN	0.81 (0.54, 1.21)
AADN vs SXN+AADN	0.57 (0.44, 0.73)
AADN vs YXDM+AADN	0.61 (0.30, 1.26)
DZHS + AADNvsSXT+AADN	0.70 (0.32, 1.48)
DZHS + AADNvsYXDM+AADN	0.75 (0.33, 1.72)
DH+AADN vs FFDS+AADN	1.53 (0.84, 2.80)
DH+AADN vs SXN+AADN	1.22 (0.69, 2.16)
DH+AADN vs XST2+AADN	1.73 (0.89, 3.34)
DS+AADN vs XST1+AADN	0.79 (0.53, 1.19)
DS+AADN vs XST2+AADN	0.75 (0.41, 1.36)
DS+AADN vs YXDM+AADN	0.64 (0.28, 1.47)
DZHS+ AADN vs SXT+AADN	0.70 (0.32, 1.48)
DZHS+ AADN vs YXDM+AADN	0.75 (0.33, 1.72)
DSCXQ+AADN vs FFDS+AADN	1.70 (0.81, 3.59)
FFDS+AADN vs SX+AADN	0.61 (0.38, 0.98)
FFDS+AADN vs SXN+AADN	0.81 (0.50, 1.31)
FFDS+AADN vs SXT+AADN	0.74 (0.51, 1.07)
FFDS+AADN vs XST1+AADN	0.76 (0.33, 1.76)
FFDS+AADN vs XST2+AADN	0.54 (0.34, 0.86)
FFDS+AADN vs YXDM+AADN	0.75 (0.53, 1.06)
HHHSS+AADN vs XST2+AADN	1.85 (0.79, 4.29)
SXT+AADN vs XST2+AADN	1.38 (0.86, 2.22)
SXT+AADN vs LI+AADN	1.47 (0.79, 2.78)
XST1+AADN vs XST2+AADN	0.65 (0.37, 1.15)
YXDM+AADN vs MLN+AADN	1.32 (0.67, 2.61)

.8 .9 1 1.1 2

Fig. 3 Forest graph of Meta-analysis on the markedly effective rate

HHHSS, SX, SXT, XST2, YXDM, and SXN were better than DS (DZXX: $OR = 8.32$, 95% $CI = 1.12–30.55$; HHHSS: $OR = 5.14$, 95% $CI = 1.48–13.28$; SX: $OR = 4.43$, 95% $CI = 1.29–11.37$; SXT: $OR = 4.96$, 95% $CI = 1.68–11.54$; XST2: $OR = 3.31$, 95% $CI = 1.25–7.23$; YXDM: $OR = 4.43$, 95% $CI = 1.57–10.1$; SXN: $OR = 5.09$, 95% $CI = 1.64–12.18$). Additionally, HHHSS, SX, SXT, XST2, YXDM, and SXN were more effective than FFDS (HHHSS: $OR = 3.76$, 95% $CI = 1.61–7.65$; SX: $OR = 3.18$, 95% $CI = 1.56–5.83$; SXT: $OR = 3.60$, 95% $CI = 2.03–5.97$; XST2: $OR = 2.47$, 95% $CI = 1.36–4.14$; YXDM: $OR = 3.24$, 95% $CI = 1.85–5.34$; SXN: $OR = 3.69$, 95% $CI = 1.97–6.31$). YXDM and SXN were more effective than XST1 (YXDM: $OR = 2.69$, 95% $CI = 1.01–5.84$; SXN: $OR = 3.04$, 95% $CI = 1.12–6.65$).

Additional file 5: Figure S2 shows the inconsistency plot used to identify heterogeneity among studies in the closed loop of this NMA. Eleven triangular loops and 25 quadratic loops were present in the NMA; 83% of IF values with 95% CIs were truncated at zero, suggesting no significant inconsistency.

Rank probability
Figure 5 shows the cumulative probabilities (SUCRA results) of CHIs that were the most effective when combined with AADN. DH had the highest likelihood of being the best treatment for the markedly effective rate (SUCRA-85.2%), followed by DZXX (SUCRA-80.4%), SXN (SUCRA-76.3%), SXT (SUCRA-75.9%), HHHSS (SUCRA-74.4%), YXDM (SUCRA-69.2%), SX (SUCRA-66.3%), XST2 (SUCRA-51.9%), DZHS (SUCRA-50.3%),

DSCXQ (SUCRA-49.2%), LI (SUCRA-36.0%), XST1 (SUCRA-24.4%), MLN (SUCRA-22.9%), FFDS (SUCRA-12.9%), and DS (SUCRA-8.2%).

Assessment of publication bias
The comparison-adjusted funnel plots (Additional file 6: Figure S3) for the markedly effective rate were asymmetric near the zero line. The result from Egger's test was $P = 0.047$. Therefore, this study may have a small sample effect and publication bias.

Bayesian network meta-analysis of the improvement of neurological impairment
According to the network of comparisons (Table 4), DH, HHHSS, SXT, YXDM, and SXN improved neurological impairment more significantly than AADN alone (DH: $SMD = - 0.71$, 95% $CI = - 1.28$ to $- 0.13$; HHHSS: $SMD = - 0.78$, 95% $CI = - 1.47$ to $- 0.09$; SXT: $SMD = - 0.81$, 95% CI = $- 1.44$ to $- 0.18$; YXDM: $SMD = - 1.14$, 95% $CI = - 1.74$ to $- 0.54$; SXN: $SMD = - 1.25$, 95% $CI = - 2.14$ to $- 0.37$). Moreover, DH, DSCXQ, DZHS, HHHSS, SX, SXT, XST2, YXDM, and SXN were more effective than FFDS (FFDS versus DH: $SMD = 0.92$, 95% $CI = 0.26–1.58$; versus DSCXQ: $SMD = 0.74$, 95% $CI = 0.01–1.47$; versus DZHS: $SMD = 0.81$, 95% $CI = 0.05–1.58$; HHHSS: $SMD = - 1$, 95% $CI = - 1.86$ to $- 0.13$; SX: $SMD = - 0.88$, 95% $CI = - 1.55$ to $- 0.21$; SXT: $SMD = - 1.03$, 95% $CI = - 1.7$ to $- 0.36$; XST2: $SMD = - 0.78$, 95% $CI = - 1.44$ to $- 0.12$; YXDM: $SMD = - 1.35$, 95% $CI = - 1.89$ to $- 0.81$;

Table 4 A summary of the meta-analysis for the improvement of neurological impairment

The table is a league (cross) table: the diagonal cells contain treatment abbreviations. The upper right corner (row < column) shows the network Meta-analysis results; the bottom left corner (row > column) shows the pairwise Meta-analysis results. Each cell gives the SMD (95% CI). Some cells are blank (—). The following is a best-effort transcription of the matrix.

	AADN	DH	DS	DSCXQ	DZHS	DZXX	FFDS	HHHSS	SX	SXT	XST1	XST2	LI	YXDM	SXN	MLN
AADN	AADN	−0.71 (−1.28,−0.13)	−0.83 (−2.21,0.56)	−0.52 (−1.15,0.1)	−0.59 (−1.26,0.07)	−0.78 (−2.19,0.63)	0.22 (−0.3,0.73)	−0.78 (−1.47,−0.09)	−0.67 (−1.34,0)	−0.81 (−1.44,−0.18)	−0.6 (−1.61,0.39)	−0.56 (−1.22,0.09)	−0.47 (−1.13,0.19)	−1.14 (−1.74,−0.54)	−1.25 (−2.14,−0.37)	−0.44 (−1.45,0.57)
DH	0.54 (0.33,0.75) I^2=13.4% P=0.32	DH	−0.12 (−1.58,1.3)	0.19 (−0.64,1.01)	0.12 (−0.74,0.96)	−0.07 (−1.57,1.41)	0.92 (0.26,1.58)	−0.07 (−0.97,0.83)	0.04 (−0.8,0.87)	−0.1 (−0.89,0.69)	0.11 (−0.97,1.16)	0.14 (−0.59,0.88)	0.24 (−0.61,1.08)	−0.43 (−1.19,0.34)	−0.54 (−1.56,0.47)	0.27 (−0.84,1.37)
DS	0.51 (−0.02,1.03) I^2=79.8% P=0.007	—	DS	0.31 (−1.18,1.8)	0.24 (−1.23,1.69)	0.05 (−1.88,1.97)	1.05 (−0.32,2.4)	0.05 (−1.49,1.58)	0.16 (−1.34,1.64)	0.02 (−1.44,1.47)	0.23 (−1.41,1.85)	0.27 (−1.22,1.75)	0.36 (−1.09,1.82)	−0.31 (−1.57,0.94)	−0.41 (−2.01,1.18)	0.39 (−1.16,1.94)
DSCXQ	1.01 (0.04,1.98) I^2=85.2% P=0.009	—	—	DSCXQ	−0.07 (−0.96,0.8)	−0.26 (−1.78,1.2)	0.74 (0.01,1.47)	−0.26 (−1.19,0.6)	−0.14 (−1.03,0.7)	−0.29 (−1.14,0.5)	−0.08 (−1.22,1.0)	−0.04 (−0.92,0.8)	0.05 (−0.84,0.9)	−0.61 (−1.43,0.2)	−0.72 (−1.79,0.3)	0.09 (−0.98,1.2)
DZHS	0.64 (0.44,0.84) I^2=87.2% P=0.000	—	—	—	DZHS	−0.19 (−1.68,1.2)	0.81 (0.05,1.58)	−0.19 (−1.16,0.7)	−0.08 (−0.99,0.8)	−0.22 (−0.99,0.5)	−0.01 (−1.16,1.1)	0.03 (−0.85,0.9)	0.12 (−0.74,0.9)	−0.55 (−1.3,0.22)	−0.65 (−1.73,0.4)	0.16 (−0.98,1.2)
DZXX	0.77 (0.43,1.11) I^2=0% P=0.60	—	—	—	—	DZXX	1.00 (−0.43,2.43)	0 (−1.57,1.57)	0.11 (−1.41,1.64)	−0.03 (−1.29,1.23)	0.18 (−1.48,1.83)	0.22 (−1.25,1.69)	0.31 (−1.16,1.79)	−0.36 (−1.82,1.12)	−0.46 (−2.09,1.17)	0.35 (−1.32,2.02)
FFDS	0.79 (0.45,1.13) I^2=0% P=1	—	—	—	0.84 (0.35,1.33)	0.03 (−0.49,0.55)	FFDS	0.07 (−0.03,0.45)	—	—	—	—	—	—	—	—
HHHSS	0.53 (0.01,1.04)	−0.61 (−1.02,−0.20)	—	—	—	—	−1 (−1.86,−0.13)	HHHSS	—	—	—	—	—	—	—	—
SX	0.83 (0.51,1.16) I^2=80.4% P=0.02	—	SX	−0.14 (−1,0.72)	−0.03 (−0.97,0.91)	0.11 (−0.85,1.08)	−0.88 (−1.55,−0.21)	−0.20 (−0.68,0.28)	SX	0.21 (−0.87,1.28)	0.06 (−1.06,1.18)	0.1 (−0.77,0.97)	0.2 (−0.71,1.1)	−0.47 (−1.28,0.33)	−0.58 (−1.63,0.48)	0.23 (−0.9,1.36)
SXT	1.03 (0.56,1.50)	0.31 (−0.20,0.81)	0.21 (−0.87,1.28)	0.18 (−1.05,1.39)	0.18 (−1.48,1.83)	0.24 (−0.10,0.58)	−1.03 (−1.7,−0.36)	−0.79 (−1.19,−0.39)	SXT	0.25 (−0.5,1)	0.04 (−0.88,0.97)	0.34 (−0.42,1.1)	−0.33 (−1.08,0.42)	−0.43 (−1.48,0.59)	0.37 (−0.73,1.48)	
XST1	—	—	—	—	—	XST1	−0.82 (−1.76,0.12)	—	0.24 (−0.10,0.58)	XST1	—	—	—	—	—	—
XST2	—	—	—	—	—	0.22 (−0.74,1.17)	−0.78 (−1.44,−0.12)	0.25 (−0.5,1)	XST2	0.04 (−0.88,0.97)	—	—	—	—	—	—
LI	0.75 (0.24,1.26)	—	—	—	0.12 (−0.74,0.9)	0.31 (−1.16,1.79)	−0.69 (−1.43,0.07)	0.34 (−0.42,1.1)	0.09 (−0.78,0.96)	0.13 (−1.01,1.28)	LI	—	—	—	—	—
YXDM	0.96 (0.51,1.42)	—	−0.31 (−1.57,0.94)	−0.61 (−1.43,0.2)	−0.55 (−1.3,0.22)	−0.36 (−1.82,1.12)	−1.35 (−1.89,−0.81)	−0.57 (−1.36,0.21)	−0.67 (−1.42,0.08)	−0.53 (−1.59,0.52)	YXDM	—	—	YXDM	—	—
SXN	2.41 (1.85,2.97)	—	−0.41 (−2.01,1.18)	−0.72 (−1.79,0.3)	−0.65 (−1.73,0.4)	−0.46 (−2.09,1.17)	−1.46 (−2.36,−0.58)	−0.77 (−1.86,0.29)	−0.68 (−1.73,0.36)	−0.64 (−1.9,0.62)	−0.11 (−1,0.88)	SXN	—	SXN	—	—
MLN	0.41 (0.15,0.66)	0.27 (−0.84,1.37)	0.39 (−1.16,1.94)	0.09 (−0.98,1.2)	0.7 (−0.22,1.62)	0.81 (−0.45,2.08)	−0.65 (−0.89,1.57)	0.03 (−1.1,1.17)	0.13 (−0.99,1.24)	0.17 (−1.14,1.48)	0.34 (−0.89,1.57)	0.37 (−0.73,1.48)	0.23 (−0.9,1.36)	0.51 (0.06,0.95)	0.44 (−0.12,1.01)	MLN

Additional values appearing in the network portion: 1.31 (−0.05,2.66) I^2=95.7% P=0; 1.15 (0.58,1.71); 0.95 (0.49,1.41); −0.67 (−1.34,0); −1.01 (−1.40,−0.62); −0.82 (−1.27,−0.37).

The upper right corner is the network Meta-analysis results. The bottom left corner is the Meta-analysis results. Results are the SMD and related 95% credibility interval (95% CI) in the row-defining treatment compared with the column-defining treatment. SMD higher than 0 favor the column-defining treatment, and vice versa. Significant effects are printed in bold. AADN aspirin + anticoagulants + dehydrant + neuroprotectant, DH Danhong injection + AADN, DS Danshen injection + AADN, DSCXQ Danshenchuangxiongqin injection + AADN, DZHS Dengzhanhuasu injection + AADN, DZXX Dengzhanxixin injection + AADN, FFDS Fufangdanshen injection + AADN, HHHSS Honghuahuangsesu injection + AADN, SX Shenxiong glucose injection + AADN, SXT Shuxuetong injection + AADN, XST1 Xueshuantong injection + AADN, XST2 Xuesetong injection + AADN, SXN Shuxuening injection + AADN, YXDM Yinxingdamo injection + AADN, LI Ligustrazine injection + AADN, YXDM Yinxingdamo injection + AADN, MLN Mailuoning injection + AADN

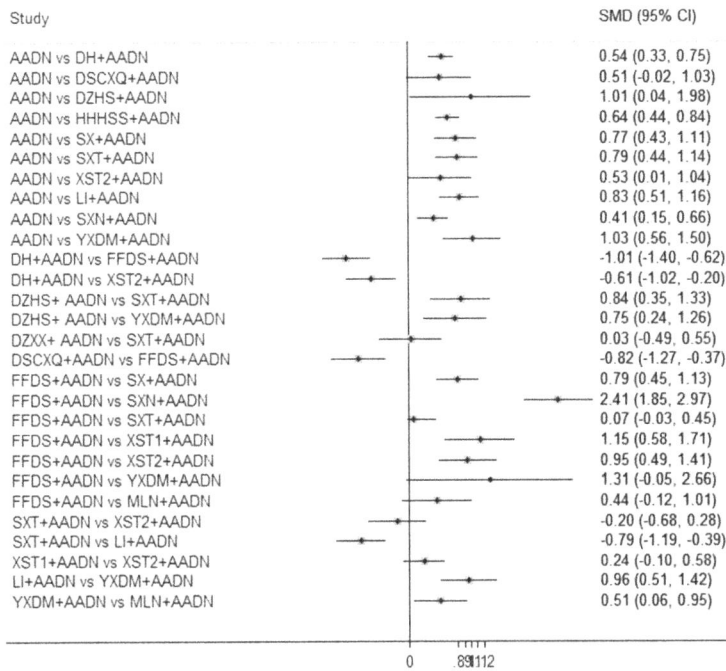

Fig. 4 Forest graph of Meta-analysis on the neurological impairment

SXN: *SMD* = − 1.46, *95% CI* = − 2.36 to − 0.58). There was no statistical significance in other treatment comparisons.

As shown in Additional file 7: Figure S4, 9 triangular loops and seventeen quadratic loops were present in the NMA; 81% of IF values with 95% CIs were truncated at zero, suggesting no significant inconsistency.

Rank probability

The cumulative probability analysis (SUCRA results) showed that SXN + AADN had the highest likelihood of improving the neurological impairment scores (SUCRA-84.7%), followed by YXDM (SUCRA-84.4%), SXT (SUCRA-63.8%), HHHSS (SUCRA-60.7%), DS

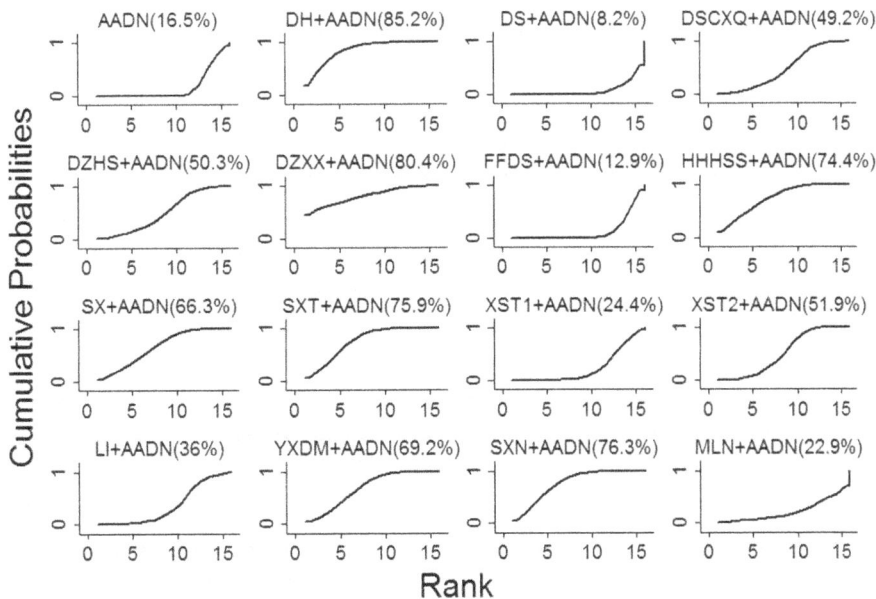

Fig. 5 SUCRA for the markedly effective rate

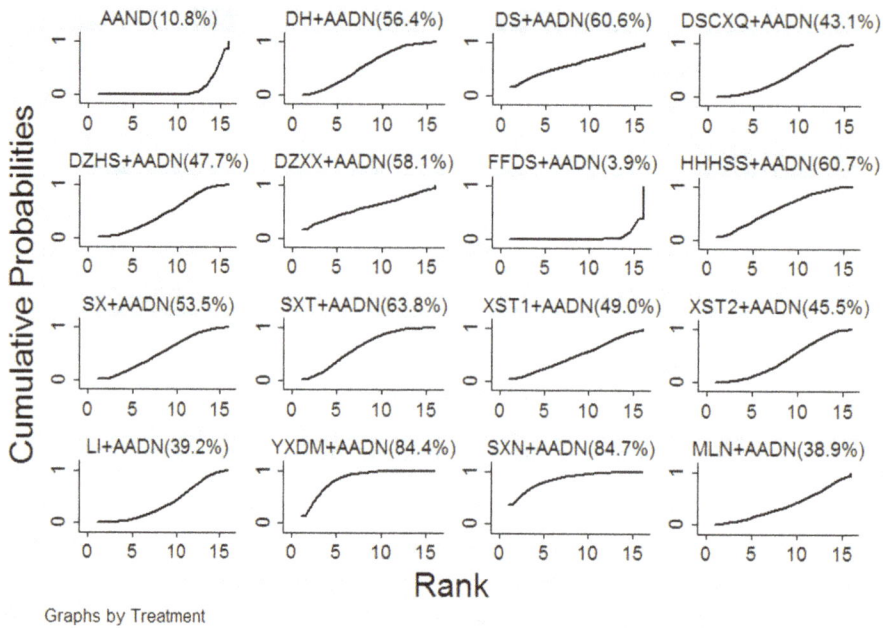

Fig. 6 SUCRA for the improvement of neurological impairment

(SUCRA-60.6%), DZXX (SUCRA-58.1%), DH (SUCRA-56.3%), SX (SUCRA-53.2%), XST1 (SUCRA-49.0%), DZHS (SUCRA-47.7%), XST2 (SUCRA-45.5%), DSCXQ (SUCRA-43.1%), LI (SUCRA-39.2%), MLN (SUCRA-38.9%), and FFDS (SUCRA-3.9%). The results are shown in Fig. 6.

Simultaneous ranking of the interventions for two outcomes

Clustered ranking plots of the network for the markedly effective rate and the improvement of neurological impairment score are shown in Fig. 7. Each color represents a group of treatments that belong to the same cluster. Treatments lying in the upper right corner are more effective than the other treatments. The upper right corner in Fig. 7 shows that SXN, YXDM, DH, SXT, HHSS, DZXX and SX produce significantly better outcomes in ACI patients.

Discussion

Considerable evidence exists regarding the clinical effectiveness of CHIs in ACI patients. Some CHIs have been

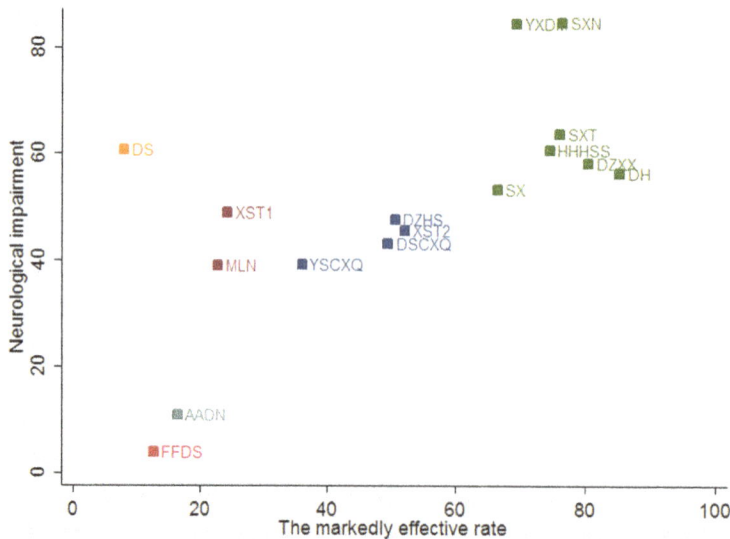

Fig. 7 Clustered ranking plot of the networks

widely used to strengthen clinical effectiveness, reduce neurological impairments and improve the patient's quality of life. However, the majority of these findings have not been analyzed in head-to-head comparisons. Clinicians must decide among several therapeutic options for ACI patients. To address the absence of comparative data, we conducted an NMA to comprehensively estimate the effectiveness of different CHIs combined with AADN for ACI.

This NMA consisted of 64 RCTs that included 6225 participants; fifteen CHIs were identified in the treatment of ACI, including injections of SXN, SXT, SX, MLN, HHHSS, FFDS, DZHS, DZXX, DSCXQ, DS, DH, YXDM, LI, XST1, and XST2. In terms of the improvement of the markedly effective rate, DH had the highest likelihood of being the best treatment in terms of the markedly effective rate. On account of improvement of neurological impairment, SXN had the highest probability of being the best treatment.

The clustered ranking according to two outcomes revealed that the markedly effective rate and the improvement of the neurological impairment cluster were best for SXN, YXDM, DH, SXT, HHHSS, DZXX and SX. SXN and YXDM are shown at the top right corner. Previous meta-analyses [106–108] found that SXN and YXDM as adjuvant treatments for ACI were beneficial compared to AADN alone. SXN and YXDM are *Ginkgo biloba* extracts (GBEs), both of which are extracted from *Ginkgo biloba* leaves. *Ginkgo biloba* leaves, the TCM for activating blood circulation, mainly contain ginkgo flavonoids, ginkgolides, and bilobalide and have been used as a therapeutic agent for managing cerebrovascular and neurological disorders [109, 110]. GBE exhibits a wide variety of biological activities, including anti-inflammation and antioxidant effects [111, 112]. ACI is the process whereby artery stenosis or blockage causes brain tissue hypoxic ischemia, resulting in brain dysfunction [6]. There is considerable evidence suggesting the active repair and recovery mechanisms following stroke, and neurogenesis is one of them [113]. GBE not only has antioxidant, anti-atherogenesis and angiogenic properties but can also strengthen repair and regeneration mechanisms and prevent cell death, protect the brain from further damage and improve neurological deficits following stroke [113–115]. The neuroprotective mechanism has been attributed to the heme oxygenase 1 (HO1)/Wnt canonical pathway as well as neuritogenic and angiogenic effects [113, 116]. HO1, a key component of the EGb 761 neuroprotective signaling pathway, activates the signaling pathway mechanisms of angiogenesis, cell survival and neuroplasticity, and neurogenesis [113]. Thus, GBE could enhance the post-stroke regeneration process to improve treatments for stroke recovery. Further research is desirable to shed more light on the mechanism underlying the effects of GBE on ACI.

A NMA was used to compare the effectiveness of different CHIs to identify the best CHIs for ACI. This study is the first indirect comparison using a network approach to compare the effectiveness of CHIs, which is valuable for clinicians selecting CHIs for ACI treatment. However, some limitations existed in this NMA.

First, all trials reported random distribution, while ten studies described the randomization methods including random number tables or the envelope method. Information about allocation concealment and blinding was not clear in the majority of trials and may have therefore affected the reliability of the results. Second, the systematic review included only published studies in the database, with no relevant gray literature, which likely caused a selection bias in the literature. Third, the study aimed to use a NMA to evaluate the clinical effectiveness of 37 CHIs combined with an AADN regimen; however, only 15 CHIs were included in the NMA. Thus, more rigorously designed RCTs focused on the 22 additional CHIs are needed to confirm the effectiveness of CHIs for ACI. Fourth, due to the original research limitation, we failed to evaluate the long-term effect of CHIs. Additionally, with the limited data extracted from the original research, we failed to evaluate the ability of CHIs to improve the activities of daily living function and reduce mortality. Fifth, our results might have limited generalizability because all of the included RCTs were conducted in China among Chinese populations. Therefore, it is uncertain whether the effect may change when CHIs are used in populations of other ethnicities and in different geographical locations. In addition, though acute phases were limited, the severities of patient were various. This point may influence the results. Sixth, a NMA compares multiple treatments by incorporating direct and indirect evidence into a general statistical framework. One issue with the validity of a NMA is the inconsistency between direct and indirect evidence. Hence, to improve the reliability of our results, we used a random-effects model within a Bayesian framework. Although, head-to-head trials provide the highest level of evidence when comparing interventions, the quantity of data for some CHI direct trials was small, such as DH versus FFDS, SXN, and XSTT. Large RCTs are needed to specifically compare CHIs with one another.

Conclusions

In summary, our evidence suggested that DH injection plus AADN was the optimum treatment regimen for patients with ACI to improve the markedly effective rate. SXN injection plus AADN was the optimum treatment

regimen for ACI to improve the neurological impairment score. Considering both the markedly effective rate and the improvement of neurological impairment, SXN, YXDM, DH, SXT, HHHSS, DZXX and SX plus AADN were the optimum treatment regimens for ACI, especially SXN + AADN and YXDM + AADN. In terms of limitations, highest levels of evidence need to support our conclusions.

Additional files

Additional file 1: Table S1. List of search terms.

Additional file 2: Search strategy.

Additional file 3: More details about the product information of CHIs.

Additional file 4: Figure S1. Risk of bias summary. Note: Green: low risk of bias; Yellow: unclear risk of bias; Red: high risk of bias. (JPEG 1934 kb)

Additional file 5: Figure S2. Inconsistency test for the markedly effective rate.

Additional file 6: Figure S3. Comparison adjusted funnel plot. (JPEG 533 kb)

Additional file 7: Figure S4. Inconsistency test for improvement of neurological impairment.

Abbreviations

AADN: Aspirin + anticoagulants + dehydrant + neuroprotectant; ACI: Acute cerebral infarction; CBM: Chinese biomedical literature database; CHIs: Chinese herbal injections; CNKI: China national knowledge infrastructure database; CI: Credible interval; CT: Computed tomography; DH: Danhong injection; DS: Danshen injection; DSCXQ: Danshenchuanxiongqin injection; DZHS: Dengzhanhuasu injection; DZXX: Dengzhanxixi injection; FFDS: Fufangdanshen injection; GBEs: *Ginkgo biloba* extracts; HHHSS: Honghuahuangsesu injection; IF: Inconsistency factor; LI: Ligustrazine injection; MeSH: Medical subject heading; MLN: Mailuoning injection; MRI: Magnetic resonance imaging; NMA: Network meta-analysis; ORs: Odds ratios; RCTs: Randomized controlled trials; SMDs: Standardized mean differences; SUCRA: Surface under the cumulative ranking probabilities; SX: Shenxiong injection; SXN: Shuxuening injection; SXT: Shuxuetong injection; TCM: traditional Chinese medicine; XST1: Xueshuantong injection; XST2: Xuesaitong injection; YXDM: Yinxingdamo injection

Funding

National Natural Science Foundation of China (Nos. 81473547 and 81673829).

Authors' contributions

Conception and design of the network meta-analysis: SL, JRW. Performance of the network meta-analysis: SL, DZ, and KHW. Quality assessment of the network meta-analysis: JRW, DZ, and BZ. Analysis of study data: XMZ, DT, and XJD. Writing of the paper: SL, YYC, and XKL. All authors read and approved the final version of the manuscript.

Competing interests

The authors declare that they have no competing interests.

References

1. Luo JN. New progress on treating acute cerebral infarction. Pract J card Cereb Pneumal. Vasc Dis. 2010;18:1546–7.
2. Hui Z, Sha DJ, Wang SL, et al. Panaxatriol saponins promotes angiogenesis and enhances cerebral perfusion after ischemic stroke in rats. BMC Complement Altern Med. 2017;17:70.
3. Wang K, Zhang D, Wu J, et al. A comparative study of Danhong injection and Salvia miltiorrhiza injection in the treatment of cerebral infarction: a systematic review and meta-analysis. Med. 2017;96:e7079.
4. Inoue T, Kobayashi M, Uetsuka Y, Uchiyama S. Pharmacoeconomic analysis of cilostazol for the secondary prevention of cerebral infarction. Circ J. 2006; 70:453–8.
5. Sun W, Ou Q, Zhang Z, et al. Chinese acute ischemic stroke treatment outcome registry (CASTOR): protocol for a prospective registry study on patterns of real-world treatment of acute ischemic stroke in China. BMC Complement Altern Med. 2017;17:357.
6. Wei J, Yang W, Yin S, et al. The quality of reporting of randomized controlled trials of electroacupuncture for stroke. BMC Complement Altern Med. 2016;16:512.
7. Wang KH, Wu JR, Liu S, Zhang D, Duan XJ, Zhang B. Meta-analysis on randomized controlled trials of xingnaojing injection for treating acute cerebral infarction. Chin J Pharmacoepidemiol. 2017;15:471–6.
8. You YN, Cho MR, Kim JH, et al. Assessing the quality of reports about randomized controlled trials of scalp acupuncture combined with another treatment for stroke. BMC Complement Altern Med. 2017;17:452.
9. Sun K, Fan J, Han J. Ameliorating effects of traditional Chinese medicine preparation, Chinese materia medica and active compounds on ischemia/ reperfusion-induced cerebral microcirculatory disturbances and neuron damage. Acta Pharm Sin B. 2015;5:8–24.
10. Cao W, Liu W. Wu T, Zhong D, Liu G. Dengzhanhua preparations for acute cerebral infarction. Cochrane Database Syst Rev. 2008;63:CD005568.
11. Liao P, Wang L, Guo L, Zeng R, Huang J, Zhang M. Danhong injection (a traditional Chinese patent medicine) for acute myocardial infarction: a systematic review and meta-analysis. Evid Based Complement Alternat Med. 2015;2015:646530.
12. Xie CL, Wang WW, Xue XD, Zhang SF, Gan J, Liu ZG. A systematic review and meta-analysis of Ginsenoside-Rg1 (G-Rg1) in experimental ischemic stroke. Sci Rep. 2015;5:7790.
13. Li B, Wang Y, Lu J, Liu J, Yuan Y, Yu Y, et al. Evaluating the effects of Danhong injection in treatment of acute ischemic stroke: study protocol for a multicenter randomized controlled trial. Trials. 2015;16:561.
14. Yu YC, Wu SZ, Hou Q. Clinical study on Xueshuantong combined with aspirinon in treatment of senium acute cerebral infarction. Drugs & Clinic. 2014;7:782–5.
15. CAST (Chinese Acute Stroke Trial) Collaborative Group. CAST: randomised placebo-controlled trial of early aspirin use in 20,000 patients with acute ischaemic stroke. Lancet. 1997;349:1641–9.
16. The International Stroke Trial (IST). A randomized trial of aspirin, subcutaneous heparin, both, or neither among 19435 patients with acute ischaemic stroke. International stroke trial collaborative group. Lancet. 1997; 349:1569–81.
17. Edaravone Acute Infarction Study Group. Effect of a novel free radical scavenger, edaravone (MCI-186), on acute brain infarction. Randomized, placebo-controlled, double-blind study at multicenters. Cerebrovasc Dis. 2003;15:222–9.
18. Gu XL, Ding XS, Di Q. Clinical study on edaravone injection in treatment of acute cerebral infarction. Chinese J New Drugs Clin Remedies. 2005;24:113–6.
19. Zhang M, Xu LJ, Deng LY. Efficacy and safety of Edaravone injection in the treatment of acute cerebral infarction: a randomized, double blind, multicenter study. Chinese J New Drugs Clin Remedies. 2007;26:105–8.
20. Davalos A, Castillo J, Alvarez-Sabin J, Secades JJ, Mercadal J, López S, et al. Oral citicoline in acute ischemic stroke: an individual patient data pooling analysis of clinical trials. Stroke. 2002;33:2850–7.

21. National Pharmacopoeia Committee. Chinese pharmacopoeia, part 1, Appendix 13. Beijing, China: Chemical Industry Press; 2005.
22. Xie YY, Xiao X, Luo J-M, Fu C, Wang Q-W, Wang Y-M, et al. Integrating qualitative and quantitative characterization of traditional Chinese medicine injection by high-performance liquid chromatography with diode array detection and tandem mass spectrometry. J Sep Sci. 2014;37:1438–47.
23. Liu J, Liu F, Li PH. Analysis of the adverse reaction of traditional Chinese medicine injections activating blood stasis. China Pharmacy. 2011;22:646–8.
24. Tan D, Wu JR, Liu S, Zhang B. Meta-analysis of efficacy of shuxuening injection in the treatment of cerebral infarction. J Pharmacoepidemiol. 2016;8:492–8.
25. Wang X, Wu JR, Zhang D, Wang KH, Zhang B. Meta-analysis of efficacy of xueshuantong injection in the treatment of acute cerebral infarction. J Pharmacoepidemiol. 2016;10:616–22.
26. Wang KH, Wu JR, Zhang D, Liu S, Zhang XM, Zhang B. Meta-analysis of efficacy of mailuoning injection in the treatment of acute cerebral infarction. J Pharmacoepidemiol. 2016;9:544–8. 590
27. Duan XJ, Wu JR, Liu S, Zhang D, Fang J, Zhang B. Meta-analysis of efficacy of danshenchuanxiongqin injection in the treatment of acute cerebral infarction. J Pharmacoepidemiol. 2017;1:27–32.
28. Liu X-T, Ren P-W, Peng L, Kang D-Y, Zhang T-L, Wen S, et al. Effectiveness and safety of ShenXiong glucose injection for acute ischemic stroke: a systematic review and GRADE approach. BMC Complement Altern Med. 2016;16:68.
29. Wu J, Zhang XM, Zhang B. Qingkailing injection for the treatment of acute stroke: a systematic review and meta-analysis. J Tradit Chin Med. 2014;34:131–9.
30. Zhang X, Wu J, Zhang B. Xuesaitong injection as one adjuvant treatment of acute cerebral infarction: a systematic review and meta-analysis. BMC Complement Altern Med. 2015;15:36.
31. Peng W, Yang J, Wang Y, Wang W, Xu J, Wang L, et al. Systematic review and meta-analysis of randomized controlled trials of Xingnaojing treatment for stroke. Evid Based Complement Altern Med. 2014;2014:210851.
32. Wu B, Liu M, Liu H, Li W, Tan S, Zhang S, et al. Meta-analysis of traditional Chinese patent medicine for ischemic stroke. Stroke. 2007;38:1973–9.
33. Jinatongthai P, Kongwatcharapong J, Foo CY, Phrommintikul A, et al. Comparative efficacy and safety of reperfusion therapy with fibrinolytic agents in patients with ST-segment elevation myocardial infarction: a systematic review and network meta-analysis. Lancet. 2017;390:747–59.
34. Sun F, Chai SB, Li LS, et al. Effects of glucagon-like peptide-1 receptor agonists on weight loss in patients with type 2 diabetes: a systematic review and network meta-analysis. J Diabetes Res. 2015;2015:157201.
35. Lu G, Ades AE. Combination of direct and indirect evidence in mixed treatment comparisons. Stat Med. 2004;23:3105–24.
36. The fourth session of the National Cerebrovascular Conference. The norm of clinical neurologic deficit score. Chin J Neurol. 1996;29:381–3.
37. Higgins JPT, Green S. Cochrane handbook for systematic reviews of interventions version 5.1.0 [EB/OL]. The Cochrane collaboration (2011). http://training.cochrane.org/handbook. Accessed 16 May 2013.
38. Moher D, Hopewell S, Schulz KF, Montori V, Gøtzsche PC, Devereaux PJ, et al. CONSORT 2010 explanation and elaboration: updated guidelines for reporting parallel group randomised trials. J Clin Epidemiol. 2010;63:e1–37.
39. Salanti G, Ades AE, Ioannidis JPA. Graphical methods and numerical summaries for presenting results from multiple-treatment meta-analysis: an overview and tutorial. J Clin Epidemiol. 2011;64:163–71.
40. Riley RD, Higgins JPT, Deeks JJ. Interpretation of random effects meta-analyses. BMJ. 2011;342:d549.
41. Egger M, Smith GD, Schneider M, Minder C. Bias in meta-analysis detected by a simple, graphical test. BMJ. 1997;315:629–34.
42. Chaimani A, Higgins JPT, Mavridis D, Spyridonos P, Salanti G. Graphical tools for network meta-analysis in STATA. PLoS One. 2013;8:e76654.
43. Yu YW, Ran ZJ. Clinical study on 58 cases acute cerebral infarction treated by Danhong injection. Pract J Card Cereb Pneum Vasc Dis. 2009;17:477–8.
44. Yu Y. Clinical study on Xueshuantong in treatment of acute cerebral infarction. Chinese Foreign Med Res. 2015;13:32–3.
45. Zhang ZJ, Cao CY. Clinical study on Shenxiong glucose injection in treatment of acute cerebral infarction and its effect on plasma endothelin. J Guangdong Med Coll. 2008;26:408–9.
46. Zheng XD. Curative effect with dipyridamole plus aspirin therapy in acute cerebral infarction. J Mod Clin Med. 2007;33:171–3.
47. Zhou SJ. Study on Shenxiong glucose injection in treatment of acute cerebral infarction. Mod. Prev Med. 2011;38:2656–9.
48. Zhou SF, Huo Y. Study on Ginkgo dipyridolum injection combined with aspirinon in treatment of acute cerebral infarction. J Mudanjiang Med Univ. 2009;20:56–8.
49. Zhou SH. Effect of Shu Xue Ning injection on serum IL - 6 and its efficacy in patients with acute cerebral infarction. Zhejiang J Tradit Chin Med. 2013;48:923.
50. Xu XY. Study on Ginkgo dipyridolum injection in treatment of acute cerebral infarction. In: Shandong province, the third integrated traditional Chinese medicine and western medicine academic symposium. Jinan; 2011. p. 268–270.
51. Xie S, Cao C. Effect of Shuxuening injection in patients with acute cerebral infarction. J Med Theory Pract. 2011;24:1891–2.
52. Xie YG, Zhou JH. Observation of effect of Suxuetong injection on acute cerebral infarction. China Trop Med. 2010;10:352–92.
53. Xu LL, Meng QY, Tian L, Liu XH, Liu T. Curative effection of tetramethylpyrazine on acute cerebral infarction. J Pract Tradit Chinese Intern Med. 2011;25:57–8.
54. Xu XQ. The observation of aplication of Ginkgo leaf extract and diphyridamole injection in the treatment of acute cerebral infarction. Chinese J Exp Tradit Med Formulae. 2012;18:211–3.
55. Yang HJ. Effect of Xuetong injection in patients with acute cerebral infarction. J Pract Med Tech. 2007;14:2157.
56. Yang YF. Study on Danhong injection combined with aspirinon in treatment of acute cerebral infarction. J Psychol Doctor. 2012;3:30.
57. Yao QY, Gong SJ. Effect of Shuxuetong injection in patients with acute cerebral infarction. Mod J Integr Tradit Chinese Western Med. 2010;19:3389–90.
58. Yao J, Lu XR. The observation of aplication of Ginkgo leaf extract and diphyridamole injection in the treatment of acute cerebral infarction. Clin Med. 2010;30:44–5.
59. Xie RP. Clinical study on Shuxuening in treatment of acute cerebral infarction. Proc Clin Med. 2010;19:758–9.
60. Tan SY, Tan ZL. Clinical study of Danhong injection in the treatment of cerebral infarction caused by branch atheromatous disease. J Shenyang Med Coll. 2016;18:18–20.
61. Wang WP. Study on Ginkgo dipyridolum injection combined with Fufangdanshen injection in treatment of acute cerebral infarction. Shenzhen J Integr Tradit Chinese and Western Med. 2015;25:21–2.
62. Ren HM. The observation of aplication of Shenxiong injection in the treatment of acute cerebral infarction. China Healthcare Innov. 2009;4:27.
63. Sun HJ, Zheng MH, Liang TS. Effects of Chuangxiongqin injection on serum sCD40L and the level of hs-CRP in patients with angina pectoris. J Shanghai Univ Tradit Chin Med. 2013;27:39–41.
64. Tang JP, Jiang P, Yang XY. Clinical efficacy and safety of safflower yellow pigment injection in the treatment of acute cerebral infarction. J Mod Med Health. 2013;29:2524–5.
65. Tang FY, Zhang GW. Clinical study on 36 cases acute cerebral infarction treated by breviscapine injection. Chinese J Pract Med. 2009;36:51–2.
66. Tang XJ. Study on Ginkgo damole injection combined with aspirinon in treatment of acute cerebral infarction. Hebei Med J. 2013;35:1188–9.
67. Wang L. Clinical study on 48 cases acute cerebral infarction treated by Shenxiong glucose injection. China Foreign Med Treat. 2010;29:116.
68. Wang YL, Zou XH, Dang LH. Expression of TNF-a and IL-6 in patients with acute cerebral infarction after clinical intervention of Shuxuetong injection and clinical significance. J Yunnan UnivTradit Chin Med. 2013;36:70–2.
69. Lan Y, Xiao JX, Zheng TY, ZX L. Effect of salvia ligustrazin injection on lysophospholipids acid, P selection and its efficacy in patients with acute cerebral infarction. Mod J Integr Tradit Chinese Western Med. 2015;24:840–2.
70. Li M, Li Q, Zhang M, Zhang XL, Hu Q, Pang Y. Effect of Dan Hong injection on serum S100B protein and neuron specific alcohol in patients with acute cerebral infarction. Herald Med. 2014;33:1596–9.
71. Liu YP, Wang ZG, Wu H. Effect of Dan Hong injection on C-reactive protein and its efficacy in patients with acute cerebral infarction. Pract J Card Cereb Pneum Vasc Dis. 2010;18:1433–4.
72. Ma J, Yu NW, Ren ZW, Chen M, Wu HH. Effect of breviscapine on serum NSE,Ang-2 and IL-6 levels and its efficacy in patients with acute cerebral infarction. Chinese J Pract Med. 2015;21:204–7.
73. Ma J, Yu NW, Wu HH, Chen M, Ren ZW, Zhao DD. Effect of Danhong injection on nerve function and hemorheology for patients with acute ischemic stroke. Chinese J Exp Tradit Med Formulae. 2015;21:204–7.

74. Chen H. Clinical study on 67 cases acute cerebral infarction treated by Shuxuetong injection. Asia-Pacific Tradit Med. 2015;11:137–8.

75. Luan T. The clinical effects of Xuesaitong injection in the treatment of acute cerebral infarction. Guide China Med. 2014;12:42–3.

76. Huang ML. Clinical study on 150 cases acute cerebral infarction treated by Xueshuangtong injection. Mod Diagn Treat. 2012;23:2254–5.

77. Li X, Zheng WW, Gao YB. Effect of carthamin yellow injection on NT-proBNP and TXB_2 for patients with acute ischemic stroke. Chinese J Integr Med Cardio/Cerebrovascular Dis. 2015;13:1900–2.

78. Ma ZL, Wu BX, Cheng DM, Zhang XL, Hu Y. Clinic observation of the curative effect of safflor yellow in the treatment of acute cerebral infarction. Chinese J Pract Nerv Dis. 2011;14:30–1.

79. Zhang Y, Hou J, Hu Y, Mu ZB, HY M. Study on Danshen Chuanxiongqin injection combined with edaravone in treatment of acute cerebral infarction. Chinese J Integr Med Cardio/Cerebrovascular Dis. 2012;10:168–9.

80. Liu M. Study on Danshen Chuanxiongqin injection combined with edaravone in treatment of acute cerebral infarction. Mod J Integr Tradit Chinese Western Med. 2014;23:2105–7.

81. Chen YC. Clinic observation of the curative effect of Ginkgo damole injection in the treatment of acute cerebral infarction. Chinese Foreign Med Res. 2011;9:45–6.

82. Yang RF. Clinical research of edaravone combined with Shuxuetong in treating acute cerebral infarction. China J Chinese Med. 2013;28:1228–9.

83. Lin YF, Wang ML, Huang ZQ, Yan P, Su Y. Clinical research of combined Ginkgo damole injection with aspirin in treating acute cerebral infarction. Proc Clin Med. 2008;17:761–2.

84. Peng T, Pang YL. Clinic observation of the curative effect of Shuxuetong injection in the treatment of acute cerebral infarction. Pract J Card Cereb Pneum Vasc Dis. 2006;14:388.

85. Li XH. Clinic observation of the curative effect of Shuxuening injection in the treatment of acute cerebral infarction. Asia-Pacific Tradit Med. 2011;7:129–30.

86. Liu L, Yang XS, Chen W, Liu ZT. Clinic observation of the curative effect of Danhong injection in the treatment of acute cerebral infarction. Clin J Tradit Chin Med. 2014;26:166–7.

87. Zhang YH, Liu WJ, Ding S. The clinical research of Danhong combined with low molecular heparin calcium to treat the acute cerebral infarction. Pract J Card Cereb Pneum Vasc Dis. 2010;18:3–5.

88. Fan J. Clinic observation of the curative effect of Ginkgo damole injection in the treatment of acute cerebral infarction. China Pharm. 2006;15:54.

89. Liu HY, Liu YM. Clinical study on 64 cases acute cerebral infarction treated by Xuesaitong injection. Jilin Med J. 2014;2014:4963–4.

90. Li FQ. Clinical study on 64 cases acute cerebral infarction treated by Ginkgo damole injection. Chinese J Ethnomed Ethnopharmacy. 2010;19:106.

91. Lian CL. Clinical observation on 46 cases of acute cerebral infarction treated with combination of traditional Chinese and western medicine. J Pract Tradit Chin Med. 2013;29:456.

92. Chen S, Jiang KW, Lu HZ. Clinic observation of the curative effect of Xuesaitong injection in the treatment of acute cerebral infarction. J Pract Med. 2006;22:1405–6.

93. Cao L. Clinic observation of the curative effect of Xueshuangtong injection in the treatment of acute cerebral infarction. Chinese J Ethnomed Ethnopharmacy. 2012;21:71.

94. Liu Y. Effective observation on acute cerebral infarction treated by Shuxuetong injection. Chinese J Med Guide. 2009;11:1157–8.

95. Luo XD, Wang P, Zeng XR. Xuesaitong injection plus routine therapy for acute cerebral infarction and the influence on plasma C-reactive protein. Pract J Clin Med. 2011;8:96–8.

96. Liao MJ, Chen ZB. Clinical study on 30 cases acute cerebral infarction treated by safflower yellow injection. Med Inf. 2014;27:109–10.

97. Shi JL, Cheng JL. The clinical research of Ginkgo-damole combinded with atorvastatin calcium to treat the acute cerebral infarction. Chinese J Pract Nerv Dis. 2010;13:52–3.

98. Ni H. Clinical study on 59 cases of Shuxuening combined with sodium ozagrel to treat the acute cerebral infarction. Jilin Med J. 2010;30:3078–9.

99. Li CP. Clinical study on 80 cases acute cerebral infarction treated by Shuxuening injection. J Shanxi Coll Tradit Chin Med. 2007;8:37–8.

100. Zhou ZP, Yang GS, Wang AY. Effect of erigeron injection on MMP- 9 in patient with acute cerebral infarction. Mod Prev Med. 2011;38:2660–1.

101. Chen C. Efficacy and safety of aspirin plus clopidogrel and Shuxuetong in treatment of patients with acute cerebral infarction. Eval Anal Drug-Use Hosp China. 2015;15:808–10.

102. Chen JY, Wang DC, Luo SW. Clinical study on 54 cases of Shuxuetong plus aspirin and clopidogrel to treat the acute cerebral infarction. China Pharmaceuticals. 2012;21:53–4.

103. Luo QY. Clinic observation of the curative effect of Ginkgo bilboa injection in the treatment of acute cerebral infarction. Youjiang Med J. 2007;35:133–4.

104. Chen J, Li SJ. Clinical observation of Ginkgo-dipyidamolum injection in treatment of acute cerebral infarction. Neural Inj Funct Reconstr. 2007;7:291–3.

105. Zhang XL, Zhang LL, Heng XL, Ma Y, Pang W. Effect of Mailuoning injection on blood rheology for patients with acute ischemic stroke. Nerv Dis Mental Health. 2015;5:216–7.

106. Ni HQ, Wu L, Li JF, Chen J. Meta-analysis of comparative study on Ginkgo dipyridolum injection in the treatment of acute cerebral infarction. China Pharm. 2008;19:1655–8.

107. Xi BC, Zhang C, Sun LL. Meta-analysis of comparative study on Shuxuening injection in the treatment of acute cerebral infarction. Pharm Care Res. 2012;12:354–7.

108. Zheng WK, Zhang L, Shang HC. Systematic review on Shuxuening injection in treating acute cerebral infarction. Chinese Licensed Pharmacist. 2012;9:33–41.

109. Rodríguez M, Ringstad L, Schäfer P, Just S, Hofer HW, Malmsten M, et al. Reduction of atherosclerotic nanoplaque formation and size by Ginkgo biloba (EGb 761) in cardiovascular high-risk patients. Atherosclerosis. 2007;192:438–44.

110. Luo Y. Alzheimer's disease, the nematode Caenorhabditis elegans, and Ginkgo biloba leaf extract. Life Sci. 2006;78:2066–72.

111. Park Y-M, Won J-H, Yun K-J, Ryu J-H, Han Y-N, Choi S-K, et al. Preventive effect of Ginkgo biloba extract (GBB) on the lipopolysaccharide-induced expressions of inducible nitric oxide synthase and cyclooxygenase-2 via suppression of nuclear factor-κB in RAW 264.7 cells. Biol Pharm Bull. 2006;29:985–90.

112. Biddlestone L, Corbett AD, Dolan S. Oral administration of Ginkgo biloba extract, EGb-761 inhibits thermal hyperalgesia in rodent models of inflammatory and post-surgical pain. Br J Pharmacol. 2007;151:285–91.

113. Nada SE, Tulsulkar J, Shah ZA. Heme oxygenase 1-mediated neurogenesis is enhanced by Ginkgo biloba (EGb 761®) after permanent ischemic stroke in mice. Mol Neurobiol. 2014;49:945–56.

114. Tulsulkar J, Shah ZA. Ginkgo biloba prevents transient global ischemia-induced delayed hippocampal neuronal death through antioxidant and anti-inflammatory mechanism. Neurochem Int. 2013;62:189–97.

115. Chen J-S, Huang P-H, Wang C-H, Lin F-Y, Tsai H-Y, Wu T-C, et al. Nrf-2 mediated heme oxygenase-1 expression, an antioxidant-independent mechanism, contributes to anti-atherogenesis and vascular protective effects of Ginkgo biloba extract. Atherosclerosis. 2011;214:301–9.

116. Shah ZA, Nada SE, Doré S. Heme oxygenase 1, beneficial role in permanent ischemic stroke and in Ginkgo biloba (EGb 761) neuroprotection. Neuroscience. 2011;180:248–55.

6

Extracts of Zuo Jin Wan, a traditional Chinese medicine, phenocopies 5-HTR1D antagonist in attenuating Wnt/β-catenin signaling in colorectal cancer cells

Jielu Pan[1†], Yangxian Xu[2†], Haiyan Song[1], Xiqiu Zhou[2], Zemin Yao[3*] and Guang Ji[1,4*] (iD)

Abstract

Background: In vitro and in vivo studies have shown that Zuo Jin Wan (ZJW), a herbal formula of traditional Chinese medicine (TCM), possessed anticancer properties. However, the underlying mechanism for the action of ZJW remains unclear. Various subtypes of 5-Hydroxytryptamine receptor (5-HTR) have been shown to play a role in carcinogenesis and cancer metastasis. 5-HTR1D, among the subtypes, is highly expressed in colorectal cancer (CRC) cell lines and tissues. The present study aimed at investigating effect of ZJW extracts on the biological function of CRC cells, the expression of 5-HTR1D, and molecules of Wnt/β-catenin signaling pathway.

Methods: In this study, the effect of ZJW extracts on 5-HTR1D expression and Wnt/β-catenin signaling pathway were investigated and contrasted with GR127935 (GR), a known 5-HTR1D antagonist, using the CRC cell line SW403. The cells were respectively treated with GR127935 and different doses of ZJW extracts. Proliferation, apoptosis, migration, and invasion of SW403 cells were compared between ZJW and GR127935 treatments. The expression of 5-HTR1D and signaling molecules involved in the canonic Wnt/β-catenin pathway were determined by Western blot analysis.

Results: After ZJW extracts treatment and GR127935 treatment, G1 arrest in cell cycle of SW403 was increased. Cell apoptosis was pronounced, and cell migration and invasion were suppressed. SW403 cells showed a dose-dependently decreased expression of 5-HTR1D, meanwhile, β-catenin level was significantly decreased in nucleus of cells cultured with GR127935. Treatment of ZJW extracts dose-dependently resulted in decreased 5-HTR1D and a concomitant reduction in the Wnt/β-catenin signal transduction, an effect indistinguishable from GR127935 treatment.

Conclusion: The anticancer activity of ZJW extracts may be partially achieved through attenuation of the 5-HTR1D-Wnt/β-catenin signaling pathway.

Keywords: 5-HTR1D, Colorectal cancer, GR127935, Zuo Jin Wan, Wnt/β-catenin pathway

Background

Colorectal cancer (CRC) is one of the most common malignancies worldwide. World Health Organization (WHO) reported that CRC ranked the third place in male and second place in female of cancer morbidity, and the fourth of the mortality rates [1]. Current treatments for CRC include surgery, radiation and chemotherapy, but the prognosis is poor [2, 3].

Zuo Jin Wan (ZJW), a herbal formula of traditional Chinese medicine (TCM), has been used in treating gastrointestinal diseases and liver diseases in China for a long history [4, 5]. It is composed of *Rhizoma Coptidis* (Huanglian in China) and *Evodia Rutaecarpa* (Wuzhuyu in China) in ratio of 6 to 1. Berberine and evodiamine are two key components of ZJW extracts that possess anti-tumorigenic activity [6]. In vitro and in vivo experiments have shown that berberine and evodiamine can arrest cell cycle, reduce

* Correspondence: zyao@uottawa.ca; jiliver@vip.sina.com
†Equal contributors
3Department of Biochemistry, Microbiology and Immunology, Ottawa Institute of Systems Biology, University of Ottawa, Ottawa, ON K1H 8M5, Canada
1Institute of Digestive Diseases, Longhua Hospital, Shanghai University of Traditional Chinese Medicine, Shanghai 200032, China
Full list of author information is available at the end of the article

expressions of some oncogenes, and inhibit tumor metasta-sis [7, 8]. Animal experiments with ZJW also show its anti-tumor effect in tumors including CRC [9, 10]. ZJW extracts can inhibit the growth of multi-drug resistant CRC cell lines, increase the sensitivity of chemotherapy, inhibit the tumor growth of xenograft mice, and reduce the P-gp pro-tein expression and reverse drug resistance of CRC cells [11]. However, to date, the mechanism whereby ZJW ex-tracts exert the anti-tumor effect is unclear.

Serotonin, also known as 5-hydroxytryptamine (5-HT), is a biogenic amine produced by enterochromaffin cells (EC) of the gastrointestinal tract [12]. It is a versatile neuro-transmitter, with a role of signal-transduction and maintenance of cell growth. 5-HT exerts its effects through the membrane-bound 5-HT receptors (5-HTRs) consisting of fourteen members [13, 14]. Over the past de-cades, accumulating preclinical and clinical evidences have pointed out that 5-HT not only plays a role in physio-logical cell mitosis, but also has a close correlation with cancers [14]. Certain subtypes of 5-HTRs have been re-ported in the process of different types of cancers, includ-ing prostate [15], colon [16], liver [17] and gallbladder cancer cells [18], breast cancer [19], and bladder cancer [20]. 5-HT and 5-HTRs may be a potential factor in the tumorigenesis and tumor progression. It has been found that the agonists of 5-HTR3, 5-HTR4 and 5-HTR1B can promote the proliferation of CRC cells [21], whereas the antagonists of 5-HTR1B can induce apoptosis [22].

Several studies have suggested a potential link between 5-HTRs and CRC. For instance, Xu et al. [23] have re-ported that a decreased risk of CRC was associated with the use of high daily doses of selective serotonin-reuptake inhibitors (SSRI) 0–5 years before a diagnosis of CRC (incidence-rate ratio 0.70 [95% CI 0·50–0·96]). In another study, it has been shown that a decrease in 5-HTR1A, 5-HTR2C, and serotonin reuptake transporter (SERT) in Caco-2 cells was associated with sulforaphane treatment in a dose-dependent manner [24]. It has been suggested that activation of 5-HTRs, followed by initi-ation of cyclic AMP signaling, might be crucial events in colon cancer progression [24]. Thus, 5-HTR-mediated signaling pathway might potentially be a novel thera-peutic target for colon cancer therapy.

The Wnt/β-catenin pathway (or canonical Wnt path-way) plays an important role in the regulation of cellular growth, apoptosis, cell adhesion, and metabolism [25, 26]. Aberrations of the Wnt/β-catenin pathway cause various diseases including cancer, and mutations in this signaling are frequently observed in cancer [27, 28]. Therefore, the Wnt/β-catenin pathway has been recently considered as the one mostly relevant to cancer [29–31]. Among all hu-man cancer types, it is only CRC for which there is un-questionable evidence that deregulated Wnt signaling drives tumorigenesis [32]. In the canonical Wnt signaling

pathway, the central player is β-catenin, a transcription cofactor that, together with T cell factor/lymphoid enhan-cer factor (TCF/LEF), controls expression of various target genes [33]. The level of β-catenin is negatively regulated by a scaffolding complex, consisting of Axin, adenomatous polyposis coli (APC) and glycogen synthase kinase 3β (GSK3β), which targets β-catenin for degradation through the ubiquitination/proteasome dependent pathway. Wnt binds to Frizzled receptor and inactivates the β-catenin destructive complex via the activation of the dishevelled (Dvl) protein [31].

Recently, higher expression of 5-HTR1D has been ob-served in human CRC tissues [34]. Experiments with a CRC cell line LoVo have shown that treatment of 5-HTR1D antagonist GR127935 resulted in decreased ex-pression of 5-HTR1D and decreased ability of CRC cell metastasis, which might be mediated by attenuating Wnt/β-catenin signaling [34]. We postulated that ZJW extracts might exert an anti-tumorigenic effect similar to that of a 5-HTR1D antagonist. In this study, we determined the ef-fect of ZJW extracts on the biological function of CRC cells, the expression of 5-HTR1D, and expression of mole-cules of Wnt/β-catenin signaling pathway.

Methods
Cell culture
Human colorectal cancer cell line, SW403, was obtained from College of Chinese Medicine, Shanghai University of Traditional Chinese Medicine (Shanghai, China). Cells were incubated in RPMI 1640 (Biowest, Nuaillé, France) supplemented with 10% (v/v) fetal bovine serum (FBS) (Gibco, Auckland, New Zealand), 2 mmol/L L-glutamine, 1 mmol/L sodium pyruvate, 100 units of penicillin, and 100 mg/mL streptomycin (Biowest). The cells were culti-vated in an atmosphere of 5% CO_2 incubator (Thermo sci-entific Heraeus, Germany) at 37 °C.

Preparation of medicines for treatment
The 5-HTR1D antagonist GR127935 (GR) (TOCRIS, Ellisville, USA) was dissolved in phosphate buffer saline (PBS) and then diluted into different concentrations. ZJW was prepared using a formula of Chinese herb *Rhi-zoma Coptidis* (60 g) and *Evodia rutaecarpa* (10 g), at a ratio of 6:1. All the herbs were purchased from Longhua Hospital herbal pharmacy department. Briefly, the mix-ture (70 g) was extracted twice for 1 h each time by refluxing in ethanol (1: 8, v/v). The filtrates were concen-trated and dried in vacuum at 60 °C. Its preparations were standardized, regulated, and quality controlled ac-cording to the guidelines defined by China Food and Drug Administration (CFDA). High-performance liquid chromatography (HPLC) was used to identify the com-ponents of ZJW extract, and confirm the final concen-tration of ZJW extract to ensure the quality and

stability. Detailed procedures were followed with the published protocol [6]. ZJW was dissolved in PBS and diluted into three different concentrations, 25, 50 and 100 μg/mL, corresponding to low, medium and high dose of ZJW (ZJW-L, ZJW-M and ZJW-H).

Western blot analysis

Cells of different treatment from three separate experiments were lysed with Radio-Immunoprecipitation Assay (RIPA) lysis buffer (Beyotime, Hangzhou, China) to extract protein. The protein in nucleus was extracted with a Kit (Beyotime, Hangzhou, China). Protein concentration was determined using a BCA protein assay kit (CoWin Bioscience, Beijing, China).The cell lysates were dissolved in a loading buffer containing 2% SDS and incubated at 95 °C for 5 min). Samples were separated by sodium dodecyl sulfate–polyacrylamide by gel electrophoresis (SDS–PAGE), subsequently transferred to polyvinylidene fluoride (PVDF) membrane, blocked with 5% non-fat dry milk in Tris-buffered saline-Tween-20 (TBST) for 1 h, and then probed with primary antibodies at 4 °C overnight. The following primary antibodies were used: 5-HTR1D (#ab13895) (Abcam, Cambridge, MA, USA), Axin1(C76H11, #2087), Dvl2 (30D2, #3224), Dvl3 (#3218), GSK-3β (27C10, #9315), phospho-GSK-3β (Ser9) (D3A4, #9322), LEF1 (C12A5, #2230), TCF4 (C48H11, #2569), cyclin D1 (92G2, #2978), c-Myc (D84C12, #5605), β-catenin ((D10A8, #8480), Bcl-2 (50E3, #2870), phospho-Bcl-2 (Ser70) (5H2, #2827), phospho-Bcl-2 (Thr56) (#2875), Bcl-xL (54H6, #2764), Mcl-1 (D35A5, #5453) (Cell Signaling Technology, Danvers, MA, USA), CDK4 (#11026–1), MMP-2 (#10373–2), MMP-7 (#10374–2), CXCR4 (#11026–1), E-cadherin (#20874–1), ICAM-1 (#10020–1) (Proteintech, Wuhan, China), β-actin (#R1102) (Hua An, Hangzhou, China) and Histone 2A (#21260) (SignalWay Antibody, College Park, MD, USA). The membrane was washed with TBST and then incubated with goat anti-rabbit or anti-mouse peroxidase-conjugated secondary antibody (Cell Signaling Technology) for 1 h. Immmunoreactive bands were visualized with enhanced chemiluminescence HRP substrate (Millipore, Billerica, MA, USA) and acquired by GBOX Chemi XT4 System (Syngene, Cambridge, UK). GeneTools software (Syngene) was used to quantify the optical density of the bands. Beta-actin was determined as a loading control for whole lysate, and Histone 2A was used as the internal control for nuclear protein.

Cell viability assay

CCK-8 assay was performed to measure the cytotoxicity of ZJW on SW403 seeded in 96-well plates with 1×10^4 cells/well. After 24 h, cells were washed with PBS gently and then exposed to either 10% FBS alone or ZJW at different concentrations (25, 50, 100, 200, 400 and 800 μg/mL). After 24 h, previous medium was replaced with

100 μl of fresh medium and 10 μl of CCK-8 reagent (Dojindo, Kumamoto, Japan), followed by 4 h of incubation. Then the optical density (OD) of the cultures was determined by the microplate reader (BioTek, Winooski, USA) at 450 nm. All experiments were done with 6 replicates per experiment and repeated at least 3 times. IC10 was defined as 10% of maximal inhibitory concentration, representing the concentration of an inhibition rate that is required for 10% of cell viability. We set IC10 as a non-cytotoxic concentration of ZJW.

Cell cycle analysis

SW403 cells were cultured with ZJW-M and ZJW-H and GR (5 μmol/L) in 6-well plates with 2×10^5 cells/well for 24 h. Then cellular total DNA contents of the cells were assessed using flow cytometry following propidium iodide (PI) staining. After 24 h, the cells were collected by trypsinization, centrifuge at 1000 rpm for 5 min, washed with cold PBS twice, and resuspended gently with 70% ethanol at 4 °C for 2 h. Fixed cells were centrifuged and washed by PBS twice. 400 μL propidium iodide (PI) was added to the cells solution, gently shaked, and stained for 30 min at 4 °C avoiding the light. Cells were conducted using FACSCalibur Flow Cytometry (BD Biosciences, USA). PI fluorescence was linearly amplified and both the area and width of the fluorescence pulse were measured. 1×10^5 cells were acquired, and the percentages of G1, S and G2 phases were determined using the DNA analysis. Fluorescence measurements were taken at excitation wavelength of 488 nm. Three separate experiments were performed in SW403 cells for cycle analysis. The results were analyzed with CellQuest Pro software.

Cell apoptosis analysis

SW403 cells were incubated with ZJW-L, ZJW-M, and ZJW-H and GR (5 μmol/L) in 6-well plates with 2×10^5 cells/well in triplicates for 24 h. The cells were collected by trypsinization, centrifuge at 1500 rpm for 5 min, washed with cold PBS twice. Then the cells were resuspended in 500 μL Binding Buffer and mixed with 5 μL Annexin V-FITC (KeyGEN Biotech, Nanjing, China) and 5 μL PI, gently shaked. After 10 min incubation at room temperature in the dark, the cell apoptosis were analyzed using FACSCalibur Flow Cytometry (BD Biosciences, USA). Apoptotic cells were represented by high FITC Annexin V and low PI fluorescence signals (Ex 488 nm/Em 530 nm). Three separate experiments were performed for cell apoptosis. The results were analyzed with CellQuest Pro software.

Cell migration and invasion assays

Cell migration was assayed in transwell chambers (Corning, Wujiang, China). SW403 cells (3×10^5/ mL) suspended in 1640 medium (100 μL, serum free) or medium with ZJW-M, ZJW-H, GR (5 μmol/L), were placed in the upper transwell chamber, and incubated for 18 h. The cells on the upper surface of the filter were completely wiped away with a cotton swab. The filter was then fixed in methanol, stained with 0.1% crystal violet (Sigma, St. Louis, MO, USA), and the cells migrated to the underside of the filter were imaged using a microscope (Olympus, Tokyo, Janpan) at a magnification of 200× (5 fields/filter). The cell number was counted through ImageJ 1.47 (NIH). Experimental procedures of in vitro invasion assay are the same as the migration assay described above except that the filter was previously coated with a layer of Matrigel (Becton-Dickinson) before cell seeding.

Statistical analysis

Values are expressed as means and standard deviation (SD) and analyzed using one-way ANOVA followed by LSD test for comparisons between groups. Statistical analysis was conducted by SPSS 18.0 and GraphPad Prism 5.0. It was considered significant difference when $P < 0.05$.

Results

5-HTR1D expression after the ZJW extracts treatment in SW403 cells

The choice of CRC model cells used in the present study is based on our initial screening for 5-HTR expression among various cell lines derived from digestive carcinoma. We found that 5-HTR1D is relatively highly expressed in

SW403 cells. In our study, the data indicated that IC50 of ZJW extracts was 382.80 μg/ml, and IC10 was 117.98 μg/ml. The 3 different doses of ZJW extracts were less than IC10 of ZJW. Thus we use 100 μg/mL, 50 μg/mL and 25 μg/mL as high, middle and low concentration of ZJW in the experiments respectively. Thus, in current experiments, concentrations at 100, 50, and 25 μg/ml of the ZJW extracts were used, representing high (ZJW-H), medium (ZJW-M), and low (ZJW-L) doses, respectively. The results showed that, treatment of SW403 cells with 5-HTR1D antagonist GR127935 (GR) at 1, 5, 10 μmol/L down-regulated 5-HTR1D protein level in a dose-dependent manner (Fig. 1a and b). Likewise, compared to control, treatment of the cells with ZJW extracts also resulted in decreased 5-HTR1D expression in a dose-dependent manner (Fig. 1c and d).

Results of cell viability assay in SW403 cells

The effect of ZJW on cell proliferation was determined by monitoring the cell viability using CCK8 assay. With increasing concentration of ZJW, SW403 cells demonstrated decreasing cell vitality in a dose-dependent manner (Fig. 2a). The effect of ZJW and GR on mitotic cycle distributions was subsequently investigated. Flow cytometry of SW403 cells showed that increased SW403 cells were arrested at G1 phase after 24 h treatment with medium or high doses of ZJW (Fig. 2b and c). The western blot results showed that the levels of cell cycle-related gene products,

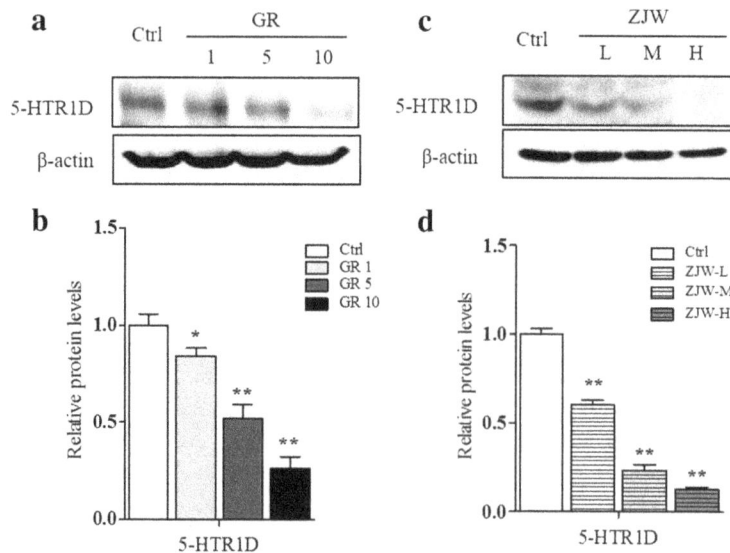

Fig. 1 Effect of the ZJW extracts treatment on 5-HTR1D expression in SW403 cell. SW403 cell was stimulated with GR (1, 5, 10 μmol/L) and ZJW at low, medium, and high dose, respectively. Cells were cultivated for 24 h. Protein expression in cells with different stimulation was determined by Western blot. Results were normalized to β-actin expression. **a** Representative western blots of 5-HTR1D protein in GR-treated SW403 cells. **b** The corresponding semi-quantification data of (**a**). **c** Representative western blots of 5-HTR1D protein in ZJW-treated and GR (5 μmol/L)-treated SW403 cells. **d** The corresponding semi-quantification data of (**c**). All values are shown as mean ± SD of three separate experiments, and significant values are indicated with asterisks (*$P < 0.05$, **$P < 0.01$ vs. control)

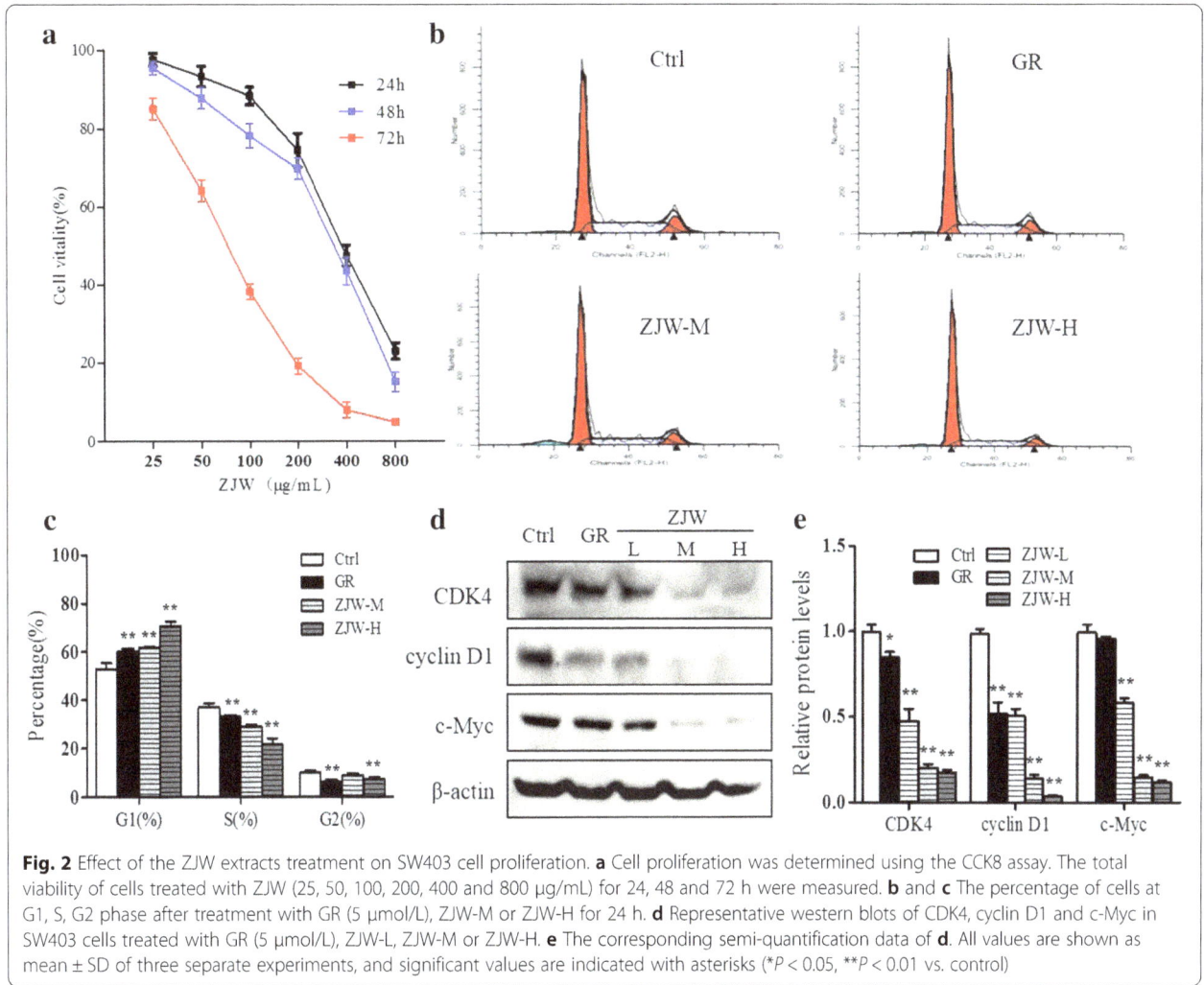

Fig. 2 Effect of the ZJW extracts treatment on SW403 cell proliferation. **a** Cell proliferation was determined using the CCK8 assay. The total viability of cells treated with ZJW (25, 50, 100, 200, 400 and 800 μg/mL) for 24, 48 and 72 h were measured. **b** and **c** The percentage of cells at G1, S, G2 phase after treatment with GR (5 μmol/L), ZJW-M or ZJW-H for 24 h. **d** Representative western blots of CDK4, cyclin D1 and c-Myc in SW403 cells treated with GR (5 μmol/L), ZJW-L, ZJW-M or ZJW-H. **e** The corresponding semi-quantification data of **d**. All values are shown as mean ± SD of three separate experiments, and significant values are indicated with asterisks (*$P < 0.05$, **$P < 0.01$ vs. control)

including cyclin D1, cyclin-dependent kinase 4 (CDK4) and c-Myc were attenuated with ZJW treatment as compared to those in control (Fig. 2d and e). The attenuation was most remarkable with ZJW-M or ZJW-H treatment.

Results of apoptosis assay in SW403 cells

We next determined the effect of ZJW extracts on cell apoptosis. Flow cytometry demonstrated that, after treating with ZJW-M and ZJW-H for 24 h, the percentage of apoptotic cells was significantly higher in ZJW treated cells than that in control (Fig. 3a and b). The levels of B-cell lymphoma-2 (Bcl-2), p-Bcl-2 (Thr70), p-Bcl-2 (Ser56) were decreased significantly under ZJW-M and ZJW-H conditions (Fig. 3b). Expression of Mcl-1 and Bcl-xL was also down-regulated in cells treated with GR127935 or ZJW. The results showed that increased cell apoptosis upon ZJW treatment was closely associated with altered mitochondrial anti-apoptosis molecules.

Results of cell migration and invasion in SW403 cells

The effect of ZJW extracts on SW403 cell migration and invasion was determined using the transwell assay. The number of cells that migrated through the chamber filter was significantly less in the group of GR or ZJW treatment than that in control group, and the effect was more profound when cells were treated with higher dose of ZJW (Fig. 4a and b). Similar results were obtained by the cell invasion assay (Fig. 4c and d). Thus, ZJW could inhibit the metastatic ability of colorectal cells.

To explore the mechanism further, we determined the level of matrix metalloproteinase 2 (MMP2), MMP7, intercellular adhesion molecule 1 (ICAM-1) and C-X-C chemokine receptor type 4 (CXCR4) that are related to metastasis. Western blot results showed that the levels of MMP2, MMP7, ICAM-1, and CXCR4 were all decreased in cells treated with ZJW in a dose-dependent manner (Fig. 4e and f).

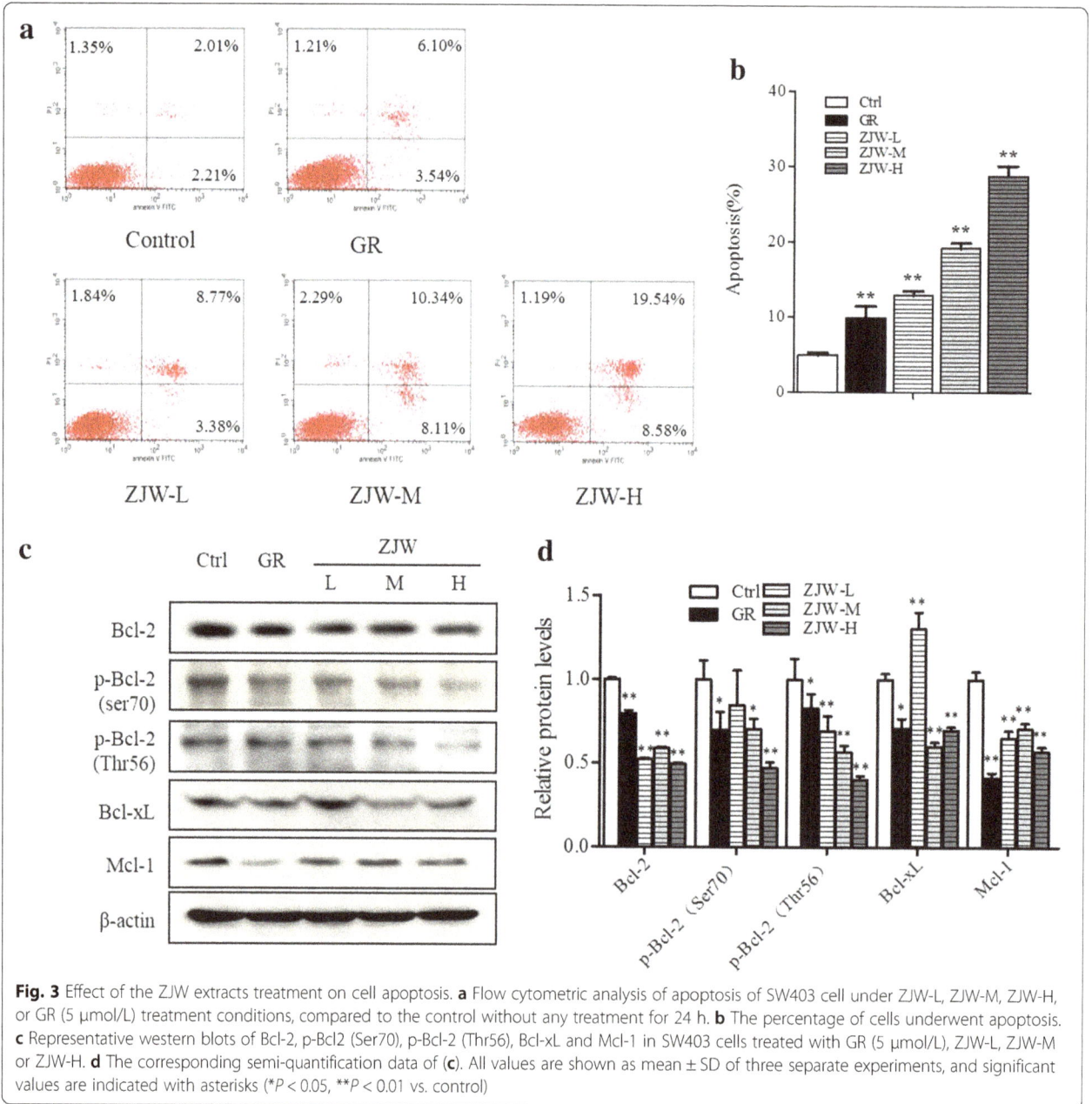

Fig. 3 Effect of the ZJW extracts treatment on cell apoptosis. **a** Flow cytometric analysis of apoptosis of SW403 cell under ZJW-L, ZJW-M, ZJW-H, or GR (5 μmol/L) treatment conditions, compared to the control without any treatment for 24 h. **b** The percentage of cells underwent apoptosis. **c** Representative western blots of Bcl-2, p-Bcl2 (Ser70), p-Bcl-2 (Thr56), Bcl-xL and Mcl-1 in SW403 cells treated with GR (5 μmol/L), ZJW-L, ZJW-M or ZJW-H. **d** The corresponding semi-quantification data of (**c**). All values are shown as mean ± SD of three separate experiments, and significant values are indicated with asterisks (*$P < 0.05$, **$P < 0.01$ vs. control)

Wnt/β-catenin signaling expression after ZJW extracts treatment in SW403 cells

In order to define the underlying mechanism of the biological effects of ZJW on CRC cells, we further examined the Wnt/β-catenin signaling pathway because it was reported recently that the Wnt/β-catenin signaling is associated with the 5-HTR1D function [34]. As shown in Fig. 5a and b, SW403 cells treated with GR exhibited increasing expression, in a GR dose-dependent manner, of Axin1 and decreasing expression of Dvl2, p-GSK-3β, LEF1 and TCF4 as compared with control. Figure 5c and d showed, with GR treatment, β-catenin level significantly was decreased in nucleus. The total β-catenin

level was decreased in cells cultured with 5 or 10 umol/L GR. Because nuclear accumulation of β-catenin is one of the key links of Wnt/β-catenin signaling transduction that promotes transcription of proliferation and metastasis related genes [35], these results suggest strongly that inhibition of 5-HTR1D can lead to suppression of Wnt/β-catenin signaling transduction.

The effect of ZJW treatment on increased Axin1 and concomitantly decreased Dvl2, Dvl3, LEF1 and TCF4 phenocopied the effect of GR treatment (Fig. 5e and f). In addition, although there was no change in the level of GSK-3β protein, ZJW treatment resulted in a significant reduction in serine-phosphorylated-GSK-3β (p-GSK-3β)

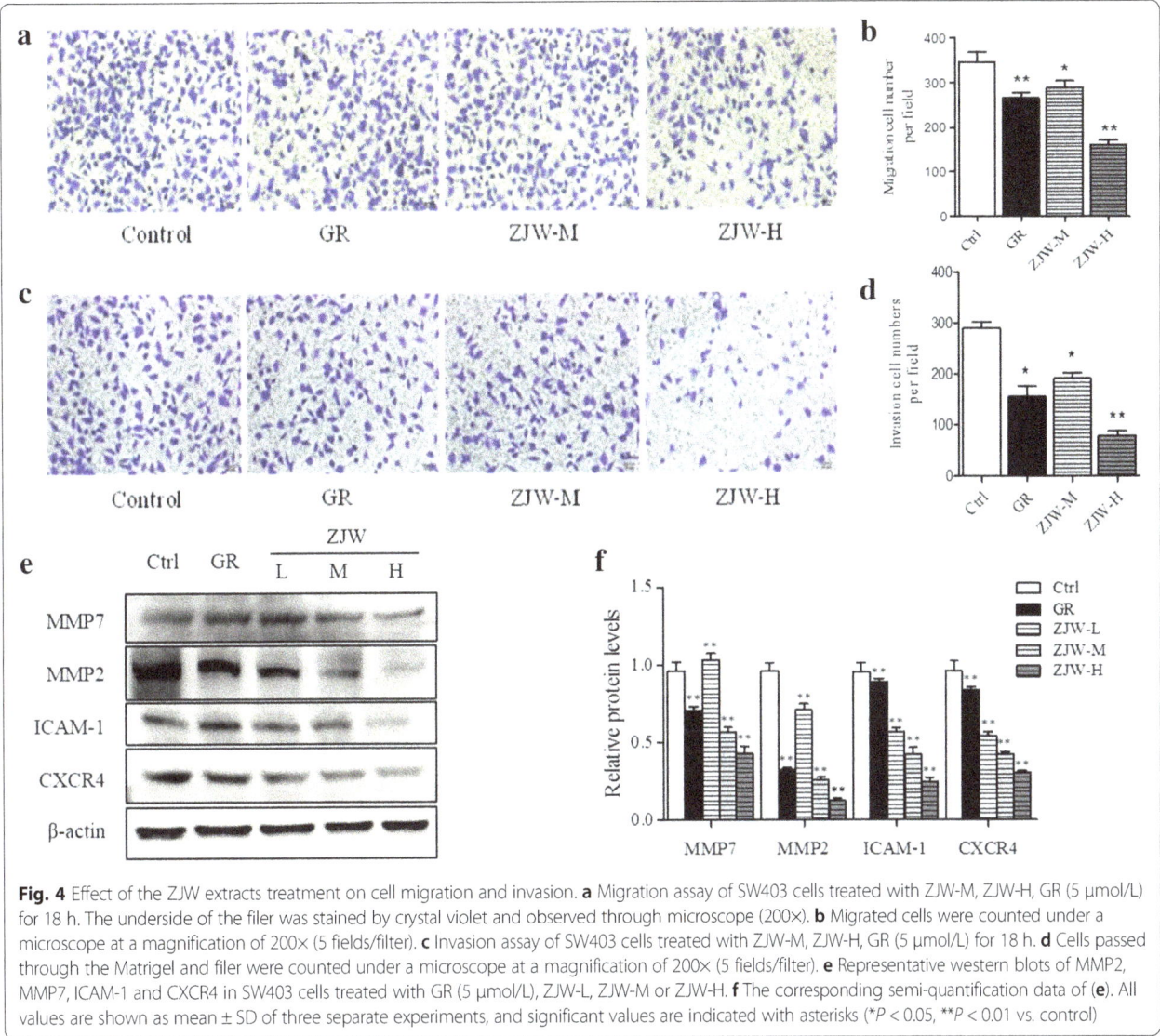

Fig. 4 Effect of the ZJW extracts treatment on cell migration and invasion. **a** Migration assay of SW403 cells treated with ZJW-M, ZJW-H, GR (5 μmol/L) for 18 h. The underside of the filer was stained by crystal violet and observed through microscope (200×). **b** Migrated cells were counted under a microscope at a magnification of 200× (5 fields/filter). **c** Invasion assay of SW403 cells treated with ZJW-M, ZJW-H, GR (5 μmol/L) for 18 h. **d** Cells passed through the Matrigel and filer were counted under a microscope at a magnification of 200× (5 fields/filter). **e** Representative western blots of MMP2, MMP7, ICAM-1 and CXCR4 in SW403 cells treated with GR (5 μmol/L), ZJW-L, ZJW-M or ZJW-H. **f** The corresponding semi-quantification data of (**e**). All values are shown as mean ± SD of three separate experiments, and significant values are indicated with asterisks (*$P < 0.05$, **$P < 0.01$ vs. control)

(Fig. 5e and f). These results suggest that effect of ZJW treatment on the Wnt/β-catenin signal transduction resembles that of the 5-HTR1D antagonist GR127935.

Discussion

Carcinogenesis is now considered as a result from a multitude of gene mutations [36], thus inhibition of a single gene product or cell signaling pathway is unlikely to prevent or treat cancer. The mechanisms vary considerably among various types of tumors. Alterations of different signaling pathways are involved in most of the pathological changes associated with these mechanisms. Many natural agents, in which TCM is included, have multi-targeting properties. We herein provide in vitro evidence that ZJW, a well-established TCM formula, has the potential for CRC intervention, which is accord to results obtained previously [6, 11]. It is a limitation not to perform cell vitality assay for ZJW in normal

colorectal cells. However, the traditional Chinese herbal medicine ZJW has been used to treat gastrointestinal disorders for over 600 years in China. Nowadays, it is widely used in clinical medicine with proved security.

The present study showed that ZJW treatment, like that of 5-HTR1D antagonist, can attenuate proliferation of SW403 cells. The IC50 and IC10 for SW403 cell of ZJW were 382.80 μg/mL and 117.98 μg/mL respectively. Previous study had showed that the dosage of IC10 in HCT116/L-OHP cell was 50 μg/mL [6, 11]. This may be because of the resistance of different cell lines. Cells treated with ZJW exhibited increased G1 arrest, which was accompanied with decreased levels of CDK4, cyclin D1 and c-Myc. It is known that CDK4 and cyclin D1 are positively relative to cell mitosis, promoting G1/S transition. Thus, overexpression of CDK4 and cyclin D1 is invariably correlated with cancer progression. Expression of c-Myc is often associated with aggressive, poorly

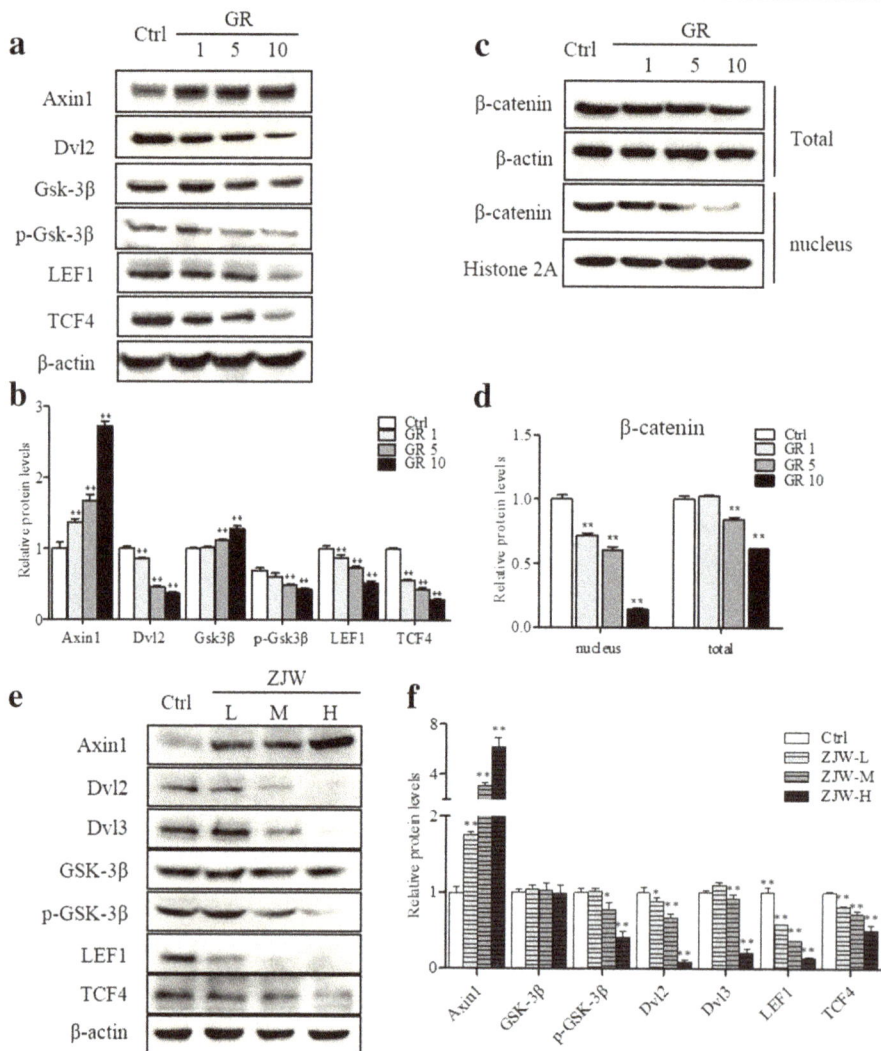

Fig. 5 Effect of GR or ZJW treatment on the Wnt/β-catenin signaling pathway. **a** SW403 cells were treated with GR (1, 5, and 10 μmol/L, respectively) for 24 h. Representative western blots of Axin1, Dvl2, Dvl3, GSK-3β, LEF1, and TCF4 were shown. **b** Semi-quantification data of the Western blot relative to β-actin. **c** Western blotting of β-catenin in total cell lysate and nucleus in SW403 cells treated as (**a**). **d** The corresponding semi-quantification data of the Western blot relative to histone 2A. **e** SW403 cells were treated with ZJW-L, ZJW-M and ZJW-H for 24 h. Representative western blots for Axin1, Dvl2, Dvl3, GSK-3β, serine-phosphorylated-GSK-3β, LEF1 and TCF4 in SW403 cells were shown. **f** The semi-quantification data of the Western blot relative to β-actin. All values are shown as mean ± SD of three separate experiments, and significant values are indicated with asterisks ($*P < 0.05$, $**P < 0.01$ vs. control)

differentiated tumors, and is also required in transduction from G1 to S phase. Down-regulation of c-Myc gene expression is regarded as a therapeutic target for cancer treatment [37–40]. The increase in the proportion of cells present in G1 phase could be attributable to a c-Myc-dependent mechanism. The treatment with ZJW extracts also resulted in increased apoptosis in SW403 cells. Expression and activation of Bcl-2 family play an important role in the regulation of apoptosis. With the intervention of ZJW or GR, the level of the anti-apoptotic members of Bcl-2 family including Bcl-2, Bcl-xL and Mcl decreased remarkably. The activation of Bcl-2 was also attenuated dose-dependently by ZJW. In addition, cell migration and

invasion were inhibited by ZJW extracts, which may be due to the significantly down-regulated expression of MMP2, MMP7, CXCR4 and ICAM-1.

Recent studies have shown that the level of 5-HTR1D expression was markedly increased in tumor as compared with normal colorectal tissue. Antagonist of 5-HTR1D, GR127935, could attenuate metastasis of CRC cell through regulating Axin1, the pivotal molecule in Wnt/β-catenin signaling pathway [34]. This suggests the relationship of 5-HTR1D and CRC. Interestingly, in the present study, we found ZJW treatment showed the same effect of inhibiting 5-HTR1D expression in CRC cells as GR did, which prompted us to propose and try to confirm that 5-HTR1D-

Wnt/β-catenin maybe one of the underlying therapeutic mechanisms of ZJW for CRC. It is noteworthy that a drastic alteration in the level of 5-HTR1D, a trans-membrane G-protein coupled receptor (GPCR), occurs in cells that are treated with 5-HTR1D antagonist GR127935 or ZJW. Although it is well understood that conformational changes occur within the trans-membrane domains of GPCRs during the receptor activation/inactivation [41], relatively little is known about regulatory mechanisms controlling GPCR synthesis or turnover. To date, few report has shown that antagonist or agonist of 5-HTR1D alters the level of this GPCR expression. The decreased level of 5-HRT1D, in cells treated with the antagonist GR127935 or ZJW extracts, may be attributable to enhanced degradation in the lysosomes after receptor/antagonist endocytosis. How the interaction between 5-HTR1D and its antagonist affects the stability and/or the functionality of the receptor protein merits further investigation.

In addition to suppressing 5-HTR1D, ZJW treatment, as mentioned above, decreased the level of proteins involved in cell proliferation, apoptosis, and metastasis, which are all target genes of the Wnt/β-catenin pathway [35]. Measurement of several key components of the Wnt/β-catenin pathway, including Dvl, Axin1, P-GSK-3β, LEF1 and TCF4, provided further evidence

suggesting that ZJW treatment attenuates cell proliferation through the Wnt/β-catenin signaling pathway. The current study has shown that Axin1 were up-regulated in cells treated with 5-HTR1D antagonist or ZJW, and the expression of Dvl2, Dvl3, P-GSK-3β, TCF4 and LEF1 were down-regulated, in an antagonist concentration dependent manner. Abnormal expression of these components is known to result in uncontrolled cell proliferation, loss of cell-cell adhesion, and increased cell migration [42]. Dvl may cause disintegration of Axin/APC/GSK-3β complex. Currently, the mechanism responsible for Axin1 upregulation is unknown, nor is it clear whether intermediary proteins are involved in signal transmission between Axin1 and Dvl. The cytoplasm β-catenin is phosphorylated by CK1 and GSK3β in the destruction complex, which could be recognized by ubiquitin E3 ligaseβ-TrCP and ubiquitylated for proteasome degradation. Prior studies have shown that Wnt signaling stimulates Akt, which in turn, in association with Dvl, enhances GSK-3β phosphorylation at Ser9, resulting in GSK-3β inactivation, causing increased β-catenin level [35]. In this study, although GSK-3β expression was not influenced by ZJW or GR, P-GSK-3β (ser9) level decreased remarkably, which means activated GSK-3β increased. Thus, ZJW or GR treatment may lead to

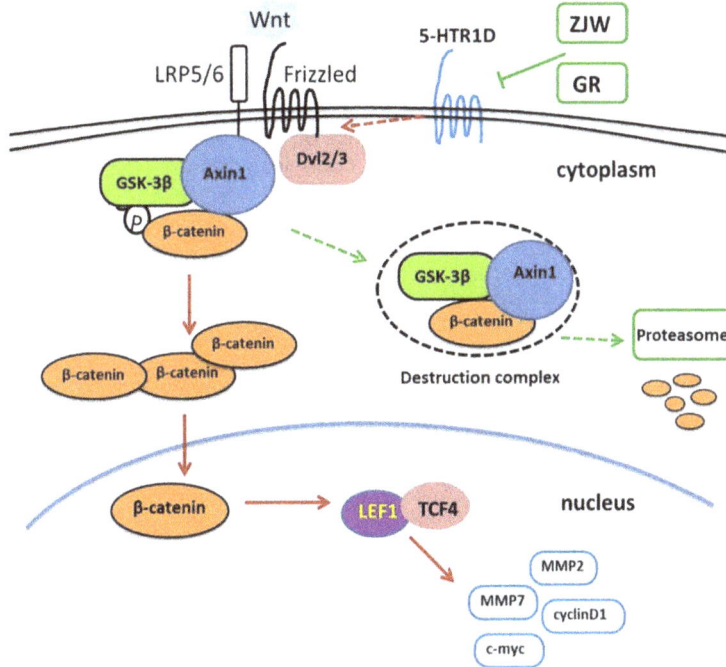

Fig. 6 A schematic model for ZJW extracts in inhibiting 5-HTR1D and attenuating Wnt/β-catenin signaling pathway. Wnt/β-catenin signaling is activated by the binding of Wnt ligand to Frizzled receptor and LRP5/6 co-receptors, leading to the recruitment of Dvl and destruction complex to the membrane, which inactivates destruction complex, causing accumulated β-catenin to enter nucleus and activate target gene transcription (red arrows). 5-HTR1D may play a role in promoting the Wnt/β-catenin signaling at upper stream, leading to stabilization of β-catenin (red arrows). The effect of ZJW extracts on Wnt/β-catenin resembles that of GR127935 (GR), an antagonist of 5-HTR1D, in inhibiting (green arrows) the Wnt/β-catenin signaling through enhanced β-catenin degradation, thus prohibiting the signaling transduction

decreased level of β-catenin and low expression of wnt target genes such as cyclin-D1, c-Myc, MMP2 and MMP7. The nuclear β-catenin was shown reduced by GR in our results, while the regulation of cytoplasmic β-catenin level as well as the effect of ZJW on β-catenin need proved in our future work. Previous studies have demonstrated that downregulation of the Wnt/β-catenin induces apoptosis in a variety of human cancer cell, suggesting that the Wnt/β-catenin pathway may be associated with cellular apoptosis. Therefore, ZJW induced apoptotic effect in CRC cell by regulating Bcl-2 proteins, possibly through Wnt/β-catenin pathway.

The current study has also shown that the transduction of Wnt/β-catenin pathway appears to be sensitive to the level of 5-HTR1D expression. Our data have indicated that 5-HTR1D might play a role in influencing the Wnt/β-catenin signaling at upper stream, leading to stabilization of β-catenin in cells. It is rather remarkable that ZJW treatment helps activate the β-catenin destruction complex, leading to degradation of β-catenin, possibly through down-regulation of 5-HTR1D. Expressions of the Wnt/β-catenin target genes, e.g., TCF4 and LEF1, were decreased by the ZJW treatment. The demonstrated effect of ZJW treatment on the expression of key components of the Wnt/β-catenin pathway and its target gene products is summarized schematically in a model depicted in Fig. 6. This model postulates that ZJW treatment attenuates CRC cell survival and metastasis through regulation of the 5-HTR1D-Axin1-TCF4/LEF1 axis of the Wnt/β-catenin signal transduction. The model also postulates that downregulation of the Wnt/β-catenin signaling might regulated by elevated Axin1, which results in increased degradation of β-catenin. However, the possibility that ZJW might exert its anti-cancer effect by directly targeting at some downstream protein factors remains to be determined.

In conclusion, the present studies thus provide experimental evidence that in the CRC cell line SW403, the level of 5-HTR1D expression can be effectively suppressed by the ZJW extracts treatment, which in turn leads to attenuated cell growth and cell invasion. The antagonizing effect of the ZJW extract in suppressing 5-HTR1D expression in SW403 cells is almost indistinguishable from that of the authentic 5-HTR1D antagonist GR127935. In addition, treatment with the ZJW extracts can achieve the same inhibitory effect on the canonical Wnt signaling pathway through suppressing the β-catenin target gene expression. Our study thus provided a possible mechanistic explanation for the potential therapeutic effectiveness of ZJW extracts in treating CRC. However, more direct evidences are required to confirm the link of ZJW-5-HTR1D and Wnt/β-catenin pathway.

Conclusions

Downregulation of 5-HTR1D expression by the ZJW extracts treatment results in suppression of CRC cell growth and invasion, which is associated with inactivated Wnt/β-catenin signaling.

Abbreviations
APC: Adenomatous polyposis coli; Bcl-2: B-cell lymphoma-2; CDK4: Cyclin-dependent kinase 4; CFDA: China Food and Drug Administration; CRC: Colorectal cancer; Dvl: Dishevelled; EC: Enterochromaffin cells; GSK3β: Glycogen synthase kinase 3β; GR: GR127935; HPLC: High-performance liquid chromatography; MMP2: Matrix metalloproteinase 2; SSRI: Selective serotonin-reuptake inhibitors; TCF/LEF: T cell factor/lymphoid enhancer factor; TCM: Traditional Chinese medicine; ZJW-L: Low dose of ZJW; ZJW-M: Medium dose of ZJW; ZJW-H: High dose of ZJW; ZJW: Zuo Jin Wan; 5-HTR: 5-hydroxytryptamine receptor ; 5-HT: 5-hydroxytryptamine

Acknowledgments
We sincerely thank other colleagues in our laboratory of Institute of Digestive Diseases for their help in this study.

Funding
This study was supported in part by the grants from National Natural Science Foundation of China (81503512), and 3-year Action Plan of Shanghai Municipal Health and Family Planning Commission (ZY3-CCCX-2-1002).

Authors' contributions
GJ conceived and designed the experiments. JP and YX performed the laboratory experiments. JP, XZ and HS participated in interpretation of the data. JP and ZY wrote and revised the manuscript. All authors read and approved the final manuscript.

Competing interests
The authors declare that they have no competing interests.

Author details
Institute of Digestive Diseases, Longhua Hospital, Shanghai University of Traditional Chinese Medicine, Shanghai 200032, China. [2]Department of General Surgery, Longhua Hospital, Shanghai University of Traditional Chinese Medicine, Shanghai 200032, China. [3]Department of Biochemistry, Microbiology and Immunology, Ottawa Institute of Systems Biology, University of Ottawa, Ottawa, ON K1H 8M5, Canada. [4]E-Institute of Shanghai Municipal Education Commission, Shanghai University of Traditional Chinese Medicine, Shanghai 201203, China.

References
1. Boyle P, Levin B. World cancer report 2008. Lyon: International Agency for Research on Cancer; 2008.
2. Nicum S, Midgley R, Kerr DJ. Colorectal cancer. Acta Oncol. 2003;42:263–75.
3. Primrose JN. Treatment of colorectal metastases: surgery, cryotherapy, or radiofrequency ablation. Gut. 2002;50:1–5.
4. Pan Y, Ran R, Wen K, Chen Y, Zhou F, Yu H. Effects of zuo jin wan and splited-zuo jin wan in gastric mucosa healing of rats of gastric ulcer and epidermal growth factor receptor expression. Chin J Integr Tradit West Med Digestion. 2008;6:368–71.
5. Chao DC, Lin LJ, Kao ST, Huang HC, Chang CS, Liang JA, Wu SL, Hsiang CY, Ho TY. Inhibitory effects of zuo-jin-wan and its alkaloidal ingredients on

activator protein 1, nuclear factor-kappab, and cellular transformation in hepg2 cells. Fitoterapia. 2011;82:696–703.

6. Sui H, Liu X, Jin BH, Pan SF, Zhou LH, Yu NA, Wu J, Cai JF, Fan ZZ, Zhu HR, et al. Zuo jin wan, a traditional chinese herbal formula, reverses p-gp-mediated mdr in vitro and in vivo. Evid Based Complement Altern Med. 2013;2013:957078.

7. Jiang J, Hu C. Evodiamine: A novel anti-cancer alkaloid from evodia rutaecarpa. Molecules. 2009;14:1852–9.

8. Park KS, Kim JB, Bae J, Park SY, Jee HG, Lee KE, Youn YK. Berberine inhibited the growth of thyroid cancer cell lines 8505c and tpc1. Yonsei Med J. 2012;53:346–51.

9. Wen B, Huang Q, Gong Y, Chen W. In vitro and in vivo anticolorectal carcinoma activities of zuojin pill and its major constituents. World Chin J Dig. 2009;17:1936–41.

10. Xu L, Qi Y, Lv L, Xu Y, Zheng L, Yin L, Liu K, Han X, Zhao Y, Peng J. In vitro anti-proliferative effects of zuojinwan on eight kinds of human cancer cell lines. Cytotechnology. 2014;66:37–50.

11. Sui H, Pan SF, Feng Y, Jin BH, Liu X, Zhou LH, Hou FG, Wang WH, Fu XL, Han ZF, et al. Zuo jin wan reverses p-gp-mediated drug-resistance by inhibiting activation of the pi3k/akt/nf-kappab pathway. BMC Complement Altern Med. 2014;14:279.

12. Modlin IM, Kidd M, Pfragner R, Eick GN, Champaneria MC. The functional characterization of normal and neoplastic human enterochromaffin cells. J Clin Endocrinol Metab. 2006;91:2340–8.

13. Pauwels P. 5-ht receptors and their ligands. Neuropharmacology. 2003;1083:38.

14. Vicaut E, Laemmel E, Stucker O. Impact of serotonin on tumour growth. Ann Med. 2000;32:187–94.

15. Dizeyi N, Bjartell A, Hedlund P, Tasken KA, Gadaleanu V, Abrahamsson PA. Expression of serotonin receptors 2b and 4 in human prostate cancer tissue and effects of their antagonists on prostate cancer cell lines. Eur Urol. 2005;47:895–900.

16. Nocito A, Dahm F, Jochum W, Jang JH, Georgiev P, Bader M, Graf R, Clavien PA. Serotonin regulates macrophage-mediated angiogenesis in a mouse model of colon cancer allografts. Cancer Res. 2008;68:5152–8.

17. Soll C, Jang JH, Riener MO, Moritz W, Wild PJ, Graf R, Clavien PA. Serotonin promotes tumor growth in human hepatocellular cancer. Hepatology. 2010;51:1244–54.

18. Coufal, M.; Invernizzi, P.; Gaudio, E.; Bernuzzi, F.; Frampton, G.; Onori, P.; Franchitto, A.; Carpino, G.; Ramirez, J.; Alvaro, D., et al. Increased local dopamine secretion has growth-promoting effects in cholangiocarcinoma. Int J Cancer 2010, 126, 2112-2122.

19. Sonier B, Arseneault M, Lavigne C, Ouellette R, Vaillancourt C. The 5-ht2a serotoninergic receptor is expressed in the mcf-7 human breast cancer cell line and reveals a mitogenic effect of serotonin. Biochem Biophys Res Commun. 2006;343:1053–9.

20. Siddiqui EJ, Shabbir MA, Mikhailidis DP, Mumtaz FH, Thompson CS. The effect of serotonin and serotonin antagonists on bladder cancer cell proliferation. BJU Int. 2006;97:634–9.

21. Ataee R, Ajdary S, Rezayat M, Shokrgozar M, Shahriari S, Zarrindast M. Study of 5ht3 and 5ht4 receptors expression in ht29 cell line and human colon adenocarcinoma tissues. Arch Iran Med. 2010;13:120–5.

22. Ataee R, Ajdary S, Zarrindast M, Rezayat M, Hayatbakhsh MR. Anti-mitogenic and apoptotic effects of 5-ht1b receptor antagonist on ht29 colorectal cancer cell line. J Cancer Res Clin Oncol. 2010;136:1461–9.

23. Xu W, Tamim H, Shapiro S, Stang M, Collet J. Use of antidepressants and risk of colorectal cancer: a nested case-control study. Lancet Oncol. 2006;7:301–8.

24. Mastrangelo L, Cassidy A, Mulholland F, Wang W, Bao Y. Serotonin receptors, novel targets of sulforaphane identified by proteomic analysis in caco-2 cells. Cancer Res. 2008;68:5487–91.

25. Behrens J. Everything you would like to know about wnt signaling. Sci Signal. 2013;6:e17.

26. Nelson W, Nusse R. Convergence of wnt, ß-catenin, and cadherin pathways. Science. 2004;303:1483–7.

27. Thiery J. Epithelial-mesenchymal transitions in tumour progression. Nat Rev Cancer. 2002;2:442–54.

28. Clevers H. Wnt/beta-catenin signaling in development and disease. Cell. 2006;127:469–80.

29. Taipale J, Beachy PA. The hedgehog and wnt signalling pathways in cancer. Nature. 2001;411:349–54.

30. Bienz M, Clevers H. Linking colorectal cancer to wnt signaling. Cell. 2000; 103:311–20.

31. Clevers H. Wnt breakers in colon cancer. Cancer Cell. 2004;5:5–6.

32. Myant K, Sansom OJ. Wnt signaling and colorectal cancer. In: Hoppler SP, Moon RT, editors. Wnt signaling in development and disease: molecular mechanisms and biological functions. New Jersey: Wiley-Blackwell; 2014. p. 359–68.

33. Cadigan KM, Nusse R. Wnt signaling: a common theme in animal development. Genes Dev. 1997;11:3286–305.

34. Sui H, Xu H, Ji Q, Liu X, Zhou L, Song H, Zhou X, Xu Y, Chen Z, Cai J, et al. 5-hydroxytryptamine receptor (5-ht1dr) promotes colorectal cancer metastasis by regulating axin1/beta-catenin/mmp-7 signaling pathway. Oncotarget. 2015;6:25975–87.

35. Gao C, Xiao G, Hu J. Regulation of wnt/beta-catenin signaling by posttranslational modifications. Cell Biosci. 2014;4:13.

36. Vogelstein B, Kinzler K. Cancer genes and the pathways they control. Nat Med. 2004;10:789–99.

37. Delmore JE, Issa GC, Lemieux ME, Rahl PB, Shi J, Jacobs HM, Kastritis E, Gilpatrick T, Paranal RM, Qi J, et al. Bet bromodomain inhibition as a therapeutic strategy to target c-myc. Cell. 2011;146:904–17.

38. Lin CY, Loven J, Rahl PB, Paranal RM, Burge CB, Bradner JE, Lee TI, Young RA. Transcriptional amplification in tumor cells with elevated c-myc. Cell. 2012;151:56–67.

39. Toyoshima M, Howie HL, Imakura M, Walsh RM, Annis JE, Chang AN, Frazier J, Chau BN, Loboda A, Linsley PS, et al. Functional genomics identifies therapeutic targets for myc-driven cancer. Proc Natl Acad Sci U S A. 2012; 109:9545–50.

40. de Souza CR, Leal MF, Calcagno DQ, Costa Sozinho EK, Borges Bdo N, Montenegro RC, Dos Santos AK, Dos Santos SE, Ribeiro HF, Assumpcao PP, et al. Myc deregulation in gastric cancer and its clinicopathological implications. PLoS One. 2013;8:e64420.

41. Millar RP, Newton CL. The year in g protein-coupled receptor research. Mol Endocrinol. 2010;24:261–74.

42. Kishida M, Koyama S, Kishida S, Matsubara K, Nakashima S, Higano K, Takada R, Takada S, Kikuchi A. Axin prevents wnt-3a-induced accumulation of beta-catenin. Oncogene. 1999;18:979–85.

7

Herbal formula Xinshuitong capsule exerts its cardioprotective effects via mitochondria in the hypoxia-reoxygenated human cardiomyocytes

Chunjiang Tan[*†], Jianwei Zeng, Yanbin Wu, Jiahui Zhang and Wenlie Chen[†]

Abstract

Background: The collapse of mitochondrial membrane potential ($\Delta\Psi$m) resulted in the cell apoptosis and heart failure. Xinshuitong Capsule (XST) could ameliorate left ventricular ejection fraction (LVEF), New York Heart Association (NYHA) classes and the quality of life in patients with chronic heart failure in our clinical study, however, its cardioprotective mechanisms remain unclear.

Methods: Primary human cardiomyocytes were subjected to hypoxia-reoxygenation and treated with XST200, 400 and 600 μg/ml. The model group was free of XST and the control group was cultured in normal conditions. Cell viability, $\Delta\Psi$m, the activity of mitochondrial respiratory chain complexes, ATPase activity, reactive oxygen species (ROS) and apoptosis cells were determined in all the groups.

Results: The cell viability in the XST-treated groups was significantly higher than that in the model group ($P < 0.05$). Coupled with the restoration of the $\Delta\Psi$m, the number of polarized cells increased dose dependently in the XST-treated groups. XST also restored the lost activities of mitochondrial respiratory chain complexes I-IV induced by the oxidative stress. The total of mitochondrial ATPase activity was significantly elevated at XST400 and 600 μg/ml compared to the model group ($P < 0.05$). The levels of mitochondrial ROS and the number of apoptosis cells declined in the XST-treated groups compared to those in the model group ($P < 0.05$).

Conclusions: XST, via restoration of $\Delta\Psi$m and the mitochondrial respiratory chain complexes I-IV activities, and suppression of mitochondrial ROS generation and the apoptosis cells, maintained the integrity of the mitochondrial membrane to exert its cardioprotective effects in the hypoxia-reoxygenated human cardiomyocytes.

Keywords: Xinshuitong capsule, Mitochondrial potential, Hypoxia-reoxygenated human cardiomyocytes

Background

Mitochondria, as the power house of the heart, are highly packed in the cardiomyocytes. Cardiac cells under prolonged hypoxia condition have been shown with the opening of mitochondrial permeability transition pore (MPTP) [1]. Due to the opening of MPTP causes a transient hyperpolarization, followed by depolarization, and subsequently the collapse of the mitochondrial membrane potential ($\Delta\Psi$m), which is characterized by mitochondrial swelling

and uncoupling. Thus, MPTP opening and mitochondrial $\Delta\Psi$m collapse have been regarded as a primary mediator of apoptosis in the ischemia-reperfusion heart injury [2, 3].

The mitochondrial electron transport chain (ETC) is found in the inner membrane, where it serves as the site of oxidative phosphorylation through the use of ATP synthase. During this chemical process, ROS can be formed as a byproduct of normal cellular aerobic metabolism in the heart [4, 5]. Thus, the major process from which the heart derives sufficient energy can also result in the production of ROS [5]. On the other hand, ROS can depress the activity of mitochondrial ETC and alter

* Correspondence: tchunj@126.com; chen.wl@163.com
†Chunjiang Tan and Wenlie Chen contributed equally to this work.
Fujian Academy of Integrative Medicine, Fujian University of Traditional Chinese Medicine, Fuzhou, Fujian, China

ion pump function in heart [6]. Mounting evidence has strongly implicated ROS signaling in the genesis of cardiac hypertrophy [7–9]. Therefore, maintaining the integrity of the mitochondrial membrane, enhancing antioxidant defense may be a therapeutic method for the protection of cardiomyocytes against the injury of ischemia or hypoxia.

Xinshuitong Capsule (XST, awarded the Invention Patent of the People's Republic of China, No.ZL201210197892.X), a Chinese herbal medicine formula for chronic heart failure (CHF), which consists of Astragali radix, Pseudostellariae radix and Salviae miltiorrhizae radix et al., has the effects of benefiting Qi and Yang, activating blood and eliminating stasis, and inducing diuresis to alleviate edema. Our previous clinical study showed that the CHF patients, who received XST treatment (3 capsules, tid.), were significantly ameliorated in left ventricular ejection fraction (LVEF), New York Heart Association (NYHA) classes, the symptoms and the quality of life compared to the control group [10]. In vitro, XST-treated hypoxia-reoxygenated human cardiomyocytes showed more tolerant to hypoxia stress. The cells exhibited more regular shape and size than the control [11]. However, the drug's cardioprotective mechanisms remain elusive, especially, its actions on MPTP and mitochondrial apoptosis pathway. Thus, in current experiments, mitochondrial $\Delta\Psi m$ and mitochondrial mass, the activities of the mitochondrial ETC and the mitochondrial ATPase, and their associations with ROS levels and apoptosis cells will be studied in the hypoxia-reoxygenated cardiomyocytes.

Methods

Hypoxia-reoxygenated cell model

Primary human cardiomyocyte (HCM) was purchased from American Science Cell Research Laboratories (San Diego. USA). When the cells reached 80–90% confluence, they ere placed on a 96-well plate or a petri dish at a density of 0.75×10^5 cells/ml in a hypoxia chamber ($80\% N_2, 10\% H_2, 10\% CO_2$ and $0.2\% O_2$) for 12 h,11 following by 2 h reoxygenation. During the process of hypoxia and reoxygenation, the study group were exposed to the water-extract of XST (200, 400 and 600 μg/ml, respectively), while the model group was cultured in the identical conditions free of XST treatment, and the control group was cultured in normal conditions. The drug's low and high concentrations used in the current experiment were comparable to the human serum levels in the previous clinical study.

Cell viability assay

As described before [12], cell viability was estimated by the assay of 3-[4,5-dimethylthiazol-2-yl]-diphenyl-tetrazolium bromide (MTT, Sigma-Aldrich). Briefly, after treatment, the cells were washed twice with phosphate-buffered saline (PBS, pH 7.4), and then added 100ul MTT in PBS (0.5 mg/ml) and incubated for 4 h at 37 °C. Followed by removing MTT and oscillating for 10 min, cell viability was estimated at absorbance 570 nm by a Tecan Infinite M200 Pro microplate reader (Tecan, Mannedorf, Swizerland).

Mitochondrial $\Delta\Psi m$ detected by JC-1 staining

As JC-1 (5,5′,6,6′-tetrachloro-1,1′,3,3′-tetraethylbenzimidazolyl-carbocyanine iodide, Beyotime, China) is a lipophilic fluorescent cation that is incorporated into the mitochondrial membrane, where it can form aggregates due to the state of the mitochondrial $\Delta\Psi m$. This aggregation changes the fluorescence properties of JC-1 from green to orange fluorescence as the $\Delta\Psi m$ increased. After treatment, cells were harvested, re-suspended and incubated with 10 μg/ml JC-1 at 37 °C for 30 min as before [13, 14]. The cells were then washed and centrifuged, the intact living cells stained the mitochondria with JC-1 would exhibit a pronounced orange fluorescence, however, the cells with a breakdown of $\Delta\Psi m$ showed a decrease of the orange fluorescence (or a increase of the green fluorescence). Thus, the intact and injured cells could be distinguished, and the cell populations will be counted according to the different fluorescence by the flow cytometry (BD Biosciences, CA) (JC-1 green: Ex/Em = 485/525 nm; JC-1 red: Ex/Em =535/590 nm).

Similarly, the fluorescence intensity of JC-1 as the index of $\Delta\Psi m$ alterations could be detected by a confocal microscope (Carl Zeiss AG, Oberkochen, Germany), and the ratio of red/green fluorescence intensity is indicated as the alterations of mitochondrial $\Delta\Psi m$.

For quantification of mitochondrial mass, we used Mitotracker Green probe (Molecular Probes), which preferentially accumulates in mitochondria regardless of the mitochondrial membrane potential and provides an accurate assessment of mitochondrial mass. Firstly, the cells were washed with PBS and incubated at 37 °C for 30 min with 100 nM MitoTracker Green FM (Molecular Probes) and then harvested using trypsin/EDTA and re-suspended in PBS. Fluorescence intensity was detected with excitation and emission wavelengths of 490 and 516 nm, respectively, and values were corrected for total protein (mg/ml).

Determination of the activities of mitochondrial respiratory chain complexes

According to manufacturer's instructions, mitochondrial isolation was performed at 4 °C using a Kit for cultured mammal cell (Thermo Scientific Rockford. USA).

The activities of mitochondrial respiratory chain complexes were analyzed by spectrophotometer (Secomam, Domont,France) as described before [13]. Briefly, complex I (NADH dehydrogenase, EC 1.6.5.3) enzyme activity was measured as a decline in absorbance from NADH oxidation by decylubiquinone before and after adding rotenone (St. Louis, MO, USA). Complex II (succinate dehydrogenase, EC 1.3.5.1) activity was determined as a function of the decrease in absorbance from 2, 6-dichloroindophenol reduction. Complex III (ubiquinone cytochrome c oxidoreductase, EC 1.10.2.2) activity was calculated as a function of increase in absorbance from cytochrome c reduction. And complex IV (cytochrome c oxidoreductase, EC 1.9.3.1) activity was measured as a function of the decrease in absorbance from cytochrome c oxidation. Mitochondrial complexes activities were normalized to whole mitochondrial protein content and expressed as arbitrary units.

Determination of mitochondrial total ATPase activity

Cell mitochondria and submitochondrial particles were prepared as described before [14]. Briefly, the mitochondrial particles were incubated at 37 °C for 60 min in a 0.5 ml medium containing 2 mmol/l ATP, 100 mmol/l NaCl, 20 mmol/l KCL, 5 mmol/l MgCl$_2$, 1 mmol/l EDTA in 50 mmol/l Tris–HCl (pH = 7.0). The tubes were chilled immediately and centrifuged at 200×g for 10 min. Inorganic phosphate liberated in the supernatant was calculated as an indication of ATPase activity according to Fiske and Subbarow [15]. Protein determination was carried out in accordance with Lowry [16] with crystalline bovine serum albumin as a standard.

Determination of mitochondrial ROS

As described before [13], mitochondrial ROS production was determined using Amplex Red (Molecular Probes, Eugene, OR, USA). Briefly, superoxide dismutase (SOD) was added at 40 units/ml to convert all superoxide into H$_2$O$_2$. Resorufin formation (Amplex Red oxidation by H$_2$O$_2$) was detected at an excitation/emission wavelength of 545/590 nm using a spectrophotometer (Secomam, Domont, France). Readings of resorufin formation were recorded every 5 min for 30 min, and a slope (i.e., rate of formation) was produced. The slope obtained was converted into the rate of H$_2$O$_2$ production with a standard curve. The assay was done at 37 °C in 96-well plates using succinate. The data was converted to nmol/mg protein/minute.

Quantitative assessment of apoptosis cells by flow cytometry

As described before [17], Annexin V-APC/7-AAD Apoptosis Detection Kits (Becton-Dickinson Biosciences) were used to detect apoptosis cells. The cells stained with annexinV+/7-AAD- were considered apoptosis cells, and the percentage of apoptosis cells was determined by flow cytometry.

Statistical analysis

Software of SPSS Version 19.0 was used for statistical analysis. Numerical data are expressed as means ± SD. The significance of differences was examined using the ANOVA method. Results with $P<0.05$ were considered to be significant.

Results

XST increased the viability of hypoxia-reoxygenated HCM

As shown in Fig. 1, the cell viability in the XST-treated 200, 400 and 600 µg/ml group were 77, 81 and 84%,

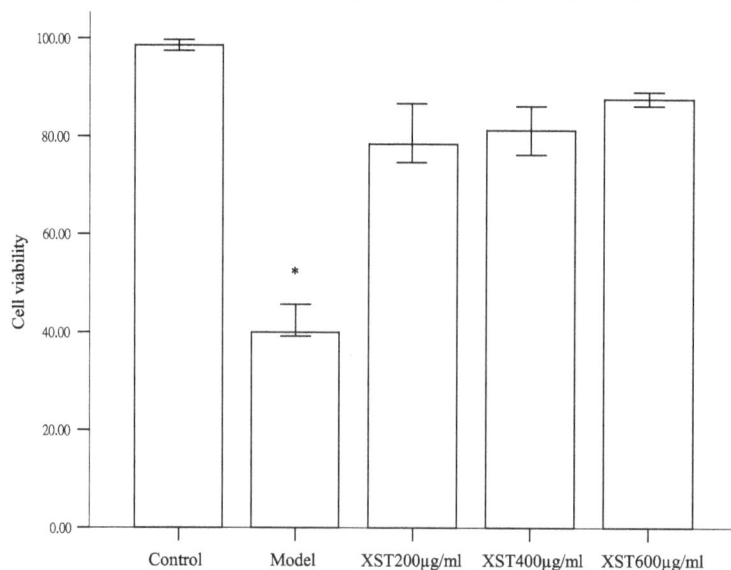

Fig. 1 Bar graphs showed the cell viability in the three XST-treated groups were significantly increased compared with the model group. No difference was found between the XST-treated groups or the XST-treated groups compared to the control group. All samples were checked in three independent experiments with three replicates each. Data are represented as the mean ± SD (*P<0.05 vs. each of the three XST-treated groups or the control group)

respectively, which showed a significant difference than the model group (42.20%, $P < 0.05$). However, the cell viability exhibited no difference between the three dosages of XST ($P > 0.05$). Under the light microscope, cells in the three XST-treated groups and the control group grew similarly well, and the cells were like in size and shape. By contrast, most of the cells in the model group showed swelling and was out of the regular shape and size (figures not shown). The data indicated that XST could protect the cells against hypoxia-induced injury.

XST dose-dependently increased the number of polarized cells

JC-1 is capable of entering selectively into mitochondria, and the color of the dye changes reversibly from green to orange as the mitochondrial membrane becomes more polarized. Based upon the specific fluorescent characteristics, the cells could be classified into two groups of cells by the flow cytometer, and the two kinds of fluorescence were indicated as the two populations of cells. Quantitative assessment was reflected by the dot plots as indicated in Fig. 2 The ratio of red/green fluorescence, as

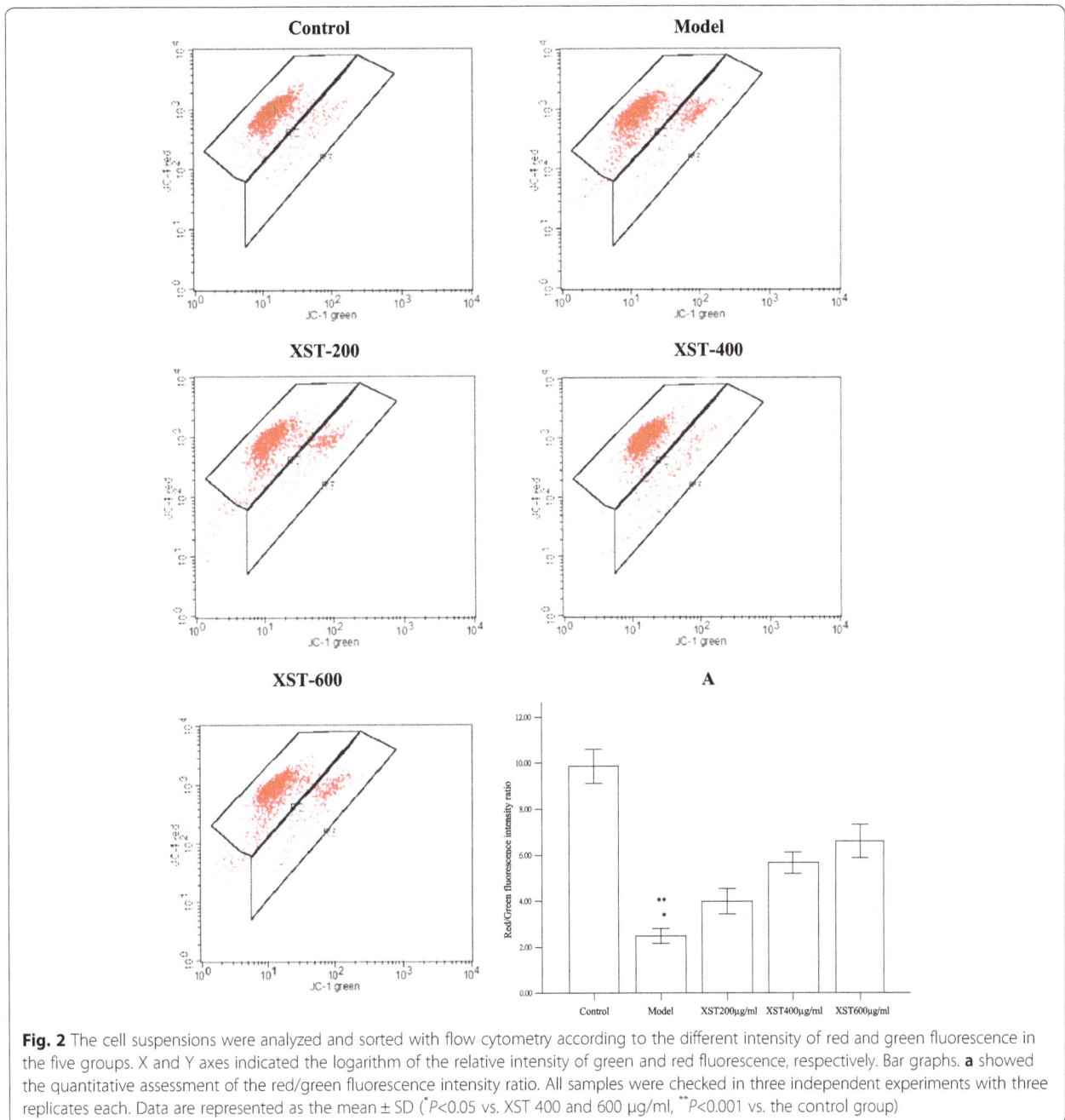

Fig. 2 The cell suspensions were analyzed and sorted with flow cytometry according to the different intensity of red and green fluorescence in the five groups. X and Y axes indicated the logarithm of the relative intensity of green and red fluorescence, respectively. Bar graphs. **a** showed the quantitative assessment of the red/green fluorescence intensity ratio. All samples were checked in three independent experiments with three replicates each. Data are represented as the mean ± SD (*$P<0.05$ vs. XST 400 and 600 μg/ml, **$P<0.001$ vs. the control group)

the index of cell populations, showed a dose-dependent increase in the three XST-treated groups. A significant difference was noted at XST400 and XST600ug/ml compared to the model group ($P < 0.05$), suggesting that XST could increase the polarized cell populations (Fig. 2a).

XST dose dependently restored the loss of ΔΨm and mitochondrial mass induced by hypoxia

The intensity of red fluorescence of JC-1 aggregates detected by confocal laser scanning microscopy decreased in the model group, however, XST could dose dependently increase the fluorescence, indicating that the drug could restore the loss of Δψm induced by hypoxia as showed in Fig. 3. Further, the red/green fluorescence ratio in XST-treated 200, 400 and 600μg/ml groups was 55, 81 and 85%, respectively, a significant difference was found in the XST-treated groups compared to the model group (18%). However, no difference was found between XST400, XST600 ug/ml and the control ($P > 0.05$) as indicated by the bar graph Fig. 3a.

Further, an accurate assessment of mitochondrial mass was conducted, showing the green fluorescence increased in the XST-treated groups (Fig. 4). A significant elevation was noted in XST-400 and 600μg/ml groups compared to that in the model group, suggesting the drug prevented the loss of mitochondria in the hypoxia cells. The data was in line with the status of mitochondrial Δψm detected in above experiments. Additionally, morphological observations showed the cells in the XST-treated groups were more uniform in shape and size compared to those in the model group.

XST restored the mitochondrial electron transport chain complexes activities

The activities of mitochondria complexes I, II, III, and IV were assessed by spectrophotometric methods. As showed in Fig. 5, the activities of complexes I- IV were reduced in varying degrees in the model group. XST could dose dependently restore the activities of complexes I, II and III, but the activity of complex IV showed no difference among XST 200, 400 and 600 μg/ml groups. Complexes I-IV activities were significantly elevated in XST 200 and 400 μg/ml groups than those in the model group ($P < 0.05$); in the XST 600 μg/ml group, the activities of complexes I-IV restored nearly to the normal levels. The data indicated that the drug could dose dependently restore the activities of the mitochondrial electron transport chain complexes I-IV.

XST increased mitochondrial total ATPase activity in the hypoxia-reoxygenated HCM

Mitochondrial total ATPase activity was determined by estimating the amount of ATP hydrolyzed in terms of inorganic phosphorus (Pi) liberated in the cell supernatant. As shown in Fig. 6, the ATPase activity in the model group

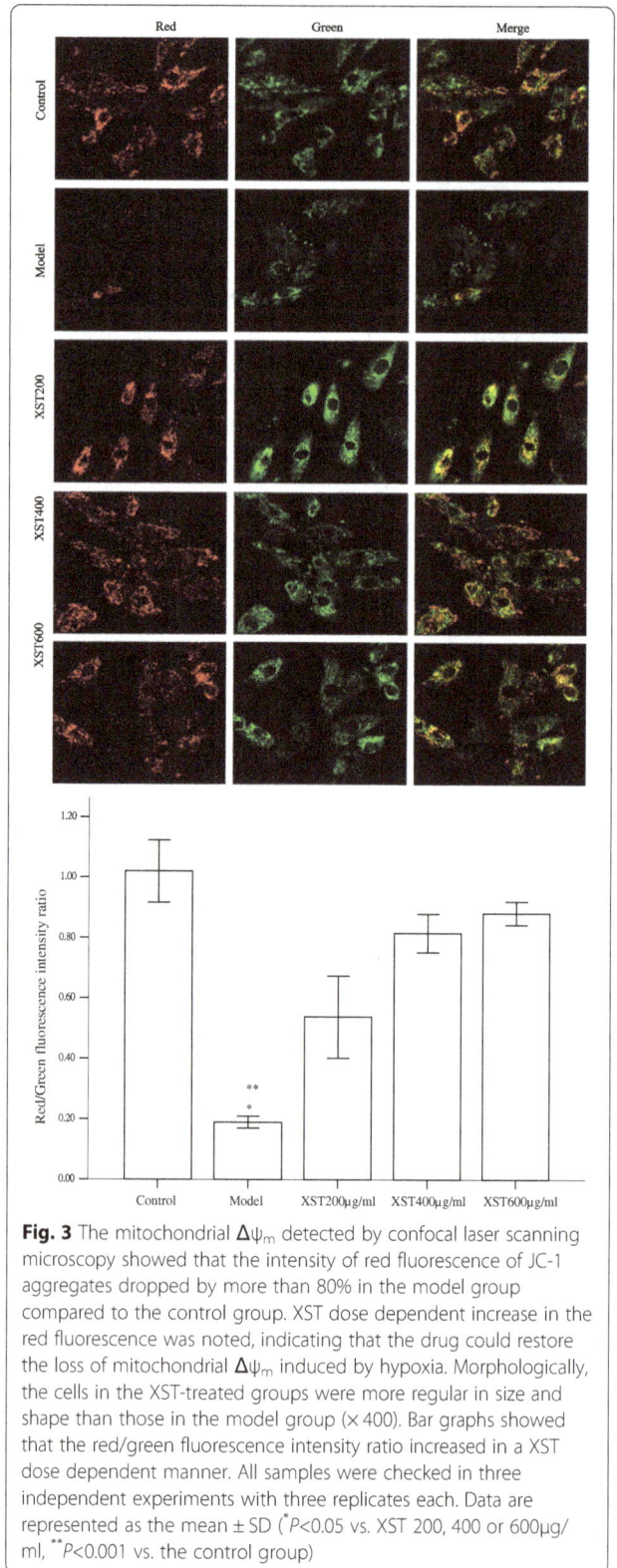

Fig. 3 The mitochondrial Δψ$_m$ detected by confocal laser scanning microscopy showed that the intensity of red fluorescence of JC-1 aggregates dropped by more than 80% in the model group compared to the control group. XST dose dependent increase in the red fluorescence was noted, indicating that the drug could restore the loss of mitochondrial Δψ$_m$ induced by hypoxia. Morphologically, the cells in the XST-treated groups were more regular in size and shape than those in the model group (× 400). Bar graphs showed that the red/green fluorescence intensity ratio increased in a XST dose dependent manner. All samples were checked in three independent experiments with three replicates each. Data are represented as the mean ± SD (*$P<0.05$ vs. XST 200, 400 or 600μg/ml, **$P<0.001$ vs. the control group)

decreased about 70% compared to the control ($P < 0.05$), however, the activity increased about 40, 52 and 60% in the XST-treated 200, 400 and 600 μg/ml groups compared to

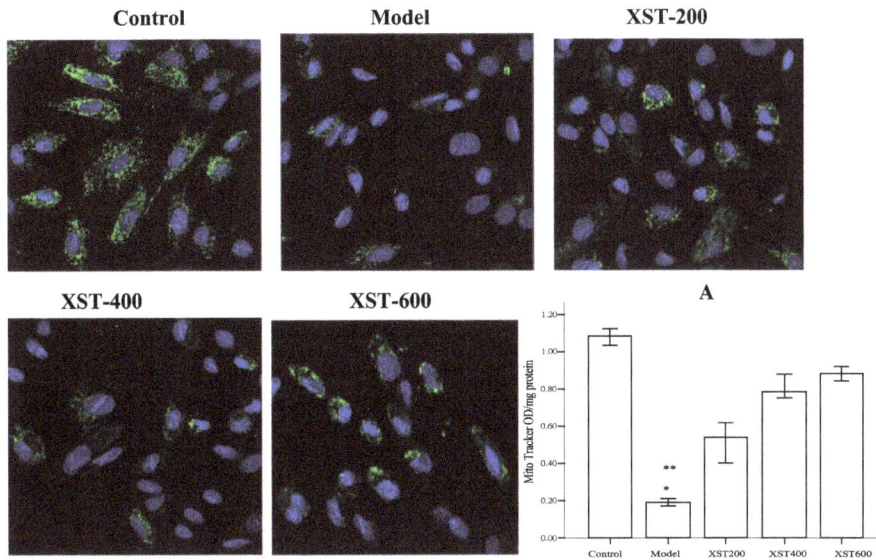

Fig. 4 Mitochondrial content (using MitoTracker Green) was detected in the five groups, showing the green fluorescence increased in a XST dose dependent manner. Quantitative assessment showed that XST-treated groups were significantly greater than that in the control (bar graphs (**a**). All samples were checked in three independent experiments with three replicates each. Data are represented as the mean ± SD (*P<0.05 vs. XST 400 and 600 μg/ml, **P<0.001 vs. the control group)

the model group ($P < 0.05$), which indicated that XST dose dependently increased the mitochondrial ATPase activity induced by hypoxia. The XST-induced elevation of ATPase activity was correlated with the increase in mitochondrial $\Delta\psi m$ and the activities of mitochondrial complexes I-IV in the XST-treated groups (Figs. 3 and 5).

XST decreasedmitochondrial ROS production in the hypoxia-reoxygenated HCM

As shown in Fig. 7, the mitochondrial ROS in the model group was about three times higher than that in the control group ($P<0.05$), however, all the three XST-treated groups exhibited a significant decrease in ROS levels compared to the model group ($P<0.05$), no difference was noted between the three dosages of XST-treated groups ($P > 0.05$). Previous studies reported that the increase in mitochondrial $\Delta\psi m$ and ATPase activity led to the decrease in mitochondrial ROS production [18]. Here, we confirmed that the XST-induced increase in $\Delta\psi m$ and ATPase activity was coupled with a decrease in ROS. The data suggested that the three dosages of XST had the similar inhibitory effects on the production of mitochondrial ROS in hypoxia-reoxygenated HCM.

XST decreased the apoptosis cells in the hypoxia-reoxygenated HCM

As detected by flow cytometry, apoptosis cells, which stained with annexinV+/7-AAD-, were significantly increased in the model group than those in the control group ($P < 0.05$) (Fig. 8). XST treatment could significantly decrease the apoptosis cells; however, no

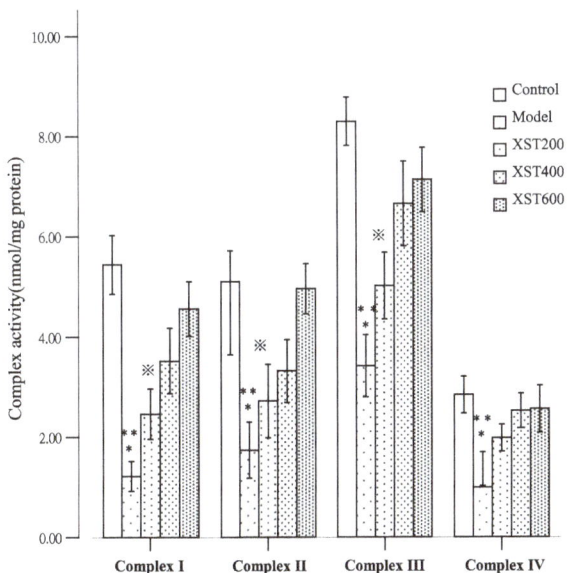

Fig. 5 The activities of complexes I-IV were decreased variable in the model group, XST could dose dependently restore the activities of complexes I, II and III, but complex IV showed no difference among the three XST-treated groups. All samples were checked in three independent experiments with three replicates each. Data are represented as the mean ± SD (*P < 0.05 vs. XST 200 μg/ml or XST400μg/ml,**P < 0.001 vs. the control or XST 600 μg/ml, ※P < 0.05 vs. XST 400 μg/ml or XST600μg/ml)

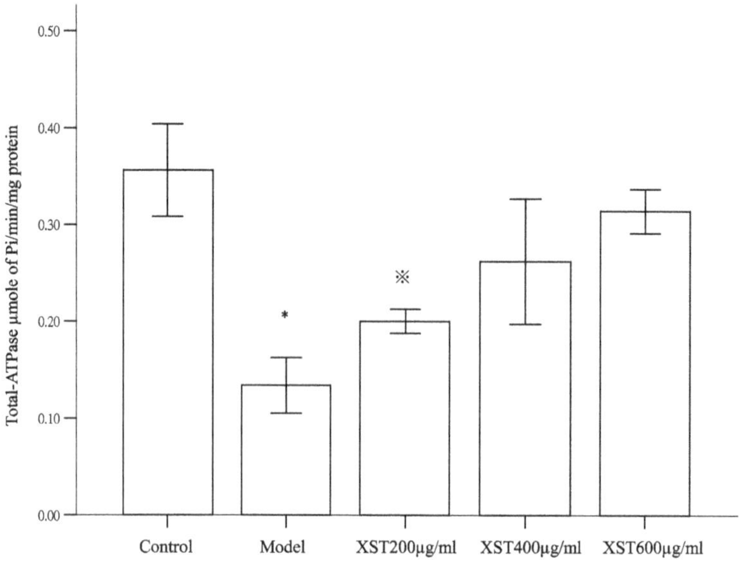

Fig. 6 Mitochondrial ATPase activity in cardiomyocytes was determined by estimating the amount of ATP hydrolysis in terms of inorganic phosphorus (Pi) liberated in the cell supernatant. A significant decrease was found in the model group compared to that in the control. Three XST-treated groups exhibited a dose-dependent increase in the activity as showed in bar graphs. All samples were checked in three independent experiments with three replicates each. Data are represented as the mean ± SD ($^*P < 0.05$ vs.XST 400 and 600 µg/ml, $^{※}P < 0.05$ vs. 600 µg/ml)

difference was noted between the three XST-treated groups ($P > 0.05$). The quantitative assessment of the apoptosis cells was indicated by bar graphs Fig. 8a.

Discussion

Mitochondria, as the dominant source of heart ATP, represent approximately one-third of the mass of the heart and play a critical role in maintaining cellular function. The mitochondrion is very susceptible to damage mediated by ischemia or ischemia/reperfusion. The damaged mitochondria cause a depletion in ATP and a release of cytochrome c, which leads to activation of caspases and onset of apoptosis [19–21]. As such, maintaining mitochondrial homeostasis is critical to cell survival.

Current experiments showed that XST could maintain the activities of mitochondrial electron transport chain

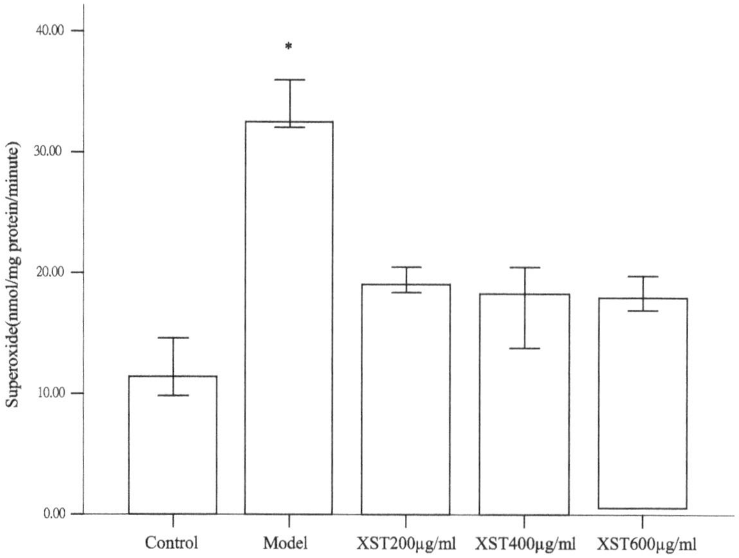

Fig. 7 Mitochondrial ROS in the model group showed significantly higher than that in the control group, however, ROS levels exhibited a significant decrease in the XST-treated groups compared to those in the model group. No difference was noted between the three XST-treated groups. All samples were tested in three independent experiments with three replicates each. Data are represented as the mean ± SD. ($^*P<0.05$ vs. each XST-treated group or the control group)

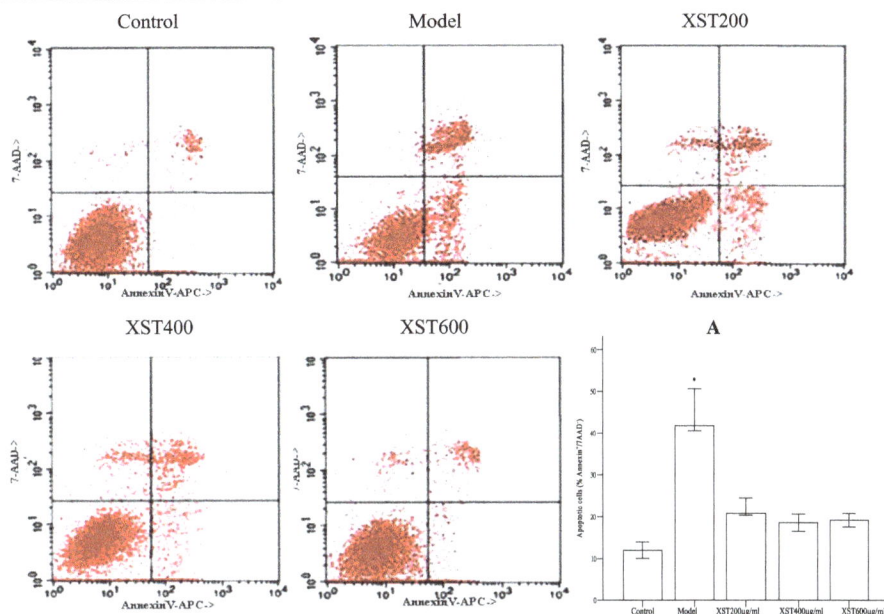

Fig. 8 Five groups were subjected to an assessment of apoptosis cells in the typical diagrams by flow cytometry (annexinV$^+$/7-AAD$^-$). The percentage of annexinV$^+$/7-AAD$^-$, as the index of the apoptosis cells, increased in the model group. XST-treated groups declined the apoptosis cells as indicated by the quantitative bar graph (**a**). All samples were tested in three independent experiments with three replicates each. Data are represented as the mean ± SD ($^*P < 0.05$ vs. the control or the XST-treated groups)

complexes I-IV, and restore the mitochondrial Δψm and mitochondria mass induced by oxidative stress in the cardiomyocytes. Further, the drug could activate mitochondrial total ATPase to supply cells energy to raise the cell viability in the anoxic conditions. On the other hand, XST could suppress the mitochondrial ROS generation and attenuate the ROS-induced damage to the cells, which may partly account for this drug's inhibition of apoptosis and the increase in cell viability. The current data suggested that XST exerted its cardioprotective effects via maintaining the integrity of mitochondria in the hypoxia-reoxygenated HCM.

Our previous clinical study showed that the CHF patients treated with XST (0.3 g each capsule, three capsules each time, tid.) showed significant improvement in LVEF, NYHA classes, as well as the symptoms (dyspnea, edema and etc.) and the patients' quality of life [22]. Further, in vitro experiments verified that dosages 200-600 μg/ml had the optimal cell protective effects in the oxidative stress conditions [11]. Based on the previous data, we used these dosages in the current study, which confirmed that XST could restore the ΔΨm and mitochondria mass to elevate the polarized cell populations. Treated at XST600μg/ml, the activities of respiratory chain complexes I-IV regained their activities nearly to the normal levels, and the total of mitochondrial ATPase activity was raised by XST. On the other hand, XST suppressed the generation of mitochondrial ROS and

cell apoptosis. The data may partly shed a light on the drug's therapeutic effects on the CHF patients.

Previous studies showed that an elevated ΔΨm was associated with the enhanced mitochondrial ROS formation [18, 23], and a slight decrease in ΔΨm could prevent ROS formation without seriously compromising cellular energetics [18, 24, 25]. However, in the isolated energized cardiac mitochondria, which were induced by hypoxia, caused the inhibition of the activity of the electron transport chain, and this mild decrease in ΔΨm led to ROS formation during reoxygenation [26]. The collapse of mitochondrial ΔΨm, regarded as an index of mitochondrial inner integrity, would go hand in hand with the dysfunctions of the mitochondrial respiratory chain and a decline of ATPase activity, which led to the elevation of mitochondrial ROS formation and cell apoptosis. The phenomena were supported in the current experiments as showed in Figs. 3, 5 and 7. XST treatment could restore the loss of ΔΨm and repaired the dysfunctions of the mitochondrial respiratory chain. Additionally, XST could activate ATPase and suppress ROS formation, resulted in the decline in apoptosis cells in the hypoxia-reoxygenated HCM. These data suggested that XST possibly exerted its cardioprotective effects partly through mitochondria. Mitochondrial respiratory chain, especially, complex I, III and III, were seen as the prime source of ROS [27–30]. ROS generations are decreased when the available electrons are limited and potential energy for the transfer is low [30].

Recent study found that when the electron transport chain functions of complexes I, III and III are at the sub optimal level, the rate of mitochondrial free radical production is inversely increasing proportional to the rate of electron transport [31], suggesting that the elevated ROS levels found under these conditions may originate extra-mitochondrially or are attributed to the defective antioxidant defense. Our experiments showed that XST-induced elevation of mitochondrial respiratory chain complexes activities was inversely correlated with the levels of mitochondria-derived ROS in the XST-treated groups (Figs. 5 and 7). Possibly, the drug suppressed ROS generation extra-mitochondrially, or through the antioxidant defense or other mechanisms. For example, other powerful sources of mitochondrial ROS production are represented by the mitochondrial NO synthase [32, 33], and the byproducts of several cellular enzymes including NADPH oxidases, xanthine oxidase [22, 23, 34]. Nevertheless, further studies should be taken to investigate the XST's specific mechanisms on inhibition of ROS generation.

Impaired $\Delta\Psi m$, a sign of the early stage of cell apoptosis [35], occurred before nucleus apoptosis characteristics (chromatin condensed and DNA rupture). Once the mitochondrial transmembrane potential collapse, apoptosis procedure is irreversible [36]. In this experiment, we confirmed that the decreased $\Delta\Psi m$ was associated with the increase in the apoptosis cells (Figs. 5 and 6). XST, via elevation of $\Delta\Psi m$ and inhibition of mitochondrial ROS generation, exerted its anti-apoptotic effects in the hypoxia-reoxygenated HCM. Conclusively, the drug, via ensuring the integrity of the mitochondrial membrane, exerted its cardioprotective effects in the hypoxia-reoxygenated HCM.

Abbreviations
CHF: Chronic heart failure; ETC: Mitochondrial electron transport chain; HCM: Primary human cardiomyocyte; LVEF: Left ventricular ejection fraction; MPTP: Mitochondrial permeability transition pore; MTT: 3-[4,5-dimethylthiazol-2-yl]-diphenyl-tetrazolium bromide; NYHA: New York Heart Association; PBS: Phosphate-buffered saline; Pi: Inorganic phosphorus; ROS: Reactive oxygen species; SOD: Superoxide dismutase; XST: Xinshuitong Capsule; $\Delta\Psi m$: Mitochondrial membrane potential

Acknowledgments
Thanks for the Molecular Biology Centre Laboratory of Fujian Academy of Integrative Medicine, Fujian Key Laboratory of Integrative Medicine on Geriatrics for the experiments.

Funding
This study is supported by the projects from Fujian Natural Science Foundation of China (No. 2013 J01334) Fujian Natural Science Foundation of Chinese-foreign cooperation Key Projects (No.2014I0012), Fujian Province Health and Family Planning Council (No.wzzy201313),Fujian University of TCM Supported Project (No.X2014137) and Fujian province health and family planning commission Foundation(No. 2017-CX-39).

Authors' contributions
CT Data collection and writing the paper, JZ and YW Drug quality inspection, JZH Cell experiments Cell viability assay, $\Delta\Psi m$ detection, mitochondrial respiratory chain complexes, total ATPase activity, mitochondrial ROS, apoptosis cells, WC Study design and experimental director, All authors have read and approved the final manuscript to submitted to this journal.

Competing interests
The authors declare that they have no competing interests.

References
1. Weiss JN, Korge P, Honda HM, Ping P. Role of the mitochondrial permeability transition in myocardial disease. Circ Res. 2003;93:292–301.
2. Crompton M. The mitochondrial permeability transition pore and its role in cell death. Biochem J. 1999;341:233–49.
3. Duchen MR, McGuinness O, Brown LA, Crompton M. On the involvement of a cyclosporin a sensitive mitochondrial pore in types are beyond the experimental reach of this study. A myocardial reperfusion injuryCardiovasc Res. 1993;27:1790–4.
4. Davies KJ. Oxidative stress: the paradox of aerobic life. Biochem Soc Symp. 1995;61:1–31.
5. Ide T, Tsutsui H, Kinugawa S, Utsumi H, Kang D, Hattori N, Uchida K, Arimura KI, Egashira K, Takeshita A. Mitochondrial electron transport complex I is a potential source of oxygen free radicals in the failing myocardium. Circ Res. 1999;85:357–63.
6. Giordano FJ. Oxygen, oxidative stress, hypoxia, and heart failure. J Clin Invest. 2005;115:500–8.
7. Kwon SH, Pimentel DR, Remondino A, Sawyer DB, Colucci WS. H₂O₂ regulates regulates cardiac myocyte phenotype via concentration dependent activation of distinct kinase pathways. J Mol Cell Cardiol. 2003;35:615–21.
8. Li JM, Gall NP, Grieve DJ, Chen M, Shah AM. Activation of NADPH oxidase during progression of cardiac hypertrophy to failure. Hypertension. 2002;40:477–84.
9. Li PC, Yang YC, Hwang GY, Kao LS, Lin CY. Inhibition of reverse-mode sodium-calcium exchanger activity and apoptosis by Levosimendan in human cardiomyocyte progenitor cell-derived cardiomyocytes after anoxia and reoxygenation. PLoS One. 2014;9:e85909.
10. Tan CJ, Chen WL, Lin JM, Lin RH, Tan LF. Clinical research of Xinshuitong capsule on chronic heart failure in patients with diuretic resistance. Chin Arch Tradit Chin Med. 2011;29:837–9.
11. Tan CJ, Wu YB, Chen WL, Lin RH. Xinshuitong capsule ameliorates hypertrophy of cardiomyocytes via aquaporin pathway in the ischemia-reperfusion rat hearts. Int J Cardiol. 2011;152:S54.
12. Xu L, Deng Y, Feng L, Li D, Chen X, Ma C, Liu X, Yin J, Yang M, Teng F, Wu W, Guan S, Jiang B, Guo D. Cardio-protection of salvianolic acid B through inhibition of apoptosis network. PLoS One. 2011;6:e24036.
13. Kavazis AN, Talbert EE, Smuder AJ, Hudson MB, Nelson WB, Powers SK. Mechanical ventilation induces diaphragmatic mitochondrial dysfunction and increased oxidant production. Free Radic Biol Med. 2009;46:842–50.
14. Alexander T. Assembly of the mitochondrial membrane system. I. Characterization of some enzymes of the inner membrane of yeast mitochondria. J Biol Chem. 1969;244:5020–6.
15. Fiske CH, Subbarow Y. The colorimetric determination of phosphorus. J Biol Chem. 1925;66:375–400.
16. Lowry OH, Rosebrough NJ, Farr AL, Randall RJ. Protein measurement with the folin phenol reagent. J Biol Chem. 1951;193:265–75.
17. Almeida A, Moncada S, Bolaños JP. Nitric oxide switches on glycolysis through the AMP protein kinase and 6-phosphofructo-2-kinase pathway. Nat Cell Biol. 2004;6:45–51.
18. Korshunov SS, Skulachev VP, Starkov AA. High protonic potential actuates a mechanism of production of reactive oxygen species in mitochondria. FEBS Lett. 1997;416:15–8.
19. Aluri HS, Simpson DC, Allegood JC, Hu Y, Szczepanek K, Gronert S, Chen Q, Lesnefsky EJ. Electron flow into cytochrome c coupled with reactive oxygen species from the electron transport chain converts cytochrome c to a cardiolipin peroxidase: role during ischemia-reperfusion. Biochim Biophys Acta. 2014;1840:9 18.
20. Lesnefsky EJ, Moghaddas S, Tandler B, Kerner J, Hoppel CL. Mitochondrial dys-function in cardiac disease: ischemia–reperfusion,aging,and heart failure. J Mol Cell Cardiol. 2001;33:1065–89.

21. Chen Q, Moghaddas S, Hoppel CL, Lesnefsky EJ. Reversible blockade of electron transport during ischemia protects mitochondria and decreases myocardial injury following reperfusion. J Pharmaco Exp Ther. 2006;319:1405 12.
22. Liu Y, Fiskum G, Schubert D. Generation of reactive oxygen species by the mitochondrial electron transport chain. J Neurochemistry. 2002;80:780–7.
23. Skulachev VP. Uncoupling: new approaches to an old problem of bioenergetics. Biochim Biophys Acta. 1998;1363:100–24.
24. Brand MD, Buckingham JA, Esteves TC, Green K, Lambert AJ, Miwa S, Murphy MP, Pakay JL, Talbot DA, Echtay KS. Mitochondrial superoxide and aging: uncoupling-protein activity and superoxide production. Biochem Soc Symp. 2004;71:203–13.
25. Brookes PS. Mitochondrial H(+) leak and ROS generation: an odd couple. Free Radic Biol Med. 2005;38:12–23.
26. Korge P, Ping P, Weiss JN. Reactive oxygen species production in energized cardiac mitochondria during hypoxia/reoxygenation: modulation by nitric oxide. Circ Res. 2008;103:873–80.
27. Petrosillo G, Ruggiero F, Di Venosa N, Paradies G. Decreased complex III activity in mitochondria isolated from rat heart subjected to ischemia and reperfusion: role of reactive oxygen species and cardiolipin. FASEB J. 2003;17:714–6.
28. Zhang J, Piantadosi CA. Mitochondrial oxidative stress after carbon monoxide hypoxia in the rat brain. J Clin Invest. 1992;90:1193–9.
29. Rustin P, Chretien D, Bourgeron T, Gerard B, Rotig A, Saudubray JM, Munnich A. Biochemical and molecular investigations in respiratory chain deficiencies. Clin Chim Acta. 1994;228:35–51.
30. Cadenas E, Davies KJ. Mitochondrial free radical generation, oxidative stress, and aging. Free Radic Biol Med. 2000;29:222–30.
31. Vinogradov AD, Grivennikova VG. Generation of superoxide-radical by the NADH: ubiquinone oxidoreductase of heart mitochondria. Biochemistry. 2005;70:120–7.
32. Poderoso JJ, Carreras MC, Lisdero C, Riobó N, Schöpfer F, Boveris A. Nitric oxide inhibits electron transfer and increases superoxide radical production in rat heart mitochondria and submitochondrial particles. Arch Biochem Biophys. 1996;328:85–92.
33. Dröge W. Free radicals in the physiological control of cell function. Physiol Rev. 2002;82:47–95.
34. Turrens JF. Mitochondrial formation of reactive oxygen species. J Physiol. 2003;552:335–44.
35. Mathur A, Hong Y, Kemp BK. Evaluation of fluorescent dyes for the detection of mitochondrial membrane potential changes in cultured cardiomyocytes. Cardiovasc Res. 2000;46:126–38.
36. Suh DH, Kim MK, Kim HS. Mitochondrial permeability transition pore as a selective target for anti-cancer therapy. Front Oncol. 2013;3:41.

8

Evaluation of the antioxidant and endothelial protective effects of *Lysimachia christinae* Hance (*Jin Qian Cao*) extract fractions

Ning-hua Wu[1†], Zhi-qiang Ke[1†], Shan Wu[2], Xiao-song Yang[1], Qing-jie Chen[1], Sheng-tang Huang[1*] and Chao Liu[1*]

Abstract

Background: *Lysimachia christinae* Hance is a traditional Chinese medicine with diuretic, detumescent, and detoxifying effects. Our aimed to optimize the extraction protocol to maximize the yield of flavonoids from *Lysimachia christinae* Hance, and evaluate the pharmacological activities of four fractions, namely, petroleum ether (PE), ethyl acetate (EA), n-butanol (NB), and aqueous (AQ) fractions, of the ethanolic extract of *Lysimachia christinae* Hance.

Methods: The flavonoid monomers in the crude extract were characterized via high performance liquid chromatography (HPLC), were used as markers for extract quality control and standardization. The total flavonoid, total phenolic, and total polysaccharide contents of each fraction were determined by spectrophotometry. Further, the in vitro free radical (diphenylpicrylhydrazyl, 2,2′-azino-bis(3-ethylbenzothiazoline-6-sulphonic acid), superoxide, and hydroxyl radicals) scavenging activities, and antioxidant capacity in endothelial cells were evaluated for each fraction.

Results: After optimizing the extraction protocol to maximize the total flavonoid yield from *L. christinae* Hance, the NB fractions had the highest total flavonoid (39.4 ± 4.55 mg RE/g), total phenolic (41.1 ± 3.07 mg GAE/g) and total polysaccharide (168.1 ± 7.07 mg GE/g); In addition, the NB fraction of the ethanolic extract of *L. christinae* Hance reveal the strongest radical-scavenging activity, antioxidant activity and protective effects against H_2O_2-induced injury in HUVECs.

Conclusions: Among the four fractions of *L. christinae* Hance, the NB fraction showed the most potent antioxidant and endothelial protective effects, which may be attributed to its high flavonoid, phenolic contents and optimal portfolio of different active ingredients of NB fractions of the ethanolic extract of *L. christinae* Hance. This study might improve our understanding of the pharmacological activities of *L. christinae* Hance, thereby facilitating its use in disease prevention and treatment.

Keywords: *Lysimachia christinae* Hance, Radical-scavenging, Antioxidant, HUVECs, Flavonoids

Background

Lysimachia christinae Hance (*Jin Qian Cao*), which belongs to the family *Primulaceae*, was recorded in the 2010 edition of the Chinese Pharmacopoeia as an herb that possesses diuretic, detumescent, and detoxifying effects. It has been widely used for treating hepatobiliary lithiasis, urolithiasis, heat stranguria, nephritis edema, damp jaundice, and carbuncle in traditional Chinese medicine (TCM) [1, 2] and is therefore being increasingly investigated for its therapeutic potential [3, 4]. Although chemical constituent analyses indicate that *L. christinae* Hance contains several bioactive constituents, flavonoids, phenols, polysaccharides, triterpenoid saponins, volatile oils, organic acids, and quinones, the identity of these constituents and their pharmacological activities remain poorly researched.

* Correspondence: shengtanghuang@mail.hbust.com.cn; tnbsys_liuchao@126.com
†Equal contributors
[1]Hubei Key Laboratory of Cardiovascular, Cerebrovascular, and Metabolic Disorders, Hubei University of Science and Technology, Xianning, China
Full list of author information is available at the end of the article

Reactive oxygen species (ROS), which include free radicals, such as superoxide anion (O_2^-) and hydroperoxyl radical ($^\bullet OH$), and non-free radicals, such as hydrogen peroxide (H_2O_2), act as signaling molecules and are constantly produced in living cells. Although they are efficiently eliminated by antioxidant defense systems under physiological conditions, an imbalance between ROS production and elimination leads to oxidative stress, which can damage biomolecules such as DNA, proteins, and lipids and greatly contribute to increased cardiovascular risk [5]. Such undesirable outcomes of oxidative stress can be effectively counteracted only by boosting endogenous antioxidant defenses or via supplementation with exogenous antioxidants [6].

The potential of naturally occurring plant flavonoids as exogenous (i.e., dietary) antioxidants and their application in the prevention and/or treatment of cardiovascular diseases over the last decades has been well-documented [7–9]. The hydroalcoholic extract of *Lysimachia clethroides*, another plant of the genus *Lysimachia*, has been reported to protect vascular function via an endothelium-dependent mechanism [10]. Further, our pilot data suggested that *L. christinae* Hance extract could inhibit ROS foramtion in HUVECs. Therefore, the present study was designed to evaluate the antioxidant potential and endothelial protective effects of *L. christinae* Hance, which was extracted with ethanol and separated into four fractions using solvents of different polarities.

Methods
Chemicals and reagents
L. christinae Hance herbs (Harvested in October 2014 from Sichuan, China, subsequently dry and stored under the condition of dark) were purchased from Kang Jin Pharmaceutical (Xianning, China). Butylated hydroxytoluene (BHT), H_2O_2, and acetylcholine (ACh) were purchased from Sigma-Aldrich (St Louis, MO, USA). Ascorbic acid (Vitamin C) and Trolox were purchased from Richu Biosciences (Shanghai, China). Diphenylpicrylhydrazyl (DPPH) and 2,2′-azino-bis(3-ethylbenzothiazoline-6 -sulphonic acid) (ABTS) were obtained from Aladdin Reagent (Shanghai, China). Rutin was purchased from Sangon Biotech (Shanghai, China). Dihydroethidium (DHE) was obtained from Thermo Fisher Scientific (MA, USA). 4′,6-diamidino-2-phenylindole (DAPI) was obtained from Calbiochem (Madrid, Spain). All other reagents used were of analytical grade. Double distilled water was used throughout the experiments.

Preparation of *L. christinae* Hance extract
The crude extract of *L. christinae* Hance was prepared in the Phytochemistry Laboratory, Department of Materia Medica, Hubei University of Science and Technology (Xianning, China). Dried herb powder (50 g) was first extracted using 75% ethanol at 60 °C for 30 min. This extraction protocol was optimized to maximize the total flavonoid yield and standardized via identification and quantification of certain markers (flavonoid monomers) in the extract by ultraviolet-high performance liquid chromatography (UV-HPLC). The crude ethanolic extract was then fractionated into the petroleum ether (PE), ethyl acetate (EA), n-butanol (NB), and aqueous (AQ) fractions. The solvents were evaporated, and the residues were dried under vacuum. Finally, the four fractions of different polarities were stored at 4 °C in the dark until use.

Qualitative and quantitative analysis of flavonoid monomers in the ethanolic extract
Certain flavonoid monomers in the crude ethanolic extract, designated as markers for quality control and standardization, were characterized by UV-HPLC. The analyses were performed on a LC-20 AD system (Shimadzu, Kyoto, Japan) equipped with an online degasser and a UV detector (G1314B, Agilent Technologies, CA, USA), using a C18 column (ZORBAX SB-C18, 4.6 × 150 mm, 5 μm, Agilent Technologies) maintained at 30 °C and a mobile phase consisting of methanol, acetonitrile, and 1% phosphoric acid in water, at a flow rate of 0.8 mL/min. The eluent was monitored at 370 nm. The most optimal chromatographic conditions were adopted to achieve the best peak resolution and shortest analysis times. The data were analyzed using LabSolutions software (version 5.51, Shimadzu).

Estimation of the total flavonoid, total phenolic, and total polysaccharide contents of the extract fractions
The total flavonoid and phenolic contents and total polysaccharide content of each fraction were determined spectrophotometrically by the protocol of Asaduzzaman [11, 12], and phenol-sulphuric acid method, respectively. All experiments were performed in triplicate. The total flavonoid, total phenolic, and total polysaccharide contents were expressed as milligrams of rutin equivalents (RE), gallic acid equivalents (GAE), and glucose equivalents (GE), respectively, per gram of extract.

Determination of the in vitro radical-scavenging activities of the extract fractions
The in vitro DPPH, ABTS, superoxide anion, and hydroxyl radical-scavenging activities of the four fractions were assayed as previously described [4, 13–15].

Cell culture and treatment
Human umbilical vein endothelial cells (HUVECs) and cell culture medium (ECM containing 5% fetal bovine serum (FBS), 1% ECGs, 100 U/mL penicillin, and

100 μg/mL streptomycin) were purchased from ScienCell Research Laboratories (San Diego, CA, USA). Cells between passages 2 and 5 were maintained at 37 ° C in a humidified atmosphere of 5% CO_2 and 95% air. Confluent cells were treated with the same dose (6.7 μg/mL) of each fraction, 2 h prior to exposure to 50 μM H_2O_2 for 5 h. Thus, using an oxidative stress model based on H_2O_2-induced injury, we compared the antioxidant activity of the four extract fractions.

Determination of cell viability

The cell viability was measured in 96-well plates via the non-radioactive cell counting kit-8 (CCK-8) assay (Dojindo Molecular Technologies, Kumamoto, Japan), according to the manufacturer's instructions.

Determination of the antioxidant activity of the extract fractions

The catalase (CAT) activity,the levels of glutathione (GSH), malondialdehyde (MDA) and Nitric Oxide (NO), and the lipid peroxidation marker, in HUVECs were measured by colorimetry using commercially available biochemical kits (Nanjing Jiancheng Bioengineering Research Institute, Nanjing, China), according to the manufacturer's instructions.

Detection of ROS production

Intracellular superoxide anions were measured using the dihydroethidium (DHE) fluorescence probe and high performance liquid chromatography (HPLC) assay. The HUVECs were washed three times with DPBS before incubation with 10 μM DHE for 30 min at 37 °C. The nuclei were counterstained with DAPI (1 μg/mL). After washed with DPBS, the HUVECs were photographed using an inverted fluorescence microscopy (Olympus IX71, Japan). The ethidium (oxidized DHE) and DAPI fluorescence were quantified using Image-Pro Plus software (version 6.0, Media Cybernetics, MD, USA). ROS production was estimated from the ratio of ethidium/DAPI fluorescence.

Statistical analysis

Statistical analyses were performed using GraphPad Prism 5 software (GraphPad Software, San Diego, CA, USA). Data are presented as the mean ± SEM. One-way analysis of variance (ANOVA) was used to determine the differences among treatment groups. Values of $P < 0.05$ were considered statistically significant.

Results

Identification of flavonoid monomers in the ethanolic extract

Since flavonoids are known to be potent radical scavengers, the extraction protocol was optimized to maximize the total flavonoid yield from *L. christinae* Hance. The plant species, source, and extraction conditions were strictly standardized to reduce the variability in phytochemical composition. Qualitative and quantitative analysis of flavonoid monomers in the crude ethanolic extract via HPLC revealed that rutin (3.36 mg/g), quercetin (0.83 mg/g), quercetin-3-methyl ether (0.17 mg/g), kaempferol (0.86 mg/g), isorhamnetin (0.35 mg/g), Isorhamnetin-robinobioside (4.11 mg/g), and chlorogenic acid (2.19 mg/g) could be used as markers for quality control and standardization.

Total flavonoid, total phenolic, and total polysaccharide contents of the extract fractions

The total flavonoid (mg RE/g), total phenolic (mg GAE/g), and total polysaccharide (mg GE/g) contents of each fraction of *L. christinae* Hance extract are shown in Table 1. The flavonoid and phenolic contents were much higher in NB and EA fractions than in PE and AQ fractions ($P < 0.05$). The NB fraction also had the highest polysaccharide content among the four fractions.

In vitro radical-scavenging activities of the extract fractions

DPPH, ABTS, superoxide anion, and hydroxyl radicals have been widely used for evaluating the antioxidant activity of chemical compounds, which is generally represented by IC_{50} (mg/mL), the concentration at which a compound shows 50% radical-scavenging activity. The IC_{50} values pertaining to the DPPH, ABTS, superoxide anion, and hydroxyl radical-scavenging activities of each extract fraction are indicated in Table 2. Collectively, the radical-scavenging activities of the four fractions decreased in the following order: NB fraction > EA fraction > PE fraction >

Table 1 Amounts of total flavonoids, phenols and polysaccharides in each fraction isolated from ethanol extract of *Lysimachia christinae* Hance

	Total flavonoids (mg RE/g)	Total phenols (mg GAE/g)	Total polysaccharide (mg GE/g)
PE fraction	15.3 ± 1.56	15.6 ± 1.03	68.9 ± 4.75
EA fraction	37.5 ± 3.07	32.4 ± 3.08	85.4 ± 4.86
NB fraction	39.4 ± 4.55	41.1 ± 3.07	168.1 ± 7.07
AQ fraction	2.3 ± 0.12	29.1 ± 2.88	135.1 ± 6.29

Values are means±SEM of three determinations. *RE* rutin, *GAE* gallic acid, *GE* glucose, *PE* petroleum ether, *EA* ethyl acetate, *NB* n-butanol, *AQ* aqueous

Table 2 In vitro radical-scavenging activities for each fraction isolated from ethanol extract of *Lysimachia christinae* Hance

Fraction/standard antioxidants	IC$_{50}$ (mg/mL)			
	DPPH radical-scavenging activity	ABTS radical-scavenging activity	Superoxide anion radical-scavenging activity	Hydroxyl radical-scavenging activity
PE fraction	0.043	2.586	***	0.451
EA fraction	0.029	1.49	0.608	0.288
NB fraction	0.026	1.288	0.191	0.214
AQ fraction	0.056	3.712	0.801	0.763
BHT	0.023	–	–	–
TROLOX	–	1.471	–	–
VC	–	–	0.118	0.187

BHT, TROLOX and VC acted as positive control. ***: Cannot be detected;——: Not used as reference. *PE* petroleum ether, *EA* ethyl acetate, *NB* n-butanol, *AQ* aqueous, *DPPH* Diphenylpicrylhydrazyl, *ABTS* 2,2'-azino-bis(3- ethylbenzothiazoline-6-sulphonic acid)

AQ fraction. Thus, the NB fraction of the ethanolic extract of *L. christinae* Hance displayed the strongest radical-scavenging activity among the four fractions.

Protective effects of the extract fractions against H$_2$O$_2$-induced oxidative stress in HUVECs

The effects of the extract fractions on cell viability and oxidant-antioxidant balance were evaluated by estimating the catalase activity and levels of GSH, NO and MDA in HUVECs subjected to H$_2$O$_2$-induced oxidative stress. The cell viability, which was significantly reduced upon exposure to H$_2$O$_2$ ($P < 0.05$), was markedly increased by

pretreatment with the NB fraction, whereas the EA, AQ, and PE fractions conferred lesser protection against H$_2$O$_2$-induced oxidative stress (Fig. 1a). Additionally, the NB fraction significantly improved the endogenous antioxidant activity and inhibited lipid peroxidation, as indicated by the increase in catalase activity and GSH, NO level (Fig. 1b–d) and decrease in MDA level (Fig. 1e) upon pretreatment with this fraction ($P < 0.05$ vs. H$_2$O$_2$ group).

Effects of the four fractions on ROS production in HUVECs

The red fluorescence of ethidium in Fig. 2 indicates the presence of ROS in the HUVECs, and blue fluorescence

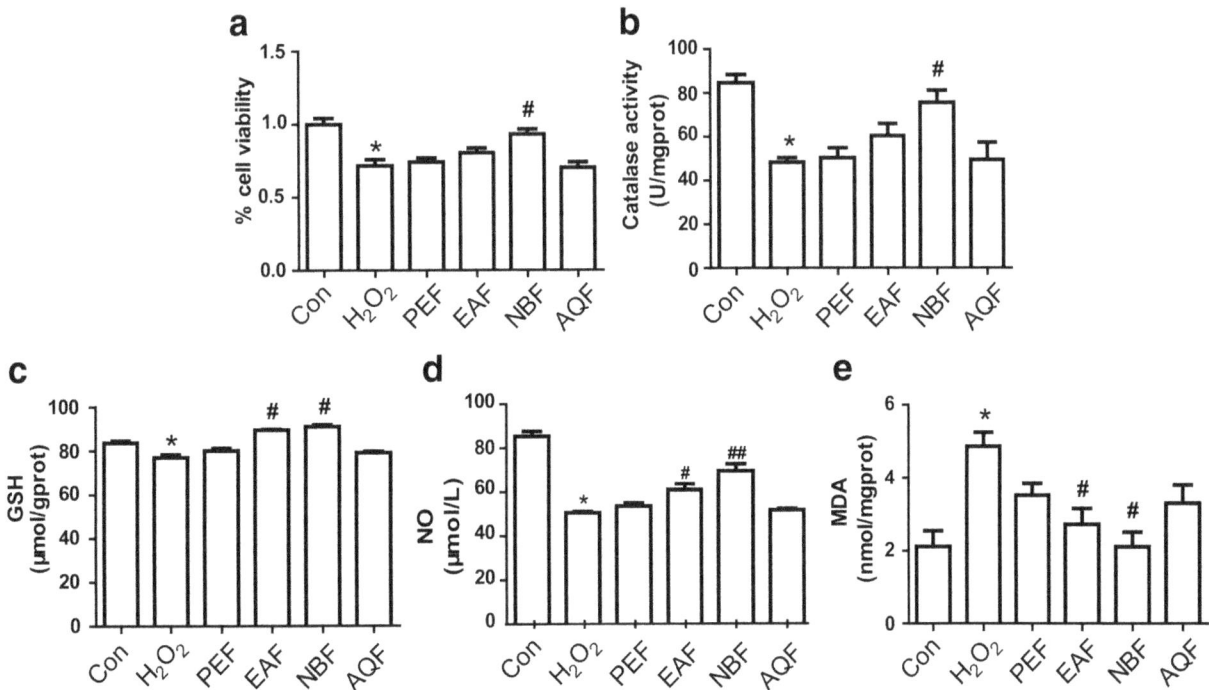

Fig. 1 Effects of the four extract fractions on cell viability (**a**), catalase activity (**b**), and levels of glutathione (GSH) (**c**), Nitric Oxide(NO) (**d**) and malondialdehyde (MDA) (**e**) in human umbilical vein endothelial cells subjected to H$_2$O$_2$-induced oxidative stress. *$P < 0.05$ vs. control. #$P < 0.05$ vs. H$_2$O$_2$ alone. $n = 12$. Con: control; PEF: petroleum ether fraction; EAF: ethyl acetate fraction; NBF: n-butanol fraction; AQF: aqueous fraction

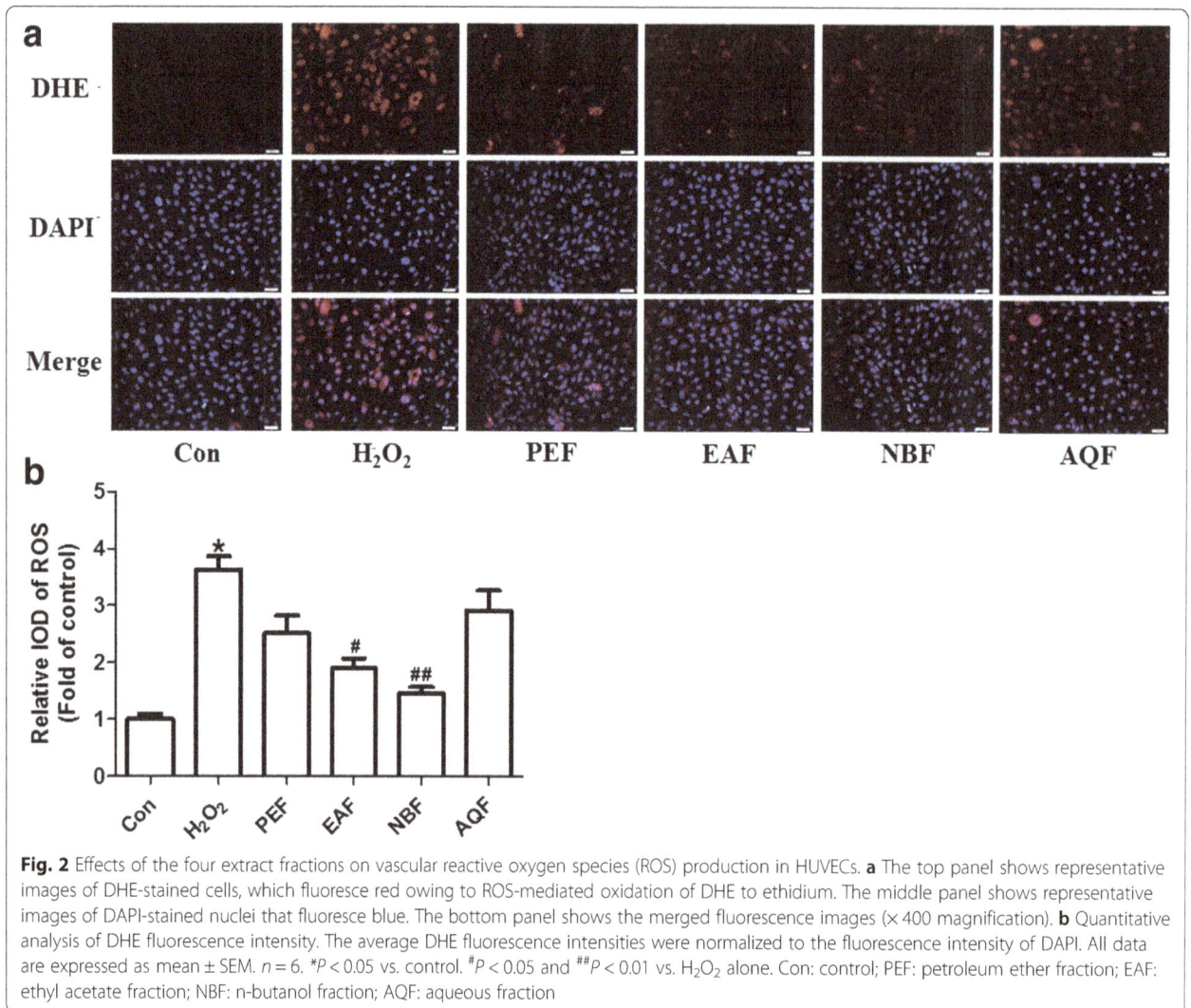

Fig. 2 Effects of the four extract fractions on vascular reactive oxygen species (ROS) production in HUVECs. **a** The top panel shows representative images of DHE-stained cells, which fluoresce red owing to ROS-mediated oxidation of DHE to ethidium. The middle panel shows representative images of DAPI-stained nuclei that fluoresce blue. The bottom panel shows the merged fluorescence images ($\times 400$ magnification). **b** Quantitative analysis of DHE fluorescence intensity. The average DHE fluorescence intensities were normalized to the fluorescence intensity of DAPI. All data are expressed as mean $\pm$ SEM. $n = 6$. *$P < 0.05$ vs. control. #$P < 0.05$ and ##$P < 0.01$ vs. H_2O_2 alone. Con: control; PEF: petroleum ether fraction; EAF: ethyl acetate fraction; NBF: n-butanol fraction; AQF: aqueous fraction

indicates the nuclear stain DAPI. The ROS production, which was dramatically increased upon treatment with H_2O_2, was mildly inhibited by the four extract fractions in the order: NB fraction > EA fraction > PE fraction > AQ fraction (Fig. 2). Thus, the NB fraction was the most competent in preventing endothelial ROS accumulation, among the four fractions.

Discussion

TCM has played a key role in protecting the health of Chinese people for over 1000 years. However, TCM formulations are generally complex mixtures composed of a variety of effective, ineffective, and even toxic ingredients. Therefore, it is essential to extract, separate, and purify the active constituents of TCM, in order to establish the intrinsic quality and improve the clinical efficacy of these medicines.

L. christinae Hance, a well-known TCM herb recorded in ancient literature, has been used to treat disease conditions such as stranguria, odynuria, brownish urine, jaundice, carbuncle, furuncle, and calculi [1, 2]. However, the active constituents responsible for these medicinal benefits have not yet been completely characterized. In the present study, the raw herb of *L. christinae* Hance was extracted with ethanol and separated into four fractions of different polarities. We then evaluated the endothelial protective effect and radical-scavenging activity of these fractions. Our results revealed that the NB fraction significantly reversed catalase activity and GSH, NO level reduced and MDA level increased by H_2O_2, suggesting that NB fraction could prevent H_2O_2-induced oxidative stress injury in HUVECs. To the best of our knowledge, this is the first study to investigate the active constituents and associated pharmacological activities of *L. christinae* Hance.

Several evidences suggest that oxidative stress plays a central role in the pathogenesis of cardiovascular diseases. Antioxidants can delay or inhibit cellular oxidative damage by blocking the initiation or propagation of the oxidative chain reaction. Thus, the use of antioxidants and free radical scavengers has been accepted as an important strategy for the prevention or treatment of various cardiovascular diseases [16]. In this study, we evaluated the radical-scavenging activities of the four extract fractions using in vitro oxidative injury models of endothelium. Our results demonstrated that the NB fraction showed the strongest radical-scavenging and antioxidant activities in the endothelium and thus the most potent endothelial protective effect among the four fractions.

The observed differences in the radical-scavenging and antioxidant activities of the four ethanolic extract fractions may be attributed to differences in their active constituents. Phenols, the most abundant antioxidants among plant secondary metabolites, have shown promising antioxidant activity both in vivo and in vitro [6]. Phenolic compounds generally contain one or more aromatic rings with one or more hydroxyl groups, and their antioxidant activity increases with an increase in the number of free hydroxyl groups and conjugation of side chains to the aromatic rings [17]. The antioxidant properties of flavonoids, a major group of polyphenols derived from 2-phenylchromone and comprising more than 10,000 compounds, have also been extensively investigated over the years [18]. In the present study, the total phenolic and total flavonoid contents were much higher in the NB fraction than in other fractions, which could well explain its higher antioxidant and radical-scavenging activities. However, the polysaccharide content of the four fractions decreased in the following order: NB fraction > AQ fraction > EA fraction > PE fraction (Table 1), which did not coincide with the orders of their radical-scavenging (Table 2) and antioxidant activities (Fig. 1b–d). Thus, the phenolic and flavonoid components of the extract fractions may be chiefly responsible for their antioxidant properties [19, 20].

Conclusions

In the present study, we separated the crude ethanolic extract of *L. christinae* Hance into four fractions of different polarities and demonstrated that the NB fraction showed the most potent antioxidant and endothelial protective effects, which may be attributed to its high phenolic and flavonoid contents. Our work has thus attempted to characterize the active ingredients and associated pharmacological activities of *L. christinae* Hance, which may aid in improving its application for disease prevention and treatment. Future research should focus on the isolation, purification, and characterization of the bioactive constituents in the NB fraction of the ethanolic extract.

Acknowledgments
Not applicable.

Funding
This research was supported by Outstanding Youth Scientific Innovation Team Project for the Universities of Hubei Province [T201213], New Century Excellent Talents Project of the Ministry of Education [NCET-13-0781], and Hubei Major Projects of Technical Innovation [2016ACA148].

Authors' contributions
LC and HST are responsible for conception and design of the study. WNH, KZQ, CQJ and WS performed the study. LC and YXS drafted, edited and revised the manuscript, and all authors had read and approved of this final manuscript.

Competing interests
The authors declare that they have no competing interests.

Author details
[1]Hubei Key Laboratory of Cardiovascular, Cerebrovascular, and Metabolic Disorders, Hubei University of Science and Technology, Xianning, China. [2]Xianning Maternal and Child Health Care Hospital, Xianning, China.

References

1. Deng J, Ren M, Dai X, Qu D, Yang M, Zhang T, Jiang B. Lysimachia christinae Hance regresses preestablished cholesterol gallstone in mice. J Ethnopharmacol. 2015;166:102–8.
2. Yang X, Wang BC, Zhang X, Liu WQ, Qian JZ, Li W, Deng J, Singh GK, Su H. Evaluation of Lysimachia christinae Hance extracts as anticholecystitis and cholagogic agents in animals. J Ethnopharmacol. 2011;137(1):57–63.
3. Wang J, Zhang Y, Zhang Y, Cui Y, Liu J, Zhang B. Protective effect of Lysimachia christinae against acute alcohol-induced liver injury in mice. Bioscience Trends. 2012;6(2):89–97.
4. Li HY, Hao ZB, Wang XL, Huang L, Li JP. Antioxidant activities of extracts and fractions from Lysimachia foenum-graecum Hance. Bioresour Technol. 2009;100(2):970–4.
5. Del Rio D, Rodriguez-Mateos A, Spencer JP, Tognolini M, Borges G, Crozier A: Dietary (poly)phenolics in human health: structures, bioavailability, and evidence of protective effects against chronic diseases. Antioxid Redox Signal 2013, 18(14):1818–1892.
6. Conti V, Izzo V, Corbi G, Russomanno G, Manzo V, De Lise F, Di Donato A, Filippelli A. Antioxidant supplementation in the treatment of aging-associated diseases. Front Pharmacology. 2016;7:24.
7. Bijak M, Saluk J, Szelenberger R, Nowak P. Popular naturally occurring antioxidants as potential anticoagulant drugs. Chem Biol Interact. 2016;257:35–45.
8. Kasote DM, Katyare SS, Hegde MV, Bae H. Significance of antioxidant potential of plants and its relevance to therapeutic applications. Int J Biol Sci. 2015;11(8):982–91.
9. Scholz EP, Zitron E, Katus HA, Karle CA. Cardiovascular ion channels as a molecular target of flavonoids. Cardiovasc Ther. 2010;28(4):e46–52.
10. Lee JO, Chang K, Kim CY, Jung SH, Lee SW, Oak MH. Lysimachia clethroides extract promote vascular relaxation via endothelium-dependent mechanism. J Cardiovasc Pharmacol. 2010;55(5):481–8.
11. Asaduzzaman M, Uddin MJ, Kader MA, Alam AH, Rahman AA, Rashid M, Kato K, Tanaka T, Takeda M, Sadik G. In vitro acetylcholinesterase inhibitory activity and the antioxidant properties of Aegle marmelos leaf extract: implications for the treatment of Alzheimer's disease. Psychogeriatrics. 2014;14(1):1–10.
12. Laghari AH, Memon S, Nelofar A, Khan KM, Yasmin A. Determination of free phenolic acids and antioxidant activity of methanolic extracts obtained from fruits and leaves of Chenopodium album. Food Chem. 2011;126(4):1850–5.
13. Machova E, Bystricky S. Antioxidant capacities of mannans and glucans are related to their susceptibility of free radical degradation. Int J Biol Macromol. 2013;61:308–11.

14. Aktumsek A, Zengin G, Guler GO, Cakmak YS, Duran A. Antioxidant potentials and anticholinesterase activities of methanolic and aqueous extracts of three endemic Centaurea L. species. Food Chem Toxicol. 2013; 55:290–6.

15. Fukumoto LR, Mazza G. Assessing antioxidant and prooxidant activities of phenolic compounds. J Agric Food Chem. 2000;48(8):3597–604.

16. Munzel T, Daiber A, Steven S, Tran LP, Ullmann E, Kossmann S, Schmidt FP, Oelze M, Xia N, Li H, et al. Effects of noise on vascular function, oxidative stress, and inflammation: mechanistic insight from studies in mice. Eur Heart J. 2017;38(37):2838–49.

17. Sakihama Y, Cohen MF, Grace SC, Yamasaki H. Plant phenolic antioxidant and prooxidant activities: phenolics-induced oxidative damage mediated by metals in plants. Toxicology. 2002;177(1):67–80.

18. Catarino MD, Alves-Silva JM, Pereira OR, Cardoso SM. Antioxidant capacities of flavones and benefits in oxidative-stress related diseases. Curr Top Med Chem. 2015;15(2):105–19.

19. Ji L, Wu J, Gao W, Wei J, Yang J, Guo C. Antioxidant capacity of different fractions of vegetables and correlation with the contents of ascorbic acid, phenolics, and flavonoids. J Food Sci. 2011;76(9):C1257–61.

20. Yen FL, Wu TH, Lin LT, Cham TM, Lin CC. Concordance between antioxidant activities and flavonol contents in different extracts and fractions of Cuscuta chinensis. Food Chem. 2008;108(2):455–62.

9

Prescription patterns of traditional Chinese medicine amongst Taiwanese children: a population-based cohort study

Hwey-Fang Liang[1,2,3]*, Yao-Hsu Yang[4,5,6], Pau-Chung Chen[7,8], Hsing-Chun Kuo[1,2,3], Chia-Hao Chang[1,2,3], Ying-Hsiang Wang[9] and Kuang-Ming Wu[10]

Abstract

Background: Traditional Chinese medicine (TCM) has been used by Chinese patients and in many other countries worldwide. However, epidemiological reports and prescription patterns on children are few.

Methods: A cohort of 178,617 children aged 18 and under from one million randomly sampled cases of the National Health Insurance Research Database was analyzed for TCM prescription patterns. SAS 9.1 was applied and descriptive medicine utilization patterns were presented.

Results: The cohort included 112,889 children treated by TCM, with adolescents (12- to 18-year-olds) as the largest group. In the children's TCM outpatient visits, Chinese herbal remedies were the main treatment. The top three categories of diseases treated with Chinese herbal remedies were respiratory system; symptoms, signs, and ill-defined conditions; and digestive system. The top three categories using acupuncture were: injury and poisoning, diseases of the musculoskeletal system and connective tissue, and diseases of the respiratory system. Of the top ten herbal medicines prescribed by TCM physicians, the top nine herbal formulae and the top ten single herbs were associated with diseases of the respiratory system.

Conclusion: This study identified patterns of TCM prescriptions for children and common disease categories treated with TCM. The results provide a useful reference for health policy makers and for those who consider the usage of TCM for children.

Keywords: Traditional Chinese medicine, Chinese herbal remedies, Herbal formulae, Single herb

Background

Traditional Chinese medicine (TCM) has generally been used not only in adults but also in pediatric patients by the Chinese population, as well as in Asia and many other countries around the world [1–4]. TCM may include acupuncture, traumatology, manipulative therapies, and moxibustion. Chinese herbal medicines are one of the most common used modes of TCM treatment [5, 6]. In Taiwan, TCM is an important part of health care and is reimbursed under the current National Health Insurance (NHI) system.

TCM application for pediatric disease is popular and widely used because most parents or caregivers believe that TCM, such as herbs, has a therapeutic effect without any harmful consequences [7]. Eighty percent of parents admitted to concurrent usage of TCM and conventional medicine for their children. In Singapore, herbal medicine was the most commonly used form of TCM, at 84.3% [8]. According to previous studies of two randomly sampled cohorts from the National Health Insurance Research Database in Taiwan, 22 and 22.5% of children used TCM in 2005 and 2010 respectively. Among them, herbal remedies were the most commonly used therapeutic approach, followed by manipulative therapy and acupuncture. In addition, there was an

* Correspondence: hfliang@gw.cgust.edu.tw
[1]Department of Nursing, Chang Gung University of Science and Technology, No.2, Sec. W., Jiapu Rd, Puzi City, Chiayi County 61363, Taiwan
[2]Chronic Diseases and Health Promotion Research Center, Chang Gung University of Science and Technology, No.2, Sec. W., Jiapu Rd, Puzi City, Chiayi County 61363, Taiwan
Full list of author information is available at the end of the article

increasing trend of using herbal remedies (from 65.6 to 74.4%) and acupuncture (from 7.5 to 11.4%) from 2005 to 2010 [6]. In another national cohort of 112,159 children < 12 years, 18.3% had used TCM; school-age children (aged 6–12 years), preschool age children (3–5 years), and toddlers (1–2 years) were more likely to use TCM than infants [9]. However, children are vulnerable to drugs [10], so the dosage varies with age and sensitivity. Little is known about patterns of use of TCM in conditions related to childhood disease and adolescent disease; further study might increase the potential for traditional medicine to be used in Western countries. Accordingly, the computerized reimbursement database of the NHI, the National Health Insurance Research Database (NHIRD), stores longitudinal data on TCM; it also provides an optimal platform for the understanding of use patterns of TCM for children. Thus, the aim of our study is to analyze a random sample of this database and to determine TCM utilization patterns for children aged 18 years and under in Taiwan by analyzing NHI claims data from 2005 to 2013.

Methods
Data source
In the health care system in Taiwan, people are free to choose between Western medicine and TCM, and are allowed to visit either primary care clinics or hospitals without referral. Furthermore, NHI covers almost the entire Taiwanese population, accounting for 99.6% of the total population (23,737,000 beneficiaries at the end of 2015) [11, 12]. All TCMs are provided and prescribed by physicians, and all are covered by NHI. In addition, only licensed TCM physicians qualify for reimbursement. The insurance coverage for TCM in Taiwan includes Chinese herbal medicine (CHM), acupuncture, and traumatology manipulative therapy. TCM medical records files include medical care facilities and specialties; drugs and other management for treatment; and patients' gender, date of birth, date of health care encounter, and unique identification number, which is used to protect the confidentiality of the patient's individually identifiable information, as is the case for Western medication [13]. According to the construct of the database, the dataset reflected primary treatment only, meaning that if children were treated with both acupuncture and herbs, only the herbal treatment was recorded. Furthermore, three major diagnoses were coded in the International Classification of Disease, 9th Revision, and Clinical Modification (ICD-9-CM) format. These databases have previously been used for epidemiologic research and information on prescription use, diagnoses, and hospitalizations. In this study, a cohort of one million patients who were beneficiaries of the NHI program from January 1, 2005, to December 31, 2013, was randomly sampled. From the sampled group, we extracted children aged 18 years and younger for whom TCM was utilized. Patients with missing data on sex or birthdate were excluded.

Following strict confidentiality guidelines in accordance with personal electronic data protection regulations, the National Health Research Institute of Taiwan maintains an anonymous database of NHI reimbursement data that is suitable for research. In addition, this study was approved by the Ethics Review Board of Chang Gung Memorial Hospital, Chiayi Branch, Taiwan.

Study subjects
For this study, we screened 178,617 eligible children aged from newborn to 18 years from the random cohort sample. The age was calculated by subtracting the birth date of the subject from December 31, 2013. We assembled a database of all outpatient department TCM records for 2005–2013 and included for final analysis the 112,889 subjects who had visited a TCM outpatient department at least once.

Products of herbal formula (HF) and single herbs (SH)
TCM has developed over the past millennia and is a well-established component of the national health system in Taiwan. Its practice includes Chinese herbal remedies (CHR), acupuncture, and traumatology manipulative therapies; these are reimbursed by the NHI of Taiwan [13]. We downloaded the list of reimbursed Chinese herbal products from the website of the Bureau of NHI. Corresponding drug information on a specific mixture or name was then obtained from the Committee on Chinese Medicine and Pharmacy (CCMP) website, including the proportions of each constituent, date and period of drug approval, drug names, and manufacturers' codes. Products of SH or HF are assigned with different drug registration numbers if produced by different manufacturers even though the constituents are the same. There are 2485 drug registration numbers for SH and 6639 drug registration numbers for HF, which involve 391 kinds of herbs based on 309 HF according to the unified formula announced by CCMP; all unified formulae were chosen from seven Chinese medicine books.

Statistical analysis
We used SAS version 9.1 software (SAS Institute Inc., Cary, NC) for data analysis and descriptive statistics of drug utilization patterns. We linked drug registration numbers from the CCMP website to outpatient visit records of the study cohort. Then we analyzed the frequencies and percentages of the most frequently used HF and SH prescriptions. We calculated average daily doses and durations for each prescription. The TCM records include data indicating which SH or HF was

prescribed, the prescription duration in days, and the dosage in grams. We used the following formula to calculate the average daily dose for SH and HF in the present study: (total dosage for SH or HF)/(total amount of prescription day for SH or HF) = average daily dose for SH or HF.

By using the ICD-9-CM of the first major diagnosis, records of visiting outpatient departments can be divided into different disease categories. We also analyzed the three most commonly used HF and SH for the five most common disease categories for the subjects.

Results

A total of 112,889 out of 178,617 (63.2%) subjects that had TCM treatments between 2005 and 2013 were analyzed. Table 1 shows there were 11,448 children (10.1%) in the 0–5-year-old age group, 43,940 children (38.9%) in the 6–11-year-old age group, and 57,501 children (50.9%) in the 12–18-year-old age group who were treated as TCM outpatients. Analyses identified a significant difference in gender and age groups ($p < 0.0001$).

Table 2 shows frequency distributions of TCM visits classified by major disease categories (according to ICD-9-CM codes). Of the 1,588,900 TCM outpatient visits among these children, 1,440,316 (90.6%) were treated with prescriptions of CHR, and 148,584 (9.4%) were treated with prescribed acupuncture and manipulative therapies. The top five categories of disease treated with TCM were: diseases of the respiratory system (42.9%); symptoms, signs, and ill-defined conditions (19.0%); diseases of the digestive system (10.6%); injury and poisoning (9.2%); and diseases of the skin and subcutaneous tissue (6.7%). These diseases or conditions accounted for more than 88.4% of all TCM visits. The top five major disease categories for which CHR was prescribed were diseases of the respiratory system (47.2%); symptoms, signs, and ill-defined conditions (21.0%); diseases of the digestive system (11.6%); diseases of the skin and subcutaneous tissue (7.4%); and disease of the genitourinary system (6.5%). These conditions accounted for more than 93.7% of CHR among all TCM visits. Moreover, injury and poisoning and diseases of the musculoskeletal system and connective tissue

accounted for more than 97.4% of TCM visits using acupuncture and traumatology.

Since CHR were the most common prescription, Table 3 displays the 10 most commonly prescribed HF and SH for children. It also includes the frequency of prescriptions, average daily doses (in grams) by age group, and average prescription duration (in days). In HF, the average daily dose was 2.5–3.1 g for children 0–5 years of age, 3.3–3.9 g for children 6–11 years of age, and 3.8–4.7 g for children 12–18 years of age; the average prescription durations were 5.5–7.2 days. The most commonly prescribed HF for children was Shin-Yi-Ching-Fey-Tang (SYCFT) (14.8%). The next four top HF were Xiao-Qing-Long-Tang (XQLT) (10.9%), Cang-Er-San (9.9%), Xin-Yi-San (XYS) (9.8%), and Ma-Xin-Gan-Shi-Tang (MXGST) (9.7%).

In SH, the average daily dose was 0.8–1.3 g for children 0–5 years of age, 0.8–1.4 g for children 6–11 years of age, and 1.0–1.5 g for children 12–18 years of age; the average prescription durations were 5.9–6.7 days. Gan-Cao (Radix Glycyrrhizae) (11.5%) was the most commonly prescribed SH for children. The next four most frequently prescribed SH were Jie-Geng (Radix Platycodi) (9.3%), Chuan-Bei-Mu (Bulbus Fritillariae Cirrhosae) (8.5%), Yu-Xing-Cao (Herba Houttuyniae) (8.2%), and Xing-Ren (Semen Armeniacae) (7.1%).

Regarding TCM used with CHR, Table 4 presents the most frequently used HF and SH for the five most common disease categories. SYCFT (25.7%), XQLT (18.8%), and XYS (18.1%) were the most common HF prescribed, and Gan-Cao (14.3%), Yu-Xing-Cao (13.3%), and Jie-Geng (13.1%) were the most common SH prescribed for respiratory system diseases. MXGST (14.1%), SYCFT (12.3%), and Xin-Su-San (11.5%) were the most frequently prescribed HF, and Jie-Geng (14%), Chuan-Bei-Mu (13.2%), and Gan-Cao (11.1%) were the most commonly prescribed SH for symptoms, signs, and ill-defined conditions. For diseases of the digestive system, Xiang-Sha-Liu-Jun-Zi-Tang (16.1%), Shen-Ling-Bai-Zhu-San (SLBZS) (16%), and Bao-He-Wan (15.2%) were the three most frequently used HF, and Shen-Qu (15.3%), Mai-Ya (14%), and Shan-Zha (11.2%) were the most commonly used SH. Xiao-Feng-San (XFS) (23.9%), Qing-Shang-Fang-Feng-Tang (QSFFT) (23.3%), and Zhen-Ren-Huo-Ming-Yin (17%) were the

Table 1 TCM used among children in different age groups ($n = 112,889$)

Age (years)	0–5(preschool and under)		6–11(school)		12–18(adolescent)		Total		p value
	n	%	n	%	n	%	n	%	< 0.0001
Boys	6223	54.4[a] (10.8)[b]	23,040	52.4 (40.0)	28,384	49.4 (49.2)	57,647	51.1 (100.0)	
Girls	5225	45.6 (9.5)	20,900	47.6 (37.8)	29,117	50.6 (52.7)	55,242	48.9 (100.0)	
Total	11,448	100.0 (10.1)	43,940	100.0 (38.9)	57,501	100.0 (50.9)	112,889	100.0 (100.0)	

Results are n and % using x^2 test
[a]Column percentage
[b]Row percentage

Table 2 Frequency distribution of TCM visits by major disease categories among children 18 years and younger

Major disease category	ICD-9-CM	Chinese herbal remedies		Acupuncture traumatology		Total of TCM	
		n (%)	Rank	n (%)	Rank	n (%)	Rank
Diseases of the Respiratory System	460–519	679,509(47.2)	1	1354(0.9)	3	680,863(42.9)	1
Symptoms, Signs, and Ill-Defined Conditions	780–799	301,712(21.0)	2	392(0.3)	7	302,104 (19.0)	2
Diseases of the Digestive System	520–579	167,701 (11.6)	3	245(0.2)	8	167,946 (10.6)	3
Diseases of the Skin and Subcutaneous Tissue	680–709	106,547 (7.4)	4	176(0.1)	10	106,723 (6.7)	5
Diseases of the Genitourinary System	580–629	94,168 (6.5)	5	2294(0.2)	4	96,462 (6.1)	6
Injury and Poisoning	800–999	25,573 (1.8)	6	121,101 (82.7)	1	146,674 (9.2)	4
Diseases of the Musculoskeletal System and Connective Tissue	710–739	24,109 (1.7)	7	21,523 (14.7)	2	45,632 (2.9)	7
Diseases of the Nervous System and Sense Organs	320–389	15,066 (1.1)	8	611(0.4)	5	15,677 (0.9)	8
Endocrine, Nutritional and Metabolic Diseases, and Immunity Disorders	240–279	7230 (0.5)	10	72(0.0)	11	7302(0.5)	10
Mental Disorders	290–319	6373 (0.4)	11	227(0.2)	9	6600(0.4)	11
Others[a]		12,328(0.9)	9	589(0.4)	6	12,917(0.8)	9
Total		1440,316(100)		148,584(100)		1,588,900 (100)	

[a]Others include ICD-9-CM code ranges 280–289, 630–677, 740–759, 760–779, V01-V82, E800-E999

most frequently used HF, and Lian-Qiao (21.6%), Jin-Yin-Hua (16.7%), and Pu-Gong-Ying (15.4%) were the most frequently used SH for diseases of the skin and sub-cutaneous tissue. For genitourinary system diseases, Jia-Wei-Xiao-Yao-San (32.2%), Dang-Gui-Shao-Yao-San (18%), and Wen-Jing-Tang (16.7%) were the three most commonly used HF, while Xiang-Fu (21.7%), Yi-Mu-Cao (21.5%), and Yan-Hu-Suo (13.6%) were the most frequently prescribed SH.

Discussion

To date, this study is the most comprehensive investigation of TCM usage among children aged 18 years and younger. The advantages of the study are in the application of a random national-level sample to analyze and document comprehensive data gathered with unrestricted access, and is particularly valid for investigating TCM. However, children may be taken for treatment to other places, such as where folk medicine is practiced, and these are not included in the database. The number of TCM patients may be underestimated. That is the limitation of this study. The integration of TCM into the health care system in Taiwan has resulted in the NHIRD providing a large database of TCM usage with de-identified patient information. Previous studies have mainly consisted of questionnaire surveys or telephone interviews from hospitals or private clinics, mostly obtaining parents' or caregivers' information [7, 8, 14, 15]. Therefore, results were limited because of small sample sizes. Additionally, young children may be unable to express ideas clearly, and most of them are protected by parents or family caregivers without the chance to present their opinions freely. Therefore, these previous studies might

only offer a limited picture of children's TCM usage. Because TCM is reimbursed by Taiwan's NHI, the results of this study could reveal a broad, less biased description and overview of children's TCM usage.

We found adolescents occupied the greatest portion (50.9%) of all TCM age groups among the 112,889 child TCM patients selected. The findings of the most common TCM use group among children is consistent with previous studies [1, 6], which showed that as a child grows older, preference for pediatric TCM use increases. However, the prevalence of TCM use was represented differently; Huang et al. [6] showed 38.4% adolescent TCM use in 2005, and 42.7% in 2010. Our study showed 50.9% adolescent TCM use in 2005–2013. Several scholars identified the role of puberty in TCM treatment of adolescents, citing the physiological and behavioral changes associated with the attainment of reproductive competence as well as nonreproductive traits, such as social, emotional, and cognitive developmental factors associated with the transition from childhood to adulthood [16, 17]. However, another investigation [9] indicated that children's age and parental TCM use were more strongly associated with TCM use, with parental TCM use being the most important factor influencing pediatric TCM use.

In our study, respiratory system diseases were the most common reason for children to visit TCM clinics, followed by symptoms, signs, and ill-defined conditions; digestive system diseases; injury and poisoning; and diseases of the skin and subcutaneous tissue. A previous study has revealed similar findings. Huang et al. [6] analyzed the use of TCM in children based on two random cohorts in 2005 and 2010 of NHIRD. The frequency

Table 3 Top ten herbal medicine prescribed by traditional Chinese physicians for children

Rank	Herbal formulae	Frequency (%)	Average daily doses (g), by age group			Average duration (days)	Single herb	Frequency (%)	Average daily doses (g), by age group			Average duration (days)
			0–5	6–11	12–18				0–5	6–11	12–18	
1	Shin-Yi-Ching-Fey-Tang	213,325 (14.8)	2.9	3.6	4.1	6.5	Gan-Cao (Radix Glycyrrhizae)	165,315 (11.5)	0.8	0.8	1.0	6.3
2	Xiao-Qing-Long-Tang	157,380 (10.9)	3.1	3.7	4.4	6.9	Jie-Geng (Radix Platycodi)	134,474 (9.3)	1.2	1.3	1.3	5.9
3	Cang-Er-San	142,826 (9.9)	2.8	3.3	3.8	6.4	Chuan-Bei-Mu (Bulbus Fritillariae Cirrhosae)	122,641 (8.5)	1.0	1.1	1.2	6.1
4	Xin-Yi-San	141,049 (9.8)	3.0	3.8	4.4	6.8	Yu-Xing-Cao (Herba Houttuyniae)	117,641 (8.2)	1.2	1.3	1.4	6.0
5	Ma-Xing-Gan-Shi-Tang	139,927 (9.7)	3.0	3.6	4.1	5.7	Xing-Ren (Semen Armeniacae)	102,099 (7.1)	1.2	1.2	1.3	6.0
6	Yin-Qiao-San	110,639 (7.7)	2.9	3.7	4.3	5.5	Huang-Qin (Radix Scutellariae)	100,846 (7.0)	1.3	1.4	1.5	6.2
7	Xin-Su-San	96,869 (6.7)	3.1	3.7	4.4	5.7	Chan-Tui (Cryptotympana atrata Fabr)	100,428 (7.0)	1.0	1.1	1.2	6.7
8	Ge-Gen-Tang	95,719 (6.6)	3.0	3.9	4.7	6.5	Bai-Zhi (Radix Angelicae Dahuricae)	94,423 (6.6)	1.2	1.3	1.4	6.6
9	Zhi-Sou-San	74,483 (5.2)	2.8	3.4	4.0	5.7	Cang-Er-Zi (Fructus Xanthii)	84,896 (5.9)	1.1	1.2	1.3	6.5
10	Jia-Wei-Xiao-Yao-San	70,066 (4.9)	2.5	3.8	4.4	7.2	Xin-Yi (Flos Magnoliae)	68,746 (4.8)	1.2	1.3	1.4	6.3

Table 4 Three most common herbal medicine for five most common disease categories in children

Diseases categories	Herbal formulae	Frequency (%)	Single herb	Frequency (%)
Diseases of the Respiratory System	Shin-Yi-Ching-Fey-Tang	166,463 (25.7)	Gan-Cao (Radix Glycyrrhizae)	92,530 (14.3)
	Xiao-Qing-Long-Tang	121,716 (18.8)	Yu-Xing-Cao (Herba Houttuyniae)	86,083 (13.3)
	Xin-Yi-San	117,546 (18.1)	Jie-Geng (Radix Platycodi)	85,060 (13.1)
Symptoms, Signs, and Ill-Defined Conditions	Ma-Xing-Gan-Shi-Tang	39,987 (14.1)	Jie-Geng (Radix Platycodi)	39,658 (14.0)
	Shin-Yi-Ching-Fey-Tang	34,987 (12.3)	Chuan-Bei-Mu (Bulbus Fritillariae Cirrhosae)	37,366 (13.2)
	Xin-Su-San	32,792 (11.5)	Gan-Cao (Radix Glycyrrhizae)	31,433 (11.1)
Diseases of the Digestive System	Xiang-Sha-Liu-Jun-Zi-Tang	24,784 (16.1)	Shen-Qu (Massa Medicata Fermentata)	23,520 (15.3)
	Shen-Ling-Bai-Zhu-San	24,642 (16.0)	Mai-Ya (Fructus Hordei Germinatus)	21,490 (14.0)
	Bao-He-Wan	23,364 (15.2)	Shan-Zha (Fructus Crataegi)	17,203 (11.2)
Diseases of the Skin and Subcutaneous Tissue	Xiao-Feng-San	22,286 (23.9)	Lian-Qiao (Fructus Forsythiae)	20,107 (21.6)
	Qing-Shang-Fang-Feng-Tang	21,723 (23.3)	Jin-Yin-Hua (Flos Lonicerae)	15,588 (16.7)
	Zhen-Ren-Huo-Ming-Yin	15,831 (17.0)	Pu-Gong-Ying (*Taraxacum officinale*)	14,355 (15.4)
Diseases of the Genitourinary System	Jia-Wei-Xiao-Yao-San	25,164 (32.2)	Xiang-Fu (Rhizoma Cyperi)	16,977 (21.7)
	Dang-Gui-Shao-Yao-San	14,102 (18.0)	Yi-Mu-Cao (Herba Leonuri)	16,833 (21.5)
	Wen-Jing-Tang	13,049 (16.7)	Yan-Hu-Suo (Rhizoma Corydalis)	10,656 (13.6)

distributions of diseases treated with TCM concurred with our study, but their study showed a different ordering of the reasons for children's TCM visits. It indicated that respiratory system diseases remained the most common reason for children to visit TCM clinics in Taiwan in 2005 and 2010, followed by symptoms, signs, and ill-defined conditions; injury and poisoning; digestive system diseases; and diseases of the skin and subcutaneous tissue. Our findings differed from the previous study [9], indicating that musculoskeletal problems were the most common underlying medical conditions among children TCM users, followed by gastrointestinal problems and respiratory problems. Our results differed slightly when compared to the entire population of TCM users in Taiwan. As Chen's study [14] showed, the top five most common reasons for TCM visits were diseases of the respiratory system; musculoskeletal system and connective tissue; symptoms, signs, and ill-defined conditions; injury and poisoning; and diseases of the digestive system. These findings could be explained by the frequency distributions of diseases for which TCM is commonly used. TCM contributes to the treatment of these diseases and plays a significant role in improving children's health.

Additionally, a high-quality, pediatric asthma outpatient TCM clinic project was administered by Taiwan's bureau of National Health Insurance and the National Union of Chinese Medical Doctors' Association, ROC. This project benefited children with asthma [18, 19]. The project was piloted in 2006 for asthmatic children under 15 years old in and was fully implemented in 2013 for children 12 years old and under [20]. As a result of this program's positive impacts for asthmatic children, the prevalence of TCM used for children may increase. Further studies are suggested to explore these potential effects.

Chinese herbal remedies (90.6%) (Table 2) comprised most TCM visits. Among them, respiratory system diseases were the leading ailment to be treated in our study. Furthermore, we found that most top ten herbal medicines including HF and SH prescribed by physicians (Table 3) were associated with treating respiratory disease. Thus, children and adolescents with respiratory disease were more likely to use TCM, especially CHR. Injury and poisoning were the most frequent conditions associated with acupuncture traumatology use, although acupuncture therapy occurred in few TCM visits (9.4%) in our study. In line with Lu, Chang, Sung, and Chen's study [21], acupuncture is one of the most common treatment modalities used in injury management, and is likely to be common in patients with dislocations, sprains, and strains because of the effectiveness of TCM modalities on pain management and function improvement. Previous studies [22, 23] have reported that acupuncture helps in alleviating pain, chronic pain, and other conditions. Although the potential for acupuncture not to be accepted among pediatric populations exists because children are often afraid of needles, some studies have depicted pediatric acupuncture as both acceptable and feasible [24, 25]. However, different characteristics of disease may indicate different patterns of acupuncture use among children. Further studies are recommended to determine these patterns.

We further determined that SYCFT, XQLT, Xin-Yi-San in HF, and Gan-Cao, Yu-Xing-Cao, and Jie-Geng in SH, were the top three herbal medicines prescribed for diseases of the respiratory system (Table 4). Gan-Cao is commonly prescribed by TCM physicians for children because of the adjustment of taste [26, 27]. Symptoms, signs, and ill-defined conditions were the second most frequent diagnoses for TCM visits with prescriptions for CHR in our study. Furthermore, we found that HF and SH often used for diseases of the respiratory system were commonly used for symptoms, signs, and ill-defined conditions. Thus, we inferred that most patients who were treated for symptoms, signs, and ill-defined conditions suffered from diseases related to the respiratory system.

Traditionally, TCM physicians always chose therapeutic principles and methods based on syndrome differentiation theory and did not make specific diagnoses based on holistic considerations in patients with many different symptoms. Syndrome differentiation is a unique method for the diagnosis of disease in TCM, using the concepts of balance and harmony to analyze the patterns within the human body and make a diagnosis [28]. However, because younger children are unable to express themselves clearly, the diagnostic process is combined with clinical treatment into a holistic approach to determine patterns of dysfunction and treatment [29]. Moreover, there is no standard methodology in the disease coding system for TCM [13]. This may be why TCM physicians use the ICD-9-CM code for symptoms, signs, and ill-defined conditions instead of using specific diagnostic codes. It is important to develop more reliable coding systems for TCM diagnostic classifications.

Jia-Wei-Xiao-Yao-San (JWXYS) was the only exception in the top ten list in that it was not related to respiratory disease. It occupied tenth position (Table 3). However, it was the top commonly prescribed HF, followed by Dang-Gui-Shao-Yao-San (DGSYS) and Wen-Jing-Tang (WJT) for treating diseases of the genitourinary system (Table 4) in our study. Our finding is similar to previous studies [30, 31] that found DGSYS was the most commonly used HF, followed by JWXYS and WJT, to treat primary dysmenorrhea for women 13–25 years old, and 20–50 years old respectively. Dysmenorrhea is a common gynecological complaint of adolescent girls who often suffer from some level of discomfort due to menstruation [31, 32]. Our results correspond to a previous study [33], which concluded JWXYS was most often used for primary dysmenorrhea, followed by DGSYS and WJT, among HF; additionally, Xiang-Fu (Cyperus rotundus L.), Yi-Mu-Cao (Leonurus heterophyllus Sweet), and Yan-Hu-Suo (Corydalis yanhusuo W. T. Wang) were the most commonly used SH to treat diseases of the genitourinary system in our study. Furthermore, SH is often used as an adjuvant to HF; however, both SH of Xiang-Fu and Yi-Mu-Cao were prescribed more frequently than the HF of DGSYS in our study. According to TCM theory, the organs work together by regulating and preserving Qi (energy) and blood through the so-called channels and collaterals. Qi stagnation usually suggests that energy and information cannot move smoothly to or from its appropriate location [29]. Xiang-Fu is used to treat qi stagnation, and Yi-Mu-Cao is used to treat blood stasis [34]. It has been used to treat dysmenorrhea and irregular menstruation [30, 35].

XSLJZT is the most commonly prescribed HF for diseases of the digestive system. It is a common Chinese herbal prescription and used for the treatment of gastrointestinal diseases in Asian countries [36]. SLBZS enhances digestive function and removes moisture to clear digestive discomforts like diarrhea and distension [37, 38]. Shen-Qu was the most commonly prescribed SH to treat diseases of the digestive system in our study. In traditional Chinese medicine, Shen-Qu is used to treat conditions such as diarrhea, abdominal distension, and lack of appetite. Shen-Qu can also inhibit the activity of 3-hydroxy-3-methylglutaryl-coenzyme A (HMG-CoA) and maintain the balance of cholesterol in the body [39].

XFS was the most commonly prescribed HF, followed by QSFFT and Zhen-Ren-Huo-Ming-Yin, for diseases of the skin and subcutaneous tissue in our study. Previous studies [40, 41] found XFS was the most commonly prescribed Chinese herbal formula for atopic dermatitis and urticaria since it has an antipruritic effect for severe, refractory, extensive, and non-exudative atopic dermatitis [42]. Chien et al. [41] found that XFS was by far the most commonly prescribed Chinese HF for subjects with urticarial by analyzing the population-based CHM database from Taiwan. Furthermore, this herbal remedy helps address weepy, itchy, red skin lesions such as eczema, urticarial, psoriasis, and diaper rash. A previous study [43] found QSFFT was the most commonly used HF, followed by Zhen-Ren-Huo-Ming-Yin, among 279,823 CHM prescriptions to treat acne. We found Lian-Qiao, Jin-Yin-Hua, and Pu-Gong-Ying, often used as antibiotics in Chinese medicine [44, 45], were the most commonly prescribed SH for the treatment of diseases of the skin and subcutaneous tissue.

Chinese herbal products were invented about 40 years ago and have been utilized ever since [13]. There are no guidelines for children's Chinese herbal product dosages. Thus, TCM doctors typically adjust the dosage according to their clinical experience, the patient's age, and/or the patient's body weight. Our research provides the average daily dose and treatment duration for the top ten herbal medicines commonly prescribed by TCM physicians for children in Taiwan.

Conclusion

We conducted a nationwide, population-based study on the use of TCM in children 18 years of age and younger based on one randomly selected cohort from the 2005–2013 NHIRD healthcare claims data in Taiwan. TCM usage is common, with approximately 63.2% of children having been treated with it. The utilization increased with age, peaking in the 12- to 18-year-old age group. Respiratory system diseases were the most common reason for TCM treatment, and Chinese herbal remedies were the most commonly used TCM modality. Shin-Yi-Ching-Fey-Tang and Gan-Cao (Radix Glycyrrhizae) were the most commonly used formula and single herb. This study provides information about the prescription patterns of TCM and disease categories treated by TCM, which should be useful for health policy makers and for those who consider the usage of TCM for children.

Abbreviations

CCMP: Committee on Chinese Medicine and Pharmacy; CHM: Chinese herbal medicine; CHR: Chinese herbal remedies; HF: Herbal formula; ICD-9-CM: International classification of disease, 9th revision, clinical modification; JWXYS: Jia-Wei-Xiao-Yao-San; MXGST: Ma-Xin-Gan-Shi-Tang; NHI: National Health Insurance; NHIRD: National Health Insurance Research Database; SH: Single herb; SLBZS: Shen-Ling-Bai-Zhu-San; SYCFT: Shin-Yi-Ching-Fey-Tang; TCM: Traditional Chinese medicine; XFS: Xiao-Feng-San; XQLT: Xiao-Qing-Long-Tang; XSLJZT: Xiang-Sha-Liu-Jun-Zi-Tang; XYS: Xin-Yi-San

Acknowledgements

The study data were obtained from the NHIRD provided by the National Health Insurance Administration, Ministry of Health and Welfare of Taiwan, and managed by the National Health Research Institutes of Taiwan. The interpretation and conclusions contained herein do not represent those of the National Health Insurance Administration, Ministry of Health and Welfare, or National Health Research Institutes of Taiwan. Furthermore, the authors would like to thank the Health Information and Epidemiology Laboratory of Chang Gung Memorial Hospital, Chiayi Branch for the technical support services.

Funding

This study was supported by a grant from Chang Gung Memorial Hospital, Chiayi Branch (CLRPG6G0041). The funding body had no involvement in the design of the study and collection, analysis and interpretation of data and in writing of this manuscript.

Authors' contributions

HFL, YHY, and KMW conceptualized the study. YHY, PCC, and CHC performed the statistical analysis. PCC, HCK, CHC, and YHW contributed to the interpretation of TCM data. HFL and YHW contributed to the interpretation of identified patterns of TCM use among children. YHY, HCK, and YHW interpreted the pharmacological mechanisms. HFL and KMW drafted the manuscript and YHY finalized the manuscript. All authors read and approved the final manuscript.

Ethics approval and consent to participate

This study was approved by Chang Gung Medical Foundation Institutional Review Board, and access to the National Health Insurance Research Database (NHIRD) was permitted by the National Health Research Institutes in Taiwan. Since the identification numbers of all subjects in the NHIRD were encrypted to protect the privacy of the individuals, the informed consents were waived. All the lack of consent forms is in accordance with Chapter II, "Information Collection, Processing and Use by a Government Agency", of the Personal Information Protection Act of Taiwan.

Competing interests

The authors declare that they have no competing interests.

Author details

[1]Department of Nursing, Chang Gung University of Science and Technology, No.2, Sec. W., Jiapu Rd, Puzi City, Chiayi County 61363, Taiwan. [2]Chronic Diseases and Health Promotion Research Center, Chang Gung University of Science and Technology, No.2, Sec. W., Jiapu Rd, Puzi County 61363, Taiwan. [3]Chang Gung Memorial Hospital, Chiayi, No.6, Sec. W., Jiapu Rd, Puzi City, Chiayi County 61363, Taiwan. [4]Department for Traditional Chinese Medicine, Chang Gung Memorial Hospital, Chiayi, Taiwan. [5]Health Information and Epidemiology Laboratory of Chang Gung Memorial Hospital, Chiayi, Taiwan. [6]School of Traditional Chinese Medicine, College of Medicine, Chang Gung University, Taoyuan, Taiwan. [7]Institute of Occupational Medicine and Industrial Hygiene, National Taiwan University College of Public Health, Taipei, Taiwan. [8]Department of Environmental and Occupational Medicine, National Taiwan University College of Medicine and National Taiwan University Hospital, Taipei, Taiwan. [9]Department of Pediatrics, Chang Gung Memorial Hospital, Chiayi, Taiwan. [10]Department of Early Childhood Education, National Chiayi University, Chiayi, Taiwan.

References

1. Shih CC, Liao CC, Su YC, Yeh TF, Lin JG. The association between socioeconomic status and traditional chinese medicine use among children in Taiwan. BMC Health Serv Res. 2012;12:27.
2. Du Y, Wolf IK, Zhuang W, Bodemann S, Knöss W, Knopf H. Use of herbal medicinal products among children and adolescents in Germany. BMC Complement Altern Med. 2014;14:218.
3. Yeh YH, Chou YJ, Huang N, Pu C, Chou P. The trends of utilization in traditional Chinese medicine in Taiwan from 2000 to 2010: a population-based study. Medicine. 2016;95(27):e4115.

4. Mitidieri A, Gurian MB, Silva AP, Tawasha K, Poli-Neto O, Nogueira A, et al. Evaluation of women with myofascial abdominal syndrome based on traditional Chinese medicine. Aust J Pharm. 2015;18(4):26–31.

5. Chen YC, Lin YH, Hu S, Chen HY. Characteristics of traditional Chinese medicine users and prescription analysis for pediatric atopic dermatitis: a population-based study. BMC Complement Altern Med. 2016;16:173.

6. Huang TP, Liu PH, Lien AS, Yang SL, Chang HH, Yen HR. A nationwide population-based study of traditional Chinese medicine usage in children in Taiwan. Complement Ther Med. 2014;22(3):500–10.

7. Hon KL, Ma KC, Wong Y, Leung TF, Fok TF. A survey of traditional Chinese medicine use in children with atopic dermatitis attending a paediatric dermatology clinic. J Dermatolog Treat. 2005;16(3):154–7.

8. Loh CH. Use of traditional Chinese medicine in Singapore children: perceptions of parents and paediatricians. Singap Med J. 2009;50(12):1162–8.

9. Chen HY, Lin YH, Wu JC, Chen YC, Thien PF, Chen TJ, et al. Characteristics of pediatric traditional Chinese medicine users in Taiwan: a nationwide cohort study. Pediatrics. 2012;129(6):e1485–92.

10. Poole RL, Carleton BC. Medication errors: neonates, infants and children are the most vulnerable. J Pediatr Pharmacol Ther. 2008;13(2):65–7.

11. Wu TY, Majeed A, Kuo KN. An overview of the healthcare system in Taiwan. London J Prim Care (Abingdon). 2010;3(2):115–9.

12. National Health Insurance Administration. Statistical annual reports, the National Health Insurance Statistics, 2015. In Edited by Ministry of Health and Welfare, Taiwan.

13. Yang YH, Chen PC, Wang JD, Lee CH, Lai JN. Prescription pattern of traditional Chinese medicine for climacteric women in Taiwan. Climacteric. 2009;12(6):541–7.

14. Chen FP, Chen TJ, Kung YY, Chen YC, Chou LF, Chen FJ, et al. Use frequency of traditional Chinese medicine in Taiwan. BMC Health Serv Res. 2007;7:26.

15. Genc RE, Senol S, Turgay AS, Kantar M. Complementary and alternative medicine used by pediatric patients with cancer in western Turkey. Oncol Nurs Forum. 2009;36(3):E159–64.

16. Walker DM, Bell MR. Adolescence and reward: making sense of neural and behavioral changes amid the chaos. J Neurosci. 2017;37(45):10855–66.

17. Lin YC, Chang TT, Chen HJ, Wang CH, Sun MF, Yen HR. Characteristics of traditional Chinese medicine usage in children with precocious puberty: a nationwide population-based study. J Ethnopharmacol. 2017;205:231–9.

18. Chung YY, Lin YT, Lin JC. Effectiveness analysis of Chinese medicine pediatric asthma trial project and future development. Taiwan J Chin Med. 2013;11(1):27–37.

19. Liao PS, Chen CL, Hsieh YH, Hou YC. Research on the health service quality in traditional Chinese medicine-ßased on traditional Chinese medical highquality outpatient clinic pilot project of pediatric asthma in remission stage. J Integr Chin West Med. 2010;12(1):11–20.

20. National Health Insurance. High-quality care to relieve pediatric asthma in TCM. In Edited by National Health Insurance. National Health Insurance Bimonthly. 2014;109:30–33.

21. Lu CY, Chang HH, Sung FC, Chen PC. Characteristics of traditional Chinese medicine use in pediatric dislocations, sprains and strains. Int J Environ Res Public Health. 2017;14(2):153.

22. Kemper KJ, Sarah R, Silver-Highfield E, Xiarhos E, Barnes L, Berde C. On pins and needles? Pediatric pain patients' experience with acupuncture. Pediatrics. 2000;105(4 Pt 2):941–7.

23. Lin YC, Tassone RF, Jahng S, Rahbar R, Holzman RS, Zurakowski D, et al. Acupuncture management of pain and emergence agitation in children after bilateral myringotomy and tympanostomy tube insertion. Paediatr Anaesth. 2009;19(11):1096–101.

24. Zeltzer LK, Tsao JC, Stelling C, Powers M, Levy S, Waterhouse M. A phase I study on the feasibility and acceptability of an acupuncture/hypnosis intervention for chronic pediatric pain. J Pain Symptom Manag. 2002;24(4):437–46.

25. Brittner M, Le Pertel N, Gold MA. Acupuncture in Pediatrics. Curr Probl Pediatr Adolesc Health Care. 2016;46(6):179–83.

26. Ho SQ. Zhang Zhongjing views of Gan-Cao. J Chin Clin. 2003;31(7):52–3.

27. Zhang Q, Ye M. Chemical analysis of the Chinese herbal medicine Gan-Cao (licorice). J Chromatogr A. 2009;1216(11):1954–69.

28. Lu AP, Jia HW, Xiao C, Lu QP. Theory of traditional Chinese medicine and therapeutic method of diseases. World J Gastroenterol. 2004;10(13):1854–6.

29. Mei MF. A systematic analysis of the theory and practice of syndrome differentiation. Chin J Integr Med. 2011;17(11):803–10.

30. Chen HY, Huang BS, Lin YH, Su IH, Yang SH, Chen JL, et al. Identifying Chinese herbal medicine for premenstrual syndrome: implications from a nationwide database. BMC Complement Altern Med. 2014;14:206.

31. Pan JC, Tsai YT, Lai JN, Fang RC, Yeh CH. The traditional Chinese medicine prescription pattern of patients with primary dysmenorrhea in Taiwan: a large-scale cross sectional survey. J Ethnopharmacol. 2014;152(2):314–9.

32. Yeh LL, Liu JY, Lin KS, Liu YS, Chiou JM, Liang KY, et al. A randomised placebo-controlled trial of a traditional Chinese herbal formula in the treatment of primary dysmenorrhoea. PLoS One. 2007;2(8):e719.

33. Chen HY, Lin YH, Su IH, Chen YC, Yang SH, Chen JL. Investigation on Chinese herbal medicine for primary dysmenorrhea: implication from a nationwide prescription database in Taiwan. Complement Ther Med. 2014;22(1):116–25.

34. Lin YR, Wu MY, Chiang JH, Yen HR, Yang ST. The utilization of traditional Chinese medicine in patients with dysfunctional uterine bleeding in Taiwan: a nationwide population-based study. BMC Complement Altern Med. 2017;17(1):427.

35. Chen Z, Wu JB, Liao XJ, Yang W, Song K. Development and validation of an UPLC-DAD-MS method for the determination of leonurine in Chinese motherwort (Leonurus japonicus). J Chromatogr Sci. 2010;48(10):802–6.

36. Xiao Y, Liu YY, Yu KQ, Ouyang MZ, Luo R, Zhao XS. Chinese herbal medicine liu jun zi tang and xiang sha liu jun zi tang for functional dyspepsia: meta-analysis of randomized controlled trials. Evid Based Complement Alternat Med. 2012;2012:936459.

37. Chang CH, Cheng PY. Treatment of diarrhea-predominant IBS with Shenling Baizhu powder a case sduty. Taiwan J Clin Chin Med. 2009;15(2):118–21.

38. Liu J. Shen Ling Bai Zhu San and its clinical application. Mintong Med J. 2014;452:14–6.

39. Chen JK, Chen T. Chinese medical herbology and pharmacology. City of Industry: Art of Medicine Press; 2004.

40. Chen HY, Lin YH, Huang JW, Chen YC. Chinese herbal medicine network and core treatments for allergic skin diseases: implications from a nationwide database. J Ethnopharmacol. 2015;168:260–7.

41. Chien PS, Tseng YF, Hsu YC, Lai YK, Weng SF. Frequency and pattern of Chinese herbal medicine prescriptions for urticaria in Taiwan during 2009: analysis of the national health insurance database. BMC Complement Altern Med. 2013;13:209.

42. Cheng HM, Chiang LC, Jan YM, Chen GW, Li TC. The efficacy and safety of a Chinese herbal product (Xiao-Feng-San) for the treatment of refractory atopic dermatitis: a randomized, double-blind, placebo-controlled trial. Int Arch Allergy Immunol. 2011;155(2):141–8.

43. Chen HY, Lin YH, Chen YC. Identifying Chinese herbal medicine network for treating acne: implications from a nationwide database. J Ethnopharmacol. 2016;179:1–8.

44. Bing-sheng X. A botanical study of the Chinese drug Jin-yin-hua (author's transl). Yao Xue Xue Bao. 1979;14(1):23–34.

45. Wong RW, Hagg U, Samaranayake L, Yuen MK, Seneviratne CJ, Kao R. Antimicrobial activity of Chinese medicine herbs against common bacteria in oral biofilm. A pilot study. Int J Oral Maxillofac Surg. 2010;39(6):599–605.

10

Extract of *Stellerachamaejasme L*(ESC) inhibits growth and metastasis of human hepatocellular carcinoma via regulating microRNA expression

Xiaoni Liu[1], Shuang Wang[1], Jianji Xu[1], Buxin Kou[1], Dexi Chen[1], Yajie Wang[2] and Xiaoxin Zhu[2*]

Abstract

Background: MicroRNAs(miRNAs)are involved in the initiation and progression of hepatocellular carcinoma. ESC, an extract of *Stellerachamaejasme L*, had been confirmed as a potential anti-tumor extract of Traditional Chinese Medicine. In light of the important role of miRNAs in hepatocellular carcinoma, we questioned whether the inhibitory effects of ESC on hepatocellular carcinoma (HCC) were associated with miRNAs.

Methods: The proliferation inhibition of ESC on HCC cells was measured with MTT assay. The migration inhibition of ESC on HCC cells was measured with transwell assay. The influences of ESC on growth and metastasis inhibition were evaluated with xenograft tumor model of HCC. Protein expressions were measured with western blot and immunofluorescence methods and miRNA profiles were detected with miRNA array. Differential miRNA and target mRNAs were verified with real-time PCR.

Results: The results showed that ESC could inhibit proliferation and epithelial mesenchymal transition (EMT) in HCC cells in vitro and tumor growth and metastasis in xenograft models in vivo. miRNA array results showed that 69 differential miRNAs in total of 429 ones were obtained in MHCC97H cells treated by ESC. hsa-miR-107, hsa-miR-638, hsa-miR-106b-5p were selected to be validated with real-time PCR method in HepG2 and MHCC97H cells. Expressions of hsa-miR-107 and hsa-miR-638 increased obviously in HCC cells treated by ESC. Target genes of three miRNAs were also validated with real-time PCR. Interestingly, only target genes of hsa-miR-107 changed greatly. ESC downregulated the MCL1, SALL4 and BCL2 gene expressions significantly but did not influence the expression of CACNA2D1.

Conclusion: The findings suggested ESC regressed growth and metastasis of human hepatocellular carcinoma via regulating microRNAs expression and their corresponding target genes.

Keywords: Hepatocellular carcinoma, microRNA, *Stellerachamaejasme L*, Target gene, MCL1, SALL4, BCL2

Background

MicroRNAs (miRNAs) are small non-coding RNAs characterized by a length of 18–25 nucleotides and capable of binding to complementary 3′UTR regions of their target genes, thereby modulating the transcription of the target mRNA [1]. Mounting evidences have demonstrated that miRNAs are involved in the initiation and progression of several types of human cancer, including hepatocellular carcinoma (HCC), which is one of the most common types of cancer and the third leading cause of cancer-related mortality worldwide [2]. It was recently demonstrated that miRNAs played critical roles in HCC progression and directly contributed to tumor cell proliferation, avoidance of apoptotic cell death and metastasis by targeting a large number of specific mRNAs. miRNAs may undergo aberrant regulation during carcinogenesis and act as oncogenes or tumor suppressor genes in HCC [3–6].

* Correspondence: zhuxx59@163.com
[2]Institute of Chinese Materia Medica, China Academy of Chinese Medical Sciences, No 16 Nan Xiao Jie, Dong Zhi Men Nei, Dong Cheng Qu, Beijing 100700, China
Full list of author information is available at the end of the article

ESC, an extract of *StellerachamaejasmeL*, rich in isomers of *Chamaejasminor, neochamaejasmine* and *Sikokianin* [7], had antitumor effects by activating apoptosis pathway and reversed EMT of tumor cells induced by TGF-β via inhibition of Smad signaling pathway in our previous studies [8, 9]. ESC had been confirmed as a potential anti-tumor extract of Traditional Chinese Medicine.

In light of the important role of miRNAs in hepatocellular carcinoma, we questioned whether the inhibitory effects of ESC on hepatocellular carcinoma were associated with miRNAs. To figure out this question, this study was performed to evaluate modulatory effect of ESC on miRNAs expression in hepatocellular carcinoma in order to clarify the molecular mechanisms of ESC on hepatocellular carcinoma.

Methods
Preparation of ESC
ESC was provided and identified by Hong Bin Xiao (China Academy of Chinese Medical Sciences, Beijing, People's Republic of China), which has been deposited in Institute of Chinese Materia Medica, China Academy of Chinese Medical Sciences(Deposition number:ICMM-001). The extract method was as follows: *Stelleracha-maejasme L* herbal medicine was extracted 3 times with ethanol. Meanwhile, the concentrated liquid (volatile to non-alcohol taste) was washed on a polyamide column with 60% ethanol, and then decompressively recycled and vacuum dried at room temperature. The final compound obtained was ESC.

Reagents and antibodies
Trypsin-ethylene-diaminetetraacetic acid and DMEM medium were purchased from Gibco (Grand Island, NY, USA); Fetal bovine serum was from China Hangzhou Sijiqing Biological Technology Co.,Ltd.; 3-(4,5-dimethyl-2-thiazolyl)-2,5-diphenyl-2-H-tetrazolium bromide (MTT) and dimethylsulfoxide (DMSO) were provided by Sigma Chemical Co. (St. Louis, MO,USA); Caspase 3, E-cadherin, Vimentin and β-actin primary monoclonal antibody were purchased from Abcam Ltd. (Cambridgem MA, USA); Matrigel was from BD Biosciences (Los Angeles, CA, USA); Crystal violet was from Beijing Solarbio Science and Technology Co., Ltd.; Trizoland SuperScript™ III Reverse Transcriptase was from Invitrogen; RT Primers were synthesized by Invitrogen Biotechnology Co. Ltd.; PCR kit was from Arraystar INC. miRCURYTM Array Power Labeling kit and miRCURY™ Array were from Exiqon.

Cell line and cell culture
HepG2, HepG2-luc and MHCC97H liver cancer cell lines were preserved in Beijing Institute of Hepatology. Cells were cultured in DMEM medium supplemented with 10% fetal bovine serum and maintained at 37 °C in a humidified incubator with 5% CO2.

Animals and animal feeding
Four-week-old male balb/c nude mice (from Beijing Vital River Laboratory Animal Technology Co. Ltd) were raised and maintained in individually ventilated cages (IVC) under specific pathogen free sterile condition.

MTT assay
Cells in the logarithmic growth phase were plated in 96-well plates in a seeding density of 2500–3000 cells per well and incubated in a 37 °C incubator with 5% CO2 overnight. After cells were treated with different concentration ESC for 24, 48, 72 h, the culture medium in each well was abandoned, incubating with 0.5 g/L MTT 100 µL for 4 h. Then each well was added with 150 µL DMSO and vibrated for 10 min, and absorbance of each well was detected with microplate reader (ELX800 type, BIO-TEX Instruments, INC, Winooski, VT, USA) at the 490 nm wave length. The inhibition rate (IR) was calculated as follows: IR (%) = $(1 - OD_{treatment}/OD_{control}) \times 100\%$. Half-maximal inhibitory concentration (IC_{50}) was determined by logistic method.

Transwell assay
The migration experiment was analyzed in 24-well transwell plates (Corning Incorporated). 2×10^4 cells in 100 µL of DMEM medium with 1% BSA and different concentrations of ESC were added to the top chamber and 500 µL of 10% serum-containing DMEM was added in the bottom chamber. The cells were then incubated at 37 °C with 5% CO2 for 24 h. After incubation, the medium was removed, and non-invading cells were scrubbed by a wet cotton swab. The invading cells were washed by PBS for three times and fixed by 4% paraformaldehyde for 15 min. Fixed cells were washed three times by PBS and stained by 0.1% crystal violet in PBS for 10 min. Excess stain was washed by distilled water for three times. The migration cells were counted in five random fields in the same area for unbiased measurement using an inverted microscope.

Western blot assay
Cells were seeded in 100 mm tissue culture dishes at the density of 2×10^6 cells per dish and incubated for overnight. Cells were then treated with various agents as indicated in figure legends, then washed with ice-cold PBS and harvested in 400 µL of cell lysis buffer. The protein concentrations of lysates were determined using the bicinchonininc acid method. Cell lysates (40 µg protein per lane) were separated using 10% SDS-PAGE and transferred electrophoretically to polyvinylidenediluoride membrane. Membranes were blocked with tris-buffered

saline/0.1% tween 20 containing 5% bovine serum albumin and then incubated overnight at 4 °C with primary antibodies (1:1000). Membranes were washed three times with TBST and incubated for 1 h at room temperature with the appropriate secondary antibody conjugated to goat anti-rabbit horseradish peroxidase (1:2000). Membranes were then washed and immunoreactive bands were developed with ECL and visualized by autoradiography. Protein loading was normalized using β-actin antibody. Gray-scale analysis of protein bands was performed using image software.

Immunofluorescence analysis

Cells were seeded into 24-well plates and treated as described as figure legends. Cells were fixed with 4% formaldehyde for 30 min, washed with PBS, blocked with 5% BSA for 30 min at room temperature, and then stained with anti-human primary antibody (1:100) at 4 °C overnight. Cells were incubated with anti-rabbit-FITC secondary antibody (1:500) for 2 h at 4 °C, and then washed with PBS. Cells were then incubated for 10 min at room temperature with DAPI to stain nuclei, washed twice with PBS, and observed using an inverted fluorescence microscope (Olympus, Japan).

Influence of ESC on Xenograft tumor models

3×10^6 HepG2-luc cells were inoculated in nude mice subcutaneously to establish xenograft tumors which must be transplanted into nude mice for 3 generations. The tumor tissues in the growth period were cut into about 1.5 mm^3 and were inoculated in the right armpit skin and liver of nude mice under the condition of sterile. 3–6 days after transplantation, the mice were divided into groups according to the tumor growth observed by in vivo imaging system. Every group contained 6 mice. Then the mice were injected intraperitoneally with ESC indifferent dose according to the MTD (maximum tolerant dosage) experiment. The sizes of subcutaneous tumors were measured with caliper and in vivo imaging and orthotopic tumors were observed by in vivo imaging. At the endpoint of the experiment, nude mice were sacrificed with cervical dislocation. The tumor samples were collected according to the follow-up experiments. The tumor growth inhibition rates and relative tumor volumes (RTV) were calculated, RTV=Vt/V0 (Vt, the volumes of tumors of every calculation; V0, the volumes of tumors of initial administration).

miRNA expression profiles of cancer cells treated with ESC

The experimental MHCC-97H cells were treated with the ESC (final concentration was 25 mg/mL) for 24 h. The control MHCC-97H cells were treated with vehicle agent for 24 h. Total RNA of cells was isolated using trizol and purified with RNeasy mini kit (QIAGEN)

according to manufacturer's instructions. RNA quality and quantity were measured by using nanodrop spectrophotometer (ND-1000, Nanodrop Technologies) and RNA integrity was determined by gel electrophoresis.

RNA labeling and array hybridization were according to Exiqon's manual.1μLRNA in 2.0 μL of water was combined with 1.0 μL of CIP buffer and CIP (Exiqon). The mixture was incubated for 30 min at 37 °C. The reaction was terminated by incubation for 5 min at 95 °C. Then 3.0 μL of labeling buffer, 1.5 μL of fluorescent label (Hy3TM), 2.0 μL of DMSO, 2.0 μL of labeling enzyme were added into the mixture. The labeling reaction was incubated for 1 h at 16 °C. Terminated by incubation for 15 min at 65 °C. After stopping the labeling procedure, the Hy3™-labeled samples were hybridized on the miR-CURYTM LNA Array (v.18.0) (Exiqon) according to array manual. The total 25 μL mixture from Hy3™-labeled samples with 25 μL hybridization buffer were first denatured for 2 min at 95 °C, incubated on ice for 2 min. Then hybridized to the microarray for 16–20 h at 56 °C in a Hybridization Systems (Hybridization System-Nimblegen Systems, Inc., Madison, WI, USA). Following hybridization, the slides were achieved, washed several times using Wash buffer kit (Exiqon). Then the slides were scanned using the Axon GenePix 4000B microarray scanner (Axon Instruments, Foster City, CA).

Evaluation of the expression level of miRNAs and target genes

The expression level of miRNAs and target genes were measured and validated with real-time PCR. The methods were described as follows: 1.0 μg RNA, 1 μL0.5 μg/μLOligo (dT), 1.6 μL DNTPs Mix (2.5 mM) and RNAase free water 10.9 μL were made into annealing mixture.

The mixture was at 65 °C for 5 min and on ice for 2 min. After brief centrifugation, centrifugal pipe was added sequentially with RT mixture (4 μL 5X First-Strand Buffer, 1 μL 0.1 μM DTT, 0.3 μL RNase Inhibitor and 0.2 μL SuperScript III RT).

Then the mixture was incubated at 37 °C for 1 min, at 50 °C for 1 min, at 70 °C for 15 min, then the cDNAs were stored – 20 °C to be used.

PCR Realtime reaction system contained 5 μL 2 × Master Mix, 0.5μL10μM PCR forward primer, 0.5μL10μM PCR Reverse primer and 4 μL ddH$_2$O. Primer sequences of validating genes were in Table 1.

After the reaction was mixed and centrifuged with 5000 rpm, 8 μl mixed solution was added into 384PCR plates, and then 2 μL cDNA was added correspondingly. The reaction system was centrifuged briefly to mix. Three hundred eighty-four plates were placed on the PCR instrument (BIO-RAD) and all indicators were carried out according to the following

Table 1

Validating genes	Primer sequences
has-miR-638	F:5'-ATCCAGTGCGTGTCGTG-3'
	R:5'-TGCTAGGGATCGCGGGCGGGTG-3'
has-miR-107	F:5'-ATACCGCTCGAGTGCCATGTGTCCACTGAAT-3'
	R:5'-ATACCGCTCGAGTTCCATGCCTCAACTCCTCT-3'
has-miR-106-5p	F:5'-GGGGGTAAAGTGCTGACAGT-3'
	R:5'-GTGCGTGTCGTGGAGTCG-3'
U6	F:5'-GCTTCGGCAGCACATATACTAAAAT-3'
	R:5'-CGCTTCACGAATTTGCGTGTCAT-3'
CDK2	F:5'-GTGGGCCCGGCAAGATTTTAG-3'
	R:5'-GCCGAAATCCGCTTGTTAGGG-3'
SOX2	F:5'-CACATGAAGGAGCACCCGGATTAT-3'
	R:5'-GTTCATGTGCGCGTAACTGTCCAT-3'
STAT3	F:5'-TGGAAATAATGGTGAAGGTGC-3'
	R:5'-ATCTGGGGTTTGGCTGTGT-3'
Bcl2	F:5'-AGTGGGATGCGGGAGATGTG-3'
	R:5'-GGGATGCGGCTGGATGGG-3'
Mcl1	F:5'-TAAGGACAAAACGGGACTGG-3'
	R:5'-ACCAGCTCCTACTCCAGCAA-3'
CACNA2D1	F:5'-GACTGACCAACACCACTCTTCAC-3'
	R:5'-CT ATCGTACCTCAGCTCCTTCC-3'
SALL4	F:5'-CCAAAGGCAACTTAAAGGTTCAC-3'
	R:5'-CCGTGAAGACCAATGAGATCTCC-3'

procedures: 95 °C, 10 min; 40 circles of PCR(95 °C, 10s;60 °C,60 s). To establish the melting curve of PCR products, after amplified reaction was over, procedures were accorded as follows: °C,10s; 60 °C,60s; 95 °C,15 s and temperature was increased slowly from 60 °C to 95 °C(0.05 °C/s). The relative increase in reporter fluorescent dye emission was monitored. The level mRNA, relative to actin, was calculated using the formula: Relative mRNA expression = $2^{\wedge}$ [ct (validating genes$_{control}$) − ct (validating genes$_{ESC}$) + ct (U6$_{ESC}$) − ct (U6$_{control}$)], where ct is defined as the number of the cycle in which emission exceeds an arbitrarily defined threshold.

Statistical analysis
All data are the means of three determinations and data were analyzed using the SPSS Package for Windows (Version 16). Statistical analysis of the data was performed with ANOVA. Differences with $P < 0.05$ were considered statistically significant.

Results
Growth inhibition of ESC in HepG2 cells and MHCC97H cells
The inhibition rates of 25–125 µg/mL ESC at 24 h in HepG2 cells were respectively – 10.28%, 28.37%, 44.82%, 54.63%, 61.33%; the inhibition rates of 25–125 µg/mL ESC at 48 h HepG2 cells were respectively 15.62%,48.59%, 54.32%,74.97%,81.52%; the inhibition rates of 25–125 µg/ mL ESC at 72 h HepG2 cells were respectively 16.16%,61.89%,74.32%,84.09%,88.23% (Fig. 1a). IC50

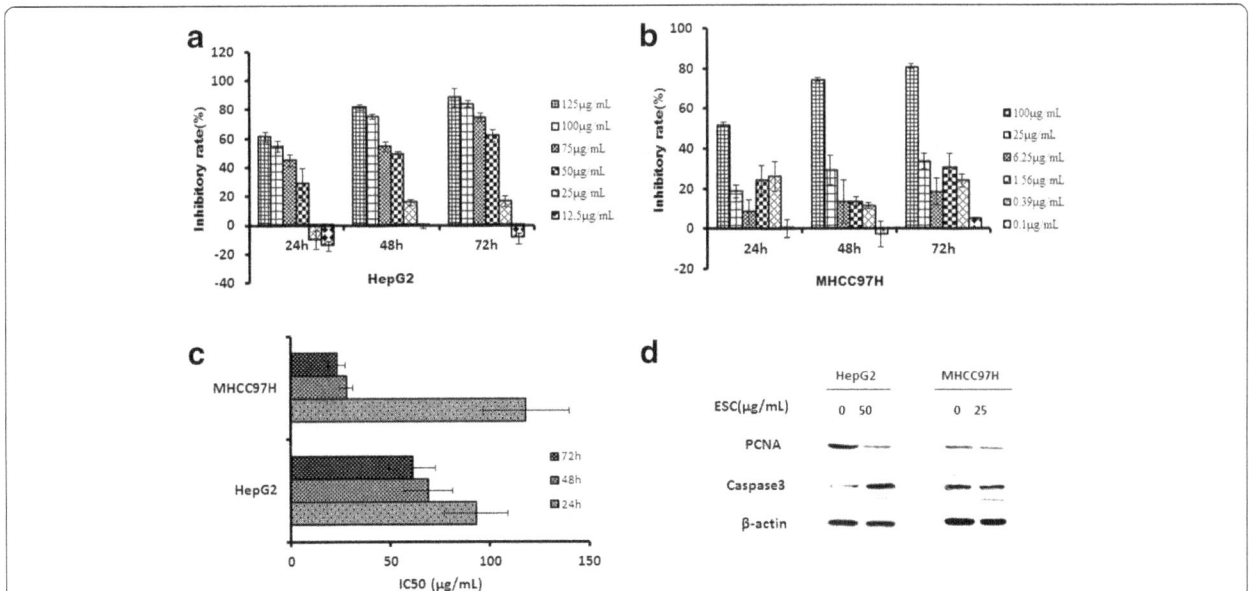

Fig. 1 Growth inhibition of ESC in HepG2 cells and MHCC97H cells. a Inhibition rates of ESC in HepG2 cells at 24, 48,72 h. b Inhibition rates of ESC in MHCC97H cells at 24, 48,72 h. c IC50 values of ESC in HepG2 and MHCC97H cells at 24, 48,72 h. d Influence of ESC on PCNA and caspases 3 expression in HepG2 cells and MHCC97H cells with western blot method

values at 24,48,72 h were respectively 92.95, 68.96, 61.06 μg/mL (Fig. 1c). These results suggested 25–125 μg/mL ESC had a significant inhibitory effect on HepG2 cells and this effect showed a certain dose and time dependence. 50 μg/mL ESC can significantly inhibit of PCNA and increase Caspase3 protein expression at 24 h in HepG2 cells (Fig. 1d). The inhibition rates of 0.39–125 μg/mL ESC at 24 h in MHCC97H cells were respectively 26.27%, 24.37%, 8.38%, 18.65%,52.03%; the inhibition rates of 0.39–125 μg/mL ESC at 48 h in MHCC97H cells were respectively 11.39%,13.63%,13.50% ,29.06%,74.30%; the inhibition rates of 25–125 μg/mL ESC at 72 h in MHCC97H cells were respectively 24.24%,30.56%,18.60%,33.67%,81.03% (Fig. 1b). IC50 values at 24,48,72 h were respectively 118.23, 27.79, 23.08 μg/mL (Fig. 1c). These results suggested 0.39–125 μg/mL ESC had a significant inhibitory effect on MHCC97H cells and this effect showed certain dose dependence. 25 μg/mL ESC can also slightly inhibit of PCNA and increase Caspase3 protein expression at 24 h in MHCC97H cells (Fig. 1d).

EMT inhibition of ESC in HepG2 cells and MHCC97H cells

Immunofluorescence results showed that 50 μg/mL ESC can obviously reduce the expression of vimentin protein inHepG2 and 25 μg/mLESC can significantly upregulate E-cadherin protein expression in MHCC97H cells (Fig. 2a). In MHCC97H, less than inhibitory concentration of 0.05 μg/mL ESC can inhibit obviously cell migration using transwell assay and the expression of vimentin with western blot method (Fig. 2b and c). These results suggested that ESC can inhibit EMT in HepG2 cells and MHCC97H cells.

Growth and metastasis inhibition of ESC on xenograft models of HepG2 cells

Nude mice bearing tumors could be tolerated 2,4 mg/kg doses of ESC, and the weight loss was always less than 20% during the whole experiment. 2,4 mg/kg ESC could significantly inhibit the relative tumor volume of subcutaneous xenograft hepatocellular carcinoma (Fig. 3a). In vivo imaging showed that 2,4 mg/kg ESC significantly inhibited fluorescence density value of tumor interior. Tumor growth inhibition rates of 2,4 mg/kg ESC were respectively 43.01% and 32.49%. Fluorescence reduction rates of 2,4 mg/kg ESC were respectively 22.29% and 14.03%(Fig. 3b). 2 mg/kg ESC could also significantly inhibit fluorescence density value of tumor interior in orthotopic xenograft nude mice and inhibited intrahepatic metastasis rate. Intrahepatic metastasis rates of control and 2 mg/kg ESC groups were respectively 67% and 16.67%. Fluorescence reduction rate of 2 mg/kg ESC was 49.30% (Fig. 3c). Pathological tissue showed severe necrosis in tumor tissues of subcutaneous xenograft nude mice and infiltration by inflammatory cells in orthotopic tumor tissues after treatment with ESC (Fig. 3d). These results suggested that ESC could inhibit the growth and metastasis of hepatocellular carcinoma.

miRNA expression profiles of HCC cells treated with ESC

RNAs ofMHCC97H cells were extracted to screen differential miRNAs after being treated with 25 μg/mL ESC. 35 up-regulated and 34 down-regulated miRNAs were detected in total of 429 miRNAs in accordance with the standard (fluorescence value change> 1.5 times and have significant difference between ESC and control group) (Fig. 4a). Among of them, 12miRNAs (hsa-miR-139-5p,

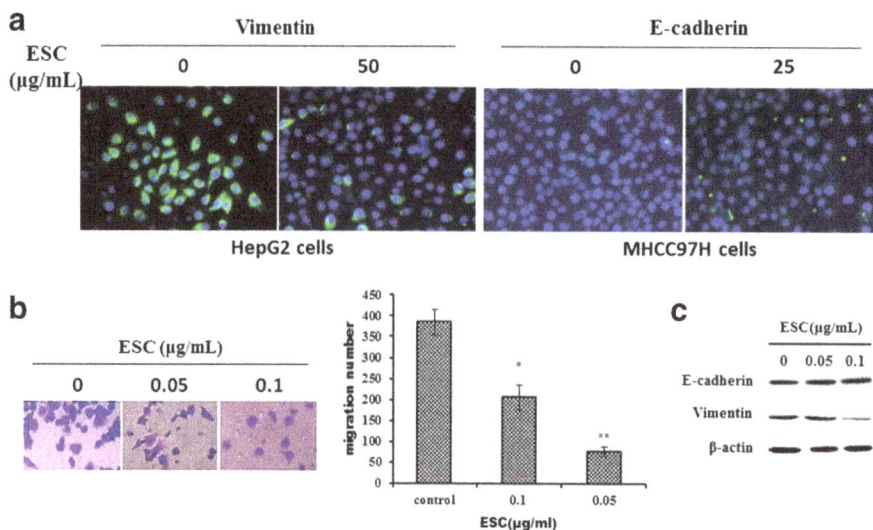

Fig. 2 EMT inhibition of ESC in HepG2 cells and MHCC97H cells. **a** Influence of ESC on Vimentin and E-cadherin expression in HepG2 cells and MHCC97H cells with immunofluorescence assay at 24 h. **b** Influence of ESC on MHCC97H cells migration with transwell assay at 24 h. **c** Influence of ESC on Vimentin and E-cadherin expression in MHCC97H cells with western blot method at 24 h. *p < 0.05, **p < 0.01vs control

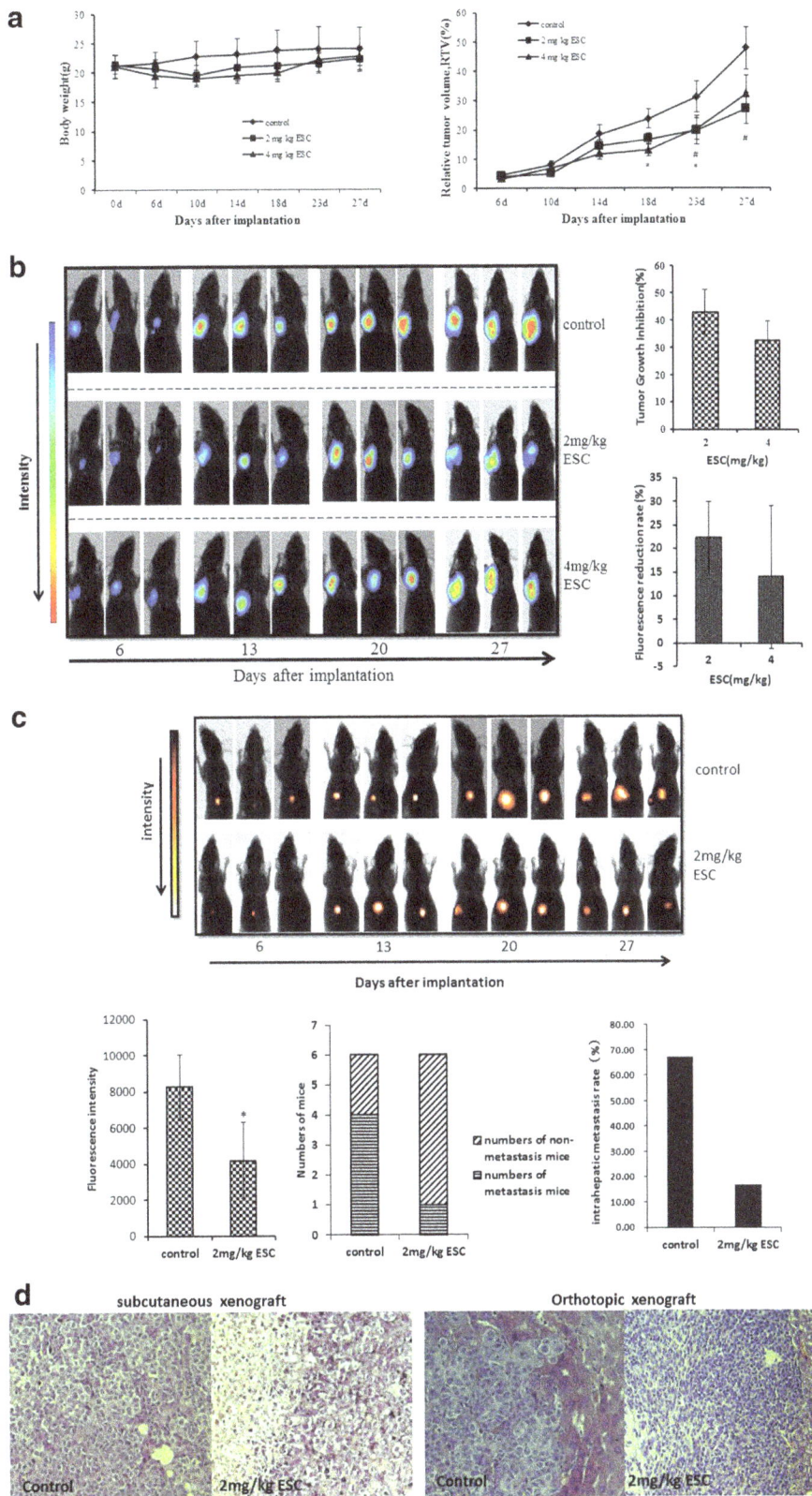

Fig. 3 (See legend on next page.)

(See figure on previous page.)
Fig. 3 Growth and metastasis inhibition of ESC on xenograft tumor models mice of HepG2 cells. **a** Changes of body weight and RTV of subcutaneous xenograft model mice of HepG2cells after treated with ESC. **b** Influence of ESC on subcutaneous xenograft tumor models mice of HepG2 cells by in vivo imaging. **c** Influence of ESC on orthotopic xenograft tumor models mice of HepG2 cells by in vivo imaging. **d** Hemetoxylin and Eosin Stains of xenograft tumor tissues (× 100)

hsa-miR-638, hsa-miR-107, hsa-miR-331-3p, hsa-miR-21-3p, hsa-miR-134-5p, hsa-miR-16-1-3p, hsa-miR-339-5p, hsa-miR-106b-5p, hsa-miR-423-3p, hsa-miR-491-3p, hsa-miR-24-3p) were related to cancers. According to the professional knowledge and literature (Table 2), 3 differential miRNAs (hsa-miR-107, hsa-miR-638, hsa-miR-106b-5p) that related to cancers were singled out for real-time PCR validation. Real-time PCR results showed that hsa-miR-107, hsa-miR-638 expressions were obviously different in MHCC97H cells and the difference of hsa-miR-107 in the HepG2 cells was obviously observed (Fig. 4b).

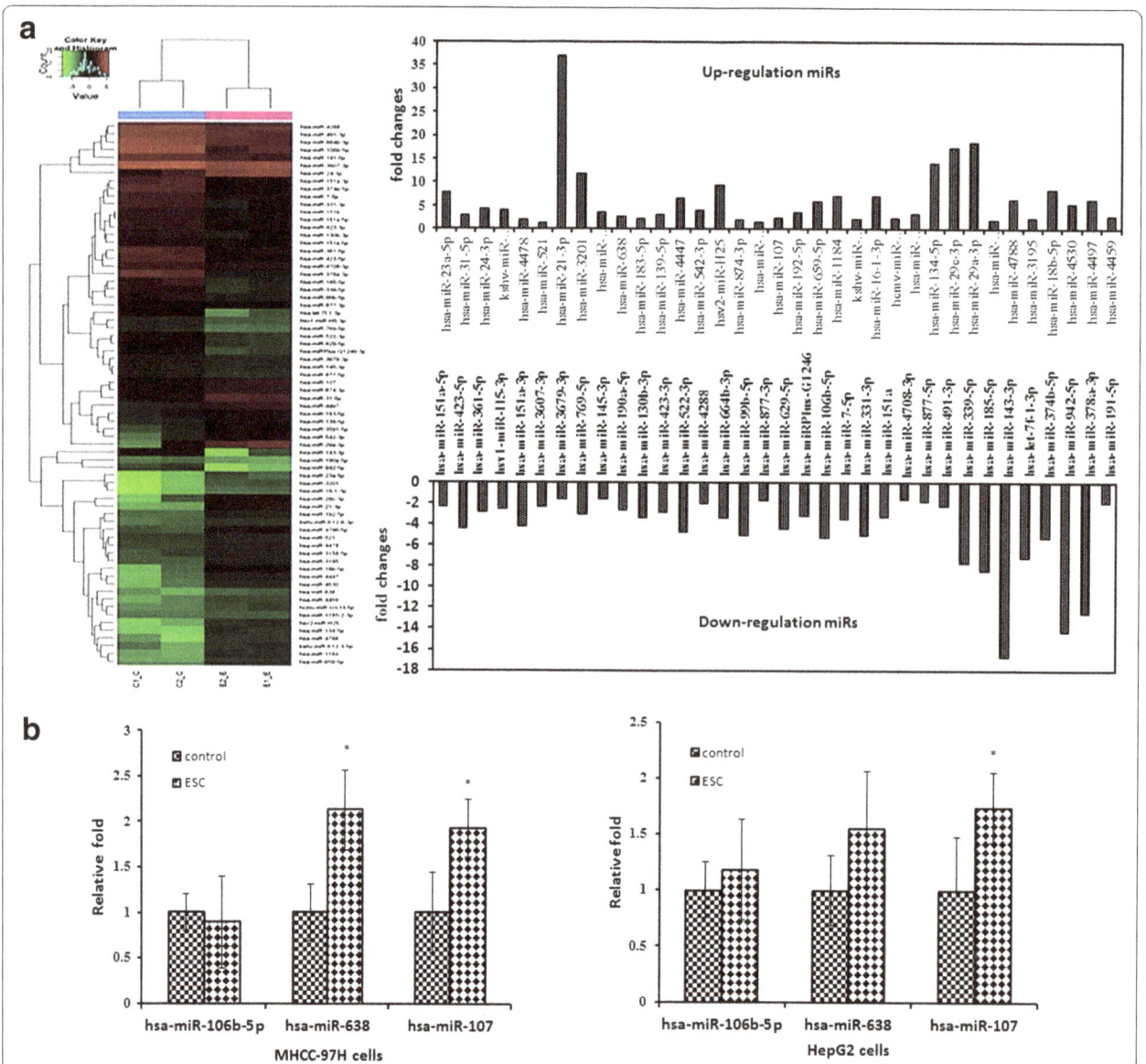

Fig. 4 miRNA expression profiles of HCC cells treated with ESC. **a** Profile of miRNAs of MHCC97H cells treated with ESC. **b** Part differential miRNA expressions were verified with realtime PCR in MHCC97H and HepG2 cells. *p < 0.05, **p < 0.01vs control

Table 2 Part differential miRNAs involving with cancers

miRNAs	Fold change	P-value	miRNA related to cancers	References
has-miR-638	2.97	0.02	Non-small cell lung cancer	[24–26]
			Melanoma	[27]
			Leukemia	[28]
			Hepatocellular cancer	[29]
			Colorectal carcinoma	[29–32, 15]
			Breast cancer	[33]
			Gastric cancer	[34]
			Cervical cancer	[35]
has-miR-107	2.56	0.04	Gastric adenocarcinoma	[36, 37]
			Glioma	[38, 39]
			Non-small cell lung cancer	[40]
			Cervical cancer	[14]
			Leukemia	[41]
			Colorectal cancer	[42]
			Neck squamous cell carcinoma	[15]
has-miR-106-5p	0.19	0.03	Pancreatic cancer	[43]
			Renal carcinoma	[44]
			Glioma	[45]
			Colorectal cancer	[13]
			Breast cancer	[46]

Evaluation of the expression level of target genes

According to the bioinformatics prediction and references (Table 3), we chose target genes STAT3, CACNA2D1, SALL4, MCL1, CDK2, SOX2 and Bcl2 for real-time PCR validation. The results showed that ESC could significantly down regulate SALL4, McL-1 and Bcl-2 genes in HCC cells (Fig. 5).

Table 3 Target genes of different miRNAs

iniRNAs	Target genes	Databases of bioinformatics prediction	References
has-miR-638	CDK2		[24–26]
	SOX2		[27]
has-miR-106-5p	STAT3	Miranda; mirbase; targetscan	[36, 37, 47]
has-miR-107	MCL1		[38, 40]
	CACNA2D1	miranda; mirbase; targetscan	[40]
	SALL4	Miranda; mirbase; targetscan	[14]
	Bcl2		[41]

Discussion

In this study, ESC showed promising inhibitory effect on growth of HepG2 and MHCC97H cells in dose and time dependent style. MHCC97H cells were more sensitive to ESC. ESC also obviously inhibited apoptotic protein caspase 3 and proliferative protein PCNA in these two cell lines. ESC inhibited EMT protein vimentin in HepG2 cells and upregulated E-cadherin in MHCC97H cells. ESC of low concentration might regress the migration of MHCC97H cells and inhibit EMT protein vimentin expression. Interestingly, the lowest dose (0.05 µg/mL) of ESC inhibited the cell migration more effectively than the highest dose (0.1 µg/mL). However, 0.1 µg/mL of ESC was more effective to increase the expression of E-cadherin and decrease that of vimentin. The contradiction result may be related to the complexity of the ESC components. No matter how, these results suggested that ESC could inhibit proliferation and EMT in HCC cells in vitro. In vivo results showed that ESC significantly inhibited tumor growth in either subcutaneous or orthotopic xenograft models mice of HepG2. ESC also had certain inhibitory effect on intrahepatic metastasis. All these results suggested that ESC was an important potential inhibitor of hepatocellular carcinoma.

Plenty of studies have shown that miRNAs play fundamental roles in many pathological processes. Meanwhile accumulating evidences in cancer diagnostics and therapeutics indicate that miRNAs involve in HCC progression, which may serve as either sensitive biomarkers for detecting carcinogenesis as well as monitoring therapies of HCC or tumor suppressors or oncogenes [10–12]. As we all know, Traditional Chinese Medicine (TCM) has the characteristics of multiple effective targets on the diseases and we reasonably hypothesized that ESC might exert anti-tumor role by regulating microRNAs. Here, the anti-cancer mechanisms of ESC targeting miRNAs have been extensively explored, and we chose miRNA array to detect the miRNA profile of MHCC97H cells treated with ESC. 69 differential miRNAs in total of 429 ones were obtained. According to the references, we selected hsa-miR-107, hsa-miR-638, hsa-miR-106b-5p to be verified with real-time PCR in MHCC97H and HepG2 cells. Expressions of hsa-miR-107, hsa-miR-638 in HCC cells treated by ESC were significantly increased. Hsa-miR-107, which functionally overlaps with miR-15, miR-16, and miR-195 due to a common 5′ sequence critical for target specificity [13]. There were opposite arguments in roles of hsa-miR-107 on cancers. Hsa-miR-107 activated ATR/Chk1 pathway, suppressed cervical cancer invasion and inhibited the tumorigenicity of head and neck squamous cell carcinoma [14, 15]. hsa-miR-107 is also confirmed to

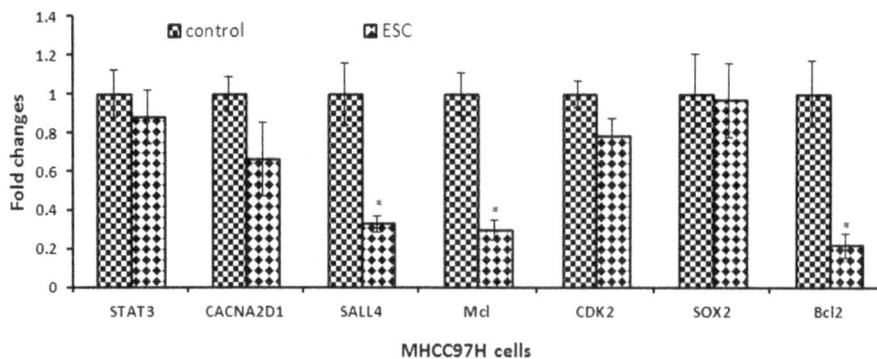

Fig. 5 Evaluation of the expression level of target genes. Target genes STAT3, CACNA2D1, SALL4, MCL1, CDK2, SOX2 and Bcl2 of miRNAs were validated with real-time PCR in MHCC-97H cells. ESC could significantly downregulate SALL4, McL-1 and Bcl-2 genes that has-miR-107 targeted in MHCC-97H cells. *p < 0.05, **p < 0.01 vs control

be involved in the progression of HCC [12, 16]. In this study, we found ESC could upregulate the expression hsa-miR-107 in both MHCC97H and HepG2 cells. Increased expression of hsa-miR-638 was only observed in MHCC97H cells treated by ESC, while the expression of hsa-miR-106b-5p did not change in any of these two cancer cell lines. These results confirmed that ESC could inhibit hepatocellular carcinoma by regulating some miRNAs.

Correspondingly, the target genes of hsa-miR-107, hsa-miR-638, hsa-miR-106b-5p were measured with PCR assay. Interestingly, only target genes of hsa-miR-107 were changed greatly. From the references and databases of bioinformatics, we have known that MCL1, CACNA2D1, SALL4 and Bcl2 were target genes of hsa-miR-107. Discovered as crucial modulators of apoptosis, anti-apoptotic Bcl-2 protein family emerged more recently as important modulators of other essential cancer processes, including cell cycle, autophagy or cell metabolism. Most cancer cell models overexpress one or more of the three major proteins: BCL-2 (B-cell lymphoma 2), BCL-xL (B-cell lymphoma-extra-large) and MCL1 (myeloid cell leukemia1). MCL1 and BCL-2 could enhance cell survival by inhibiting apoptosis [17, 18]. CACNA2D1(calcium voltage-gated channel auxiliary subunit alpha2delta 1) genes was critical for HCC TIC (tumor initiating cell) stemness and was predictive of poor prognosis for HCC patients [19, 20]. SALL4 (spalt like transcription factor 4), a member of a family of zinc finger transcription factors, was a marker for a progenitor subclass of HCC with an aggressive phenotype and a regulator of embryogenesis, organogenesis, pluripotency. Upregulation of SALL4 was also associated with poor prognosis in HCC [21–23]. The real-time PCR validation showed that ESC downregulated the MCL1, SALL4 and BCL2 gene expression significantly, but did not influence the expression of CACNA2D1. These results illustrated that ESC might regulate target genes of miRNAs, but

what regulating style, direct or indirect, was still needed to be further explored in future.

Conclusion

ESC regressed growth and metastasis of human hepatocellular carcinoma. ESC obviously upregulated hsa-miR-107 and hsa-miR-638 expression, but only target genes of hsa-miR-107, MCL1, SALL4 and Bcl2, were changed greatly. These findings suggested that regulating microRNAs expression and their corresponding target genes might the one of important molecular mechanisms of ESC treatment with HCC.

Abbreviations
BCL2: B-cell lymphoma 2; CACNA2D1: Calcium voltage-gated channel auxiliary subunit alpha2 delta 1; CDK2: Cyclin-dependent kinase 2; DMSO: Dimethyl sulfoxide; EMT: Epithelial mesenchymal transition; ESC: Extract of Stellerachamaejasme; HCC: Hepatocellular carcinoma; IC50: Half-maximal inhibitory concentration; IR: Inhibition rate; IVC: Individually ventilated cage; MCL1: Myeloid cell leukemia-1; MTT: 3-(4,5-dimethyl- 2-thiazolyl)-2,5-diphenyl-2-H-tetrazolium bromide; PCR: Polymeras chain reaction; RT: Reverse transcription; RTV: Relative tumor volume; SALL1: Spalt like transcription factor 4; SOX2: Sex determining region Y box 2; STAT: Signal transducers and activators of transcription; TGF: Transforming growth factor; TIC: Tumor initiating cell

Funding
This work was supported by National Major Scientific and Technological Special Project for "Significant New Drugs Development"during the Twelfth Five-year Plan Period (No. 2013ZX09301307001004), Training plan for high level of health technical personnel of Beijing health system (2015–3-101), Foundation of Beijing Institute of Hepatology(No. BJIH-01604)and National Natural Science Foundation of China (No. 81303273), Beijing Municipal Institute of Public Medical Research Development and Reform Pilot Project (No. 2016–2) and Beijing Precision Medicine and Transformation Engineering Technology Research Center of Hepatitis and Liver Cancer.

Authors' contributions
XL was the main experimental investigator and designer. XL had drafted the manuscript. SW carried out the cell culture. JX and BK participated the animal experiments. DC helped to complete the molecular experiments. YW helped to analyze the data. XZ supervised the study and the manuscript. All authors read and approved the final manuscript.

Competing interests

The authors declared no potential conflicts of interest with respect to the research, authorship, and/or publication of this article.

Author details

[1]Beijing Institute of Hepatology and Beijing YouAn Hospital, Capital Medical University, No 8 Xi TouTiao, You An Men Wai, Feng Tai Qu, Beijing 100069, China. [2]Institute of Chinese Materia Medica, China Academy of Chinese Medical Sciences, No 16 Nan Xiao Jie, Dong Zhi Men Nei, Dong Cheng Qu, Beijing 100700, China.

References

1. Bartel DP. MicroRNAs: target recognition and regulatory functions. Cell. 2009;136(2):215–33.
2. Wang L, Yue Y, Wang X, Jin H. Function and clinical potential of microRNAs in hepatocellular carcinoma. Oncol Lett. 2015;10(6):3345–53.
3. Laudadio I, Manfroid I, Achouri Y, Schmidt D, Wilson MD, Cordi S, Thorrez L, Knoops L, Jacquemin P, Schuit F, Pierreux CE, Odom DT, Peers B, Lemaigre FP. A feedback loop between the liver-enriched transcription factor network and miR-122 controls hepatocyte differentiation. Gastroenterology. 2012;142(1):119–29.
4. Chai ZT, Kong J, Zhu XD, Zhang YY, Lu L, Zhou JM, Wang LR, Zhang KZ, Zhang QB, Ao JY, Wang M, Wu WZ, Wang L, Tang ZY, Sun HC. MicroRNA-26a inhibits angiogenesis by down-regulating VEGFA through the PIK3C2α/Akt/HIF-1α pathway in hepatocellular carcinoma. PLoS One. 2013;8(10):e77957.
5. Yang H, Cho ME, Li TW, Peng H, Ko KS, Mato JM, Lu SC. MicroRNAs regulate methionine adenosyltransferase 1A expression in hepatocellular carcinoma. J Clin Invest. 2013;123(1):285–98.
6. Zhang Y, Yang P, Wang XF. Microenvironmental regulation of cancer metastasis by miRNAs. Trends Cell Biol. 2014;24(3):153–60.
7. Liu X, Yang Q, Zhang G, Li Y, Chen Y, Weng X, Wang Y, Wang Y, Zhu X. Anti-tumor pharmacological evaluation of extracts from stellerachamaejasme L based on hollow fiber assay. BMC Complement Altern Med. 2014;14:116.
8. Liu XN, Wang S, Yang Q, Wang YJ, Chen DX, Zhu XX. ESC reverses epithelial mesenchymal transition induced by transforming growth factor-β via inhibition of Smad signal pathway in HepG2 liver cancer cells. Cancer Cell Int. 2015;15:114.
9. Liu X, Yang Q, Zhang G, Li Y, Chen Y, Weng X, Wang Y, Wang Y, Zhu X. Anti-tumor pharmacological evaluation of extracts from stellerachamaejasme L based on hollow fiber assay. BMC Complement Altern Med. 2014;14(1):116.
10. Hong M, Wang N, Tan HY, Tsao SW, Feng Y. MicroRNAs and Chinese medicinal herbs: new possibilities in cancer therapy. Cancers (Basel). 2015;7(3):1643–57.
11. Yang N, Ekanem NR, Sakyi CA, Ray SD. Hepatocellular carcinoma and microRNA: new perspectives on therapeutics and diagnostics. Adv Drug Deliv Rev. 2015;81:62–74.
12. Mao B, Wang G. MicroRNAs involved with hepatocellular carcinoma (review). Oncol Rep. 2015;34(6):2811–20.
13. Zheng L, Zhang Y, Liu Y, Zhou M, Lu Y, Yuan L, Zhang C, Hong M, Wang S, Li X. MiR-106b induces cell radioresistance via the PTEN/PI3K/AKT pathways and p21 in colorectal cancer. J Transl Med. 2015;13:252.
14. Zhou C, Li G, Zhou J, Han N, Liu Z, Yin J. miR-107 activates ATR/Chk1 pathway and suppress cervical cancer invasion by targeting MCL1. PLoS One. 2014;9(11):e111860.
15. Piao L, Zhang M, Datta J, Xie X, Su T, Li H, Teknos TN, Pan Q. Lipid-based nanoparticle delivery of pre-miR-107 inhibits the tumorigenicity of head and neck squamous cell carcinoma. Mol Ther. 2012;20(6):1261–9.
16. Zhang JJ, Wang CY, Hua L, Yao KH, Chen JT, Hu JH. miR-107 promotes hepatocellular carcinoma cell proliferation by targeting Axin2. Int J Clin Exp Pathol. 2015;8(5):5168–74.
17. Hardwick JM, Soane L. Multiple functions of BCL-2 family proteins. Cold Spring Harb Perspect Biol. 2013;5(2):a008722.
18. Cerella C, Muller F, Gaigneaux A, Radogna F, Viry E, Chateauvieux S, Dicato M, Diederich M. Early downregulation of Mcl-1 regulates apoptosis triggered by cardiac glycoside UNBS1450. Cell Death Dis. 2015;6:e1782.
19. Zhao W, Wang L, Han H, Jin K, Lin N, Guo T, Chen Y, Cheng H, Lu F, Fang W, Wang Y, Xing B, Zhang Z. 1B50-1, a mAb raised against recurrent tumor cells, targets liver tumor-initiating cells by binding to the calcium channel α2δ1 subunit. Cancer Cell. 2013;23(4):541–56.
20. Han H, Du Y, Zhao W, Li S, Chen D, Zhang J, Liu J, Suo Z, Bian X, Xing B, Zhang Z. PBX3 is targeted by multiple miRNAs and is essential for liver tumour-initiating cells. Nat Commun. 2015;6:8271.
21. Tanaka Y, Aishima S, Kohashi K, Okumura Y, Wang H, Hida T, Kotoh K, Shirabe K, Maehara Y, Takayanagi R, Oda Y. Spalt-like transcription factor 4 immunopositivity is associated with epithelial cell adhesion molecule expression in combined hepatocellular carcinoma and cholangiocarcinoma. Histopathology. 2016;68(5):693–701.
22. Han SX, Wang JL, Guo XJ, He CC, Ying X, Ma JL, Zhang YY, Zhao Q, Zhu Q. Serum SALL4 is a novel prognosis biomarker with tumor recurrence and poor survival of patients in hepatocellular carcinoma. J Immunol Res. 2014;2014:262385.
23. Oikawa T, Kamiya A, Zeniya M, Chikada H, Hyuck AD, Yamazaki Y, Wauthier E, Tajiri H, Miller LD, Wang XW, Reid LM, Nakauchi H. Sal-like protein 4 (SALL4), a stem cell biomarker in liver cancers. Hepatology. 2013;57(4):1469–83.
24. Wang F, Lou JF, Cao Y, Shi XH, Wang P, Xu J, Xie EF, Xu T, Sun RH, Rao JY, Huang PW, Pan SY, Wang H. miR-638 is a new biomarker for outcome prediction of non-small cell lung cancer patients receiving chemotherapy. ExpMol Med. 2015;8(47):e162.
25. Xia Y, Wu Y, Liu B, Wang P, Chen Y. Downregulation of miR-638 promotes invasion and proliferation by regulating SOX2 and induces EMT in NSCLC. FEBS Lett. 2014;588(14):2238–45.
26. Wang WX, Kyprianou N, Wang X, Nelson PT. Dysregulation of the mitogen granulin in human cancer through the miR-15/107 microRNA gene group. Cancer Res. 2010;70(22):9137–42.
27. Bhattacharya A, Schmitz U, Raatz Y, Schönherr M, Kottek T, Schauer M, Franz S, Saalbach A, Anderegg U, Wolkenhauer O, Schadendorf D, Simon JC, Magin T, Vera J, Kunz M. miR-638 promotes melanoma metastasis and protects melanoma cells from apoptosis and autophagy. Oncotarget. 2015;6(5):2966–80.
28. Lin Y, Li D, Liang Q, Liu S, Zuo X, Li L, Sun X, Li W, Guo M, Huang Z. miR-638 regulates differentiation and proliferation in leukemic cells by targeting cyclin-dependent kinase 2. J Biol Chem. 2015;290(3):1818–28.
29. Kubota S, Chiba M, Watanabe M, Sakamoto M, Watanabe N. Secretion of small/microRNAs including miR-638 into extracellular spaces by sphingomyelin phosphodiesterase 3. Oncol Rep. 2015;33(1):67–73.
30. Zhang J, Fei B, Wang Q, Song M, Yin Y, Zhang B, Ni S, Guo W, Bian Z, Quan C, Liu Z, Wang Y, Yu J, Du X, Hua D, Huang Z. MicroRNA-638 inhibits cell proliferation, invasion and regulates cell cycle by targeting tetraspanin 1 in human colorectal carcinoma. Oncotarget. 2014;5(23):12083–96.
31. Tay Y, Tan SM, Karreth FA, Lieberman J, Pandolfi PP. Characterization of dual PTEN and p53-targeting microRNAs identifies microRNA-638/Dnm2 as a two-hit oncogenic locus. Cell Rep. 2014;8(3):714–22.
32. Ma K, Pan X, Fan P, He Y, Gu J, Wang W, Zhang T, Li Z, Luo X. Loss of miR-638 in vitro promotes cell invasion and a mesenchymal-like transition by influencing SOX2 expression in colorectal cancer cells. Mol Cancer. 2014;13:118.
33. Tan X, Peng J, Fu Y, An S, Rezaei K, Tabbara S, Teal CB, Man YG, Brem RF, Fu SW. miR-638 mediated regulation of BRCA1 affects DNA repair and sensitivity to UV and cisplatin in triple-negative breast cancer. Breast Cancer Res. 2014;16(5):435.
34. Zhao LY, Yao Y, Han J, Yang J, Wang XF, Tong DD, Song TS, Huang C, Shao Y. miR-638 suppresses cell proliferation in gastric cancer by targeting Sp2. Dig Dis Sci. 2014;59(8):1743–53.
35. Wilting SM, Verlaat W, Jaspers A, Makazaji NA, Agami R, Meijer CJ, Snijders PJ, Steenbergen RD. Methylation-mediated transcriptional repression of microRNAs during cervical carcinogenesis. Epigenetics. 2013;8(2):220–8.
36. Zhang M, Wang X, Li W, Cui Y. miR-107 and miR-25 simultaneously target LATS2 and regulate proliferation and invasion of gastric adenocarcinoma (GAC) cells. Biochem Biophys Res Commun. 2015;460(3):806–12.
37. Wang S, Lv C, Jin H, Xu M, Kang M, Chu H, Tong N, Wu D, Zhu H, Gong W, Zhao Q, Tao G, Zhou J, Zhang Z, Wang M. A common genetic variation in the promoter of miR-107 is associated with gastric adenocarcinoma susceptibility and survival. Mutat Res. 2014;769:35–41.
38. Ji Y, Wei Y, Wang J, Ao Q, Gong K, Zuo H. Decreased expression of microRNA-107 predicts poorer prognosis in glioma. Tumour Biol. 2015;36(6):4461–6.
39. He J, Zhang W, Zhou Q, Zhao T, Song Y, Chai L, Li Y. Low-expression of microRNA-107 inhibits cell apoptosis in glioma by upregulation of SALL4. Int J Biochem Cell Biol. 2013;45(9):1962–73.

40. Zhang Z, Zhang L, Yin ZY, Fan XL, Hu B, Wang LQ, Zhang D. miR-107 regulates cisplatin chemosensitivity of A549 non small cell lung cancer cell line by targeting cyclin dependent kinase. Int J Clin Exp Pathol. 2014;7(10):7236–41.

41. Ruan J, Liu X, Xiong X, Zhang C, Li J, Zheng H, Huang C, Shi Q, Weng Y. miR-107 promotes the erythroid differentiation of leukemia cells via the downregulation of Cacna2d1. Mol Med Rep. 2015;11(2):1334–9.

42. Molina-Pinelo S, Carnero A, Rivera F, Estevez-Garcia P, Bozada JM, Limon ML, Benavent M, Gomez J, Pastor MD, Chaves M, Suarez R, Paz-Ares L, de la Portilla F, Carranza-Carranza A, Sevilla I, Vicioso L, Garcia-Carbonero R. MiR-107 and miR-99a-3p predict chemotherapy response in patients with advanced colorectal cancer. BMC Cancer. 2014;14:656.

43. Luo ZL, Luo HJ, Fang C, Cheng L, Huang Z, Dai R, Li K, Tian FZ, Wang T, Tang LJ. Negative correlation of ITCH E3 ubiquitin ligase and miRNA-106b dictates metastatic progression in pancreatic cancer. Oncotarget. 2016;7(2):1477–85.

44. Xiang W, He J, Huang C, Chen L, Tao D, Wu X, Wang M, Luo G, Xiao X, Zeng F, Jiang G. miR-106b-5p targets tumor suppressor gene SETD2 to inactive its function in clear cell renal cell carcinoma. Oncotarget. 2015;6(6):4066–79.

45. Liu F, Gong J, Huang W, Wang Z, Wang M, Yang J, Wu C, Wu Z, Han B. MicroRNA-106b-5p boosts glioma tumorigensis by targeting multiple tumor suppressor genes. Oncogene. 2014;33(40):4813–22.

46. Liu Y, Zhang J, Sun X, Li M. EMMPRIN down-regulating miR-106a/b modifies breast cancer stem-like cell properties via interaction with fibroblasts through STAT3 and HIF-1α. Sci Rep. 2016;6:28329.

47. Maimaiti A, Maimaiti A, Yang Y, Ma Y. MiR-106b exhibits an anti-angiogenic function by inhibiting STAT3 expression in endothelial cells. Lipids Health Dis. 2016;15:51.

11

Coix lacryma-jobi var. ma-yuen Stapf sprout extract has anti-metastatic activity in colon cancer cells in vitro

Eun Suk Son[1†], Young Ock Kim[2†], Chun Geon Park[2], Kyung Hun Park[2], Sung Hwan Jeong[1], Jeong-Woong Park[1*] and Se-Hee Kim[3*] (iD)

Abstract

Background: *Coix lacryma-jobi var. ma-yuen* (Rom.Caill.) Stapf has been used in China as an herbal medicine. Many studies of this plant have reported anti-proliferative and apoptotic activities on human cancer cell lines. Therefore, this study of the anti-metastatic effect of *Coix lacryma-jobi var. ma-yuen* Stapf sprout extract (CLSE) in colorectal cancer cells may provide a scientific basis for exploring anti-cancer effects of edible crops.

Methods: To evaluate the effect of CLSE on cell proliferation and signaling, we performed a Cell Counting Kit-8 (CCK-8) assay in HCT116 cells and used western blot analysis. Furthermore, scratch-wound healing, transwell migration, matrigel invasion, and adhesion assays were conducted to elucidate the anti-metastatic effects of CLSE under hypoxic conditions in colon cancer cells.

Results: First, CLSE decreased deferoxamine (DFO)-induced migration of colon cancer cells by 87%, and blocked colon cancer cell migration by 80% compared with hypoxia control cells. Second, CLSE treatment resulted in a 54% reduction in hypoxia-induced invasiveness of colon cancer cells, and 50% inhibition of adhesive potency through inactivation of the extracellular signal-regulated kinase (ERK) 1/2 and protein kinase b (AKT) pathways. Third, conditioned medium collected from CLSE-treated HCT116 cells suppressed tube formation of human umbilical vein endothelial cells (HUVECs) by 91%.

Conclusions: CLSE inhibited migration, invasion, and adhesion of colon cancer cells and tube formation by HUVECs via repression of the ERK1/2 and AKT pathways under hypoxic conditions. Therefore, CLSE may be used to treat patients with colon cancer.

Keywords: *Coix*, Colon cancer, Metastasis, Invasion, Hypoxia

Background

Worldwide, colon cancer is one of the most deadly cancers because it is highly metastatic and invasive. An important determinant of the prognosis of cancer patients is the progression of tumor cell metastasis and invasion. The ability for metastasis and invasion enables cancer cells to find new areas of the body to occupy when space and nutrients become limited in their current location. The metastatic cascade can be separated into three processes: invasion, intravasation, and extravasation. First, the process of invasion involves the dissociation of tumor cells from the primary tumor mass and subsequent invasion into the surrounding tissue. Next, intravasation occurs when detached cells are transported via blood vessels to distant sites. Finally, tumor cells interact with endothelial cells to form stronger bonds, and penetrate the endothelium and basement membrane. Consequently, the new tumor cells can proliferate in secondary sites. Therefore, the metastatic spread of tumor tissue requires the growth of a vascular network [1].

* Correspondence: jwpark@gilhospital.com; sehee0423@gilhospital.com
†Equal contributors
[1]Department of Internal Medicine, Gachon University Gil Medical Center, 21 Namdong-daero 774 beon-gil, Namdong-gu, Incheon 405-760, Republic of Korea
[3]Gachon medical research institute, Gachon University Gil Medical Center, 21 Namdong-daero 774 beon-gil, Namdong-gu, Incheon 405-760, Republic of Korea
Full list of author information is available at the end of the article

The growth of new blood vessels (angiogenesis) is required for primary tumor growth as well as tumor invasion and metastasis [1]. The vasculature that supplies oxygen and nutrients is important for cancer cell survival [2].

Tumor hypoxia results from an imbalance between the oxygen supply and demand due to uncontrolled tumor cell proliferation [3]. Because cancer cells rapidly proliferate, the tumor quickly exhausts the nutrient and oxygen supply from the normal vasculature, and becomes hypoxic. This hypoxic condition upregulates the production of angiogenic factors from hypoxic tumor sites [4]. Therefore, hypoxia signaling can contribute to tumor progression by promoting tumor cell migration, invasion, metastasis, and angiogenesis [5].

Coix lacryma-jobi var. ma-yuen (Rom.Caill.) Stapf, which is an important cereal crop for many indigenous groups in upland areas, is characterized by having a similar appearance and taste to rice, with a standing crop comparable with corn. This plant is utilized as a rice alternative, health-promoting staple crop, and as an alternative livelihood and income source through value-added products. An increase in the number of health-conscious individuals has also contributed to the popularity of *Coix*, with the market currently growing due to increased acceptance of this product. *Coix* is largely consumed for household food security as a rice alternative or used to make porridge, champorado, and other recipes.

Previous studies have reported that *Coix* extract has anti-proliferative and apoptotic activities on human lung cancer, histolytic lymphoma, and colon cancer cells, as well as chemopreventive effects on lung cancer in vivo [6–9]. Although a few studies have reported that *Coix* has anti-cancer effects in terms of regulating the proliferation and cell cycle of cancer cells, the effects of *Coix lacryma-jobi var. ma-yuen* Stapf sprout extract (CLSE) on cancer metastasis are unknown. Therefore, this study aimed to explore the anti-cancer effects of CLSE in colorectal cancer cells.

Methods
Reagents
CLSE was manufactured in the herbarium of the Herbal Crop Research Institute (Eumseong, Republic of Korea).

Deferoxamine (DFO), Phorbol 12-myristate 13-acetate (PMA), and SC79 were obtained from Sigma-Aldrich (St. Louis, MO, USA). CLSE and DFO were dissolved in water. PMA and SC79 were dissolved in the solvent dimethyl sulfoxide (DMSO).

CLSE preparation
Coix cultivars were obtained from the National Institute of Crop Science (Miryang, Republic of Korea). *Coix* were germinated in a modified commercial soil bed (0.7–1.0 mg/m^3 soil bulk density, 450–650 mg/L available phosphate, 800–1000 mg/kg nitrogen) (Punong Bed Soil, Gyeongju, Republic of Korea). The germinated *Coix* was grown at 22–23 °C with humidity of 60% in a 900–1000 lx environment. Between 15 and 22 d after germination, young barley leaves about 8–13-cm long were harvested and freeze-dried [10]. We used a water extraction method because most traditional Oriental herbs are decocted in boiling water. In addition, some components are more soluble in water than in organic solvents. Crushed plant materials (200 g each) were extracted three times under reflux with distilled water. The water extracts were combined and lyophilized. The yield was 25% (wt/wt) of the dried *Coix* sprouts. Extracts were stored at –20 °C until usage. A voucher specimen (HPR-208) was deposited in the herbarium of Herbal Crop Research Institute (Eumseong, Republic of Korea).

Cell lines and cell culture conditions
HCT116 and CCD-18Co cells were obtained from the Korean Cell Line Bank (Seoul, Republic of Korea). Human umbilical vein endothelial cells (HUVECs) were obtained from the Lonza (San Diego, CA, USA). HCT116 cells were cultured in McCoy's medium (Gibco Cell Culture, Carlsbad, CA, USA) supplemented with 10% fetal bovine serum (FBS) (Gibco) and 1% penicillin-streptomycin (Gibco). CCD-18Co cells were cultured in MEM (Gibco) with 10% FBS (Gibco) and 1% penicillin-streptomycin (Gibco), and were used between passages 5 and 6. HUVECs were grown in EBM-2 (Lonza) supplemented with an EGM™-2 SingleQuots™ kit (Lonza), and used between passages 2 and 4 for experiments. Cells were incubated at 37 °C in a humidified atmosphere with 5% CO_2. A hypoxia incubator (New Brunswick Scientific, Edison, NJ, USA) containing 1% O_2, 5% CO_2, and 94% N_2 was used to create hypoxic conditions.

Cell counting Kit-8 (CCK-8) assay
Cells were seeded into 96-well plates and exposed to various concentrations of CLSE for 24–72 h prior to the addition of 10 μL CCK-8 solution (Dojindo Molecular Technologies, Inc., Rockville, MD, USA) containing 2-(2-methoxy-4-nitrophenyl0–3-(4-nitrophenyl)-5-(2,4-disulfophenyl)-2H–tetrazolium, monosodium salt (WST-8) to each well. After 1 h of incubation at 37 °C in a humidified atmosphere with 5% CO_2, the absorbance was determined at 450 nm.

Scratch-wound healing assay
Cells were seeded in 60-mm plates and then scratched using a pipette tip after 24-h incubation. After washing with phosphate buffered saline (PBS), cells were incubated in medium containing CLSE and/or 100 μM DFO

for 24 h. Images were then obtained at 0 and 24 h with an Olympus CFX41 microscope (Hamburg, Germany) at 40× magnification. The area of cell migration was quantified using ImageJ software (https://imagej.nih.gov/ij/) and the percentage of wound closure was calculated as described previously [11].

Transwell migration assay

The experiment was performed as described previously [11]. Briefly, cells in CLSE-containing serum-free medium were seeded into the inner chamber with the lower surface coated with 0.2% gelatin. The cells were incubated in normoxic or hypoxic conditions for 24 h. 20% FBS-containing medium in the bottom chamber was used as a chemoattractant. Cells on the upper membrane were wiped off using wet cotton swabs after fixation with methanol and crystal violet staining. Cells on the lower surface were mounted using mounting solution (Vectashield®; Vector Laboratories Burlingame, CA, USA). Stained cells were counted under a light microscope (DP72; Olympus, Hamburg, Germany) and images were taken at 200× magnification. All of the experiments were independently repeated in triplicate.

Matrigel invasion assay

The matrigel invasion assay was performed as previously described [11]. Briefly, the lower surface were coated with 0.2% gelatin, and then the upper surfaces were coated with Matrigel® (BD Biosciences, San Jose, CA, USA) at 37 °C for 2 h. Cells in CLSE-containing serum-free medium were plated into the inner chamber and incubated in normoxic or hypoxic conditions for 48 h with 20% FBS in the bottom chamber as the chemoattractant. The cells were processed as described for the transwell migration assay. All of the experiments were independently repeated in triplicate.

Adhesion assay

Cells were treated with or without CLSE and/or DFO for 24 h, suspended in serum-free McCoy's medium, and then seeded in a 96-well plate that had been pre-coated with Matrigel® (BD Biosciences). After incubation at 37 °C for 90 min, the cells were washed with PBS and treated with 0.5 mg/mL 3-(4,5-Dimethylthiazol-2-yl)-2,5-diphenyltetrazolium bromide (MTT). The absorbance of formazan crystals dissolved in 100 μL DMSO was determined at 570 nm using a microplate reader. The experiments were independently performed in triplicate.

Western blot analysis

Cells were harvested with lysis buffer [50 mM Tris-HCl (pH 8.0), 0.5% sodium deoxycholate, 150 mM NaCl, 0.1% sodium dodecyl sulfate (SDS), and 1% NP-40]. Antibodies to p65, phospho-p65, extracellular signal-regulated kinase (ERK) 1/2, phospho-ERK1/2, protein kinase B (AKT), phospho-AKT, c-Jun N-terminal kinase (JNK), phospho-JNK, p38, phospho-p38, Signal transducer and activator of transcription 3 (STAT3), and phospho-STAT3 were all purchased from Cell Signaling Technology (Beverly, MA, USA). β-actin antibody was obtained from Santa Cruz Biotechnology (Santa Cruz, CA, USA). Immunoblot bands were quantified as a ratio of phosphorylated protein/total protein using ImageJ software.

Generation of conditioned medium

HCT116 cells were treated with or without CLSE (0.5, 1 mg/mL) and/or DFO (100 μM) for 24 h in complete medium, and then the supernatant was saved. The supernatant, called conditioned medium, was filtered and stored at −70 °C.

Tube formation assay

HUVECs were diluted in conditioned medium and seeded in a 48-well plate that had been pre-coated with Matrigel®. After a 12-h incubation period, images of formed tubules were taken at 40× magnification and quantified by determining the number of branching points. The experiments were independently performed in triplicate.

Statistical analysis

All data were analyzed with GraphPad Prism® software using a two-tailed Student t test. P values less than 0.05 were significantly considered.

Results

CLSE inhibits colon cancer cell migration under hypoxic conditions

To examine effects on the viability of colon cancer cells, HCT116, and of normal cells, CCD-18Co, caused by CLSE treatment, we performed a CCK-8 assay. As shown in Fig. 1, CLSE strongly decreased the viability of HCT116 cells compared to CCD-18Co cells. Next, we performed scratch-wound healing assays to determine if CLSE had an effect on the migratory potency of HCT116 cells. For this assay, we used DFO, a reagent used to simulate hypoxic conditions. As shown in Fig. 2a and b, DFO enhanced the migration of colon cancer cells ($p < 0.05$). However, HCT116 cells co-treated with DFO and CLSE had 47–87% less healing ability than cells treated with DFO only ($p < 0.05$). Furthermore, to confirm the inhibitory effect of CLSE on HCT116 cell migration, we plated CLSE-treated HCT116 cells in a Transwell® chamber and incubated the cells for 24 h under hypoxic conditions. The results showed that CLSE inhibited the migration of hypoxic HCT116 cells in the Transwell® chamber by 48–80% compared with the hypoxia control group ($p < 0.01$) (Fig. 2c, d). These results

A HCT116

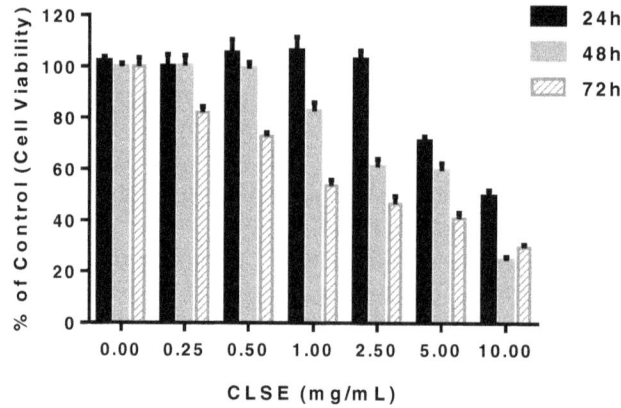

B CCD-18Co

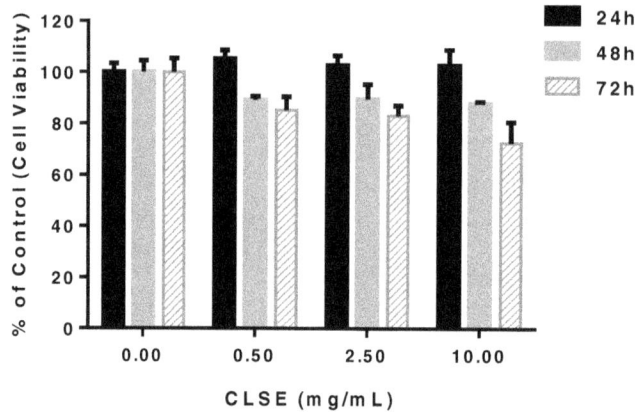

Fig. 1 Cytotoxic effect of CLSE on HCT116 and CCD-18Co cells. **a, b**. A Cell Counting Kit (CCK)-8 assay was used to measure HCT116 and CCD-18Co cells proliferation for 24–72 h after treatment with various concentrations of CLSE. Data are mean ± SD. CLSE, *Coix lacryma-jobi var. ma-yuen* Strapt sprout extract; SD, Standard Deviation

imply that CLSE has the potential to inhibit HCT116 cell migration under hypoxic conditions.

CLSE inhibits invasion and adhesion of colon cancer cells in hypoxia

In cancer cell metastasis, invasion is as important as migration. To investigate the effects of CLSE on colon cancer cell invasion, we performed an invasion assay using a Transwell® coated with Matrigel®. As we showed, hypoxia promoted the invasion of HCT116 cells ($p < 0.01$). However, CLSE-treated cells under hypoxic conditions showed a 21–54% reduction in invasion compared with the hypoxia control group ($p < 0.05$) (Fig. 3a, b).

Metastatic cancer cells have high adhesion potency to migrate to secondary sites for new tumor growth. Therefore, cell adhesion assays are used to examine the metastatic potency of cancer cells. As shown in Fig. 3c, DFO-treated cells had increased adhesion compared with untreated cells ($p < 0.05$); however, cells co-treated with DFO and CLSE showed a 19–50% reduction in

adhesive ability compared with cells treated with DFO only ($p < 0.001$, $p < 0.01$). Taken together, these results suggest that CLSE regulates the invasion and adhesion of HCT116 cells under hypoxic conditions.

CLSE inactivates ERK1/2 and AKT activities in hypoxic conditions

To identify the cellular signaling pathways regulated by CLSE during colon cancer cell metastasis under hypoxic conditions, we examined the expression of signaling markers using Western blot analysis. Among the various signaling markers investigated, hypoxia-induced activation of ERK1/2 and AKT were downregulated by 1 mg/mL CLSE (Fig. 4a). To confirm whether the activation of ERK1/2 and AKT were repressed by CLSE in HCT116 cells, we performed western blot and scratch-wound healing assay at earlier stage in the presence of the ERK1/2 and AKT activators, PMA and SC79, respectively. As shown in Fig. 4b, inhibition of the ERK1/2 and AKT pathways by CLSE was reversed in CLSE-treated

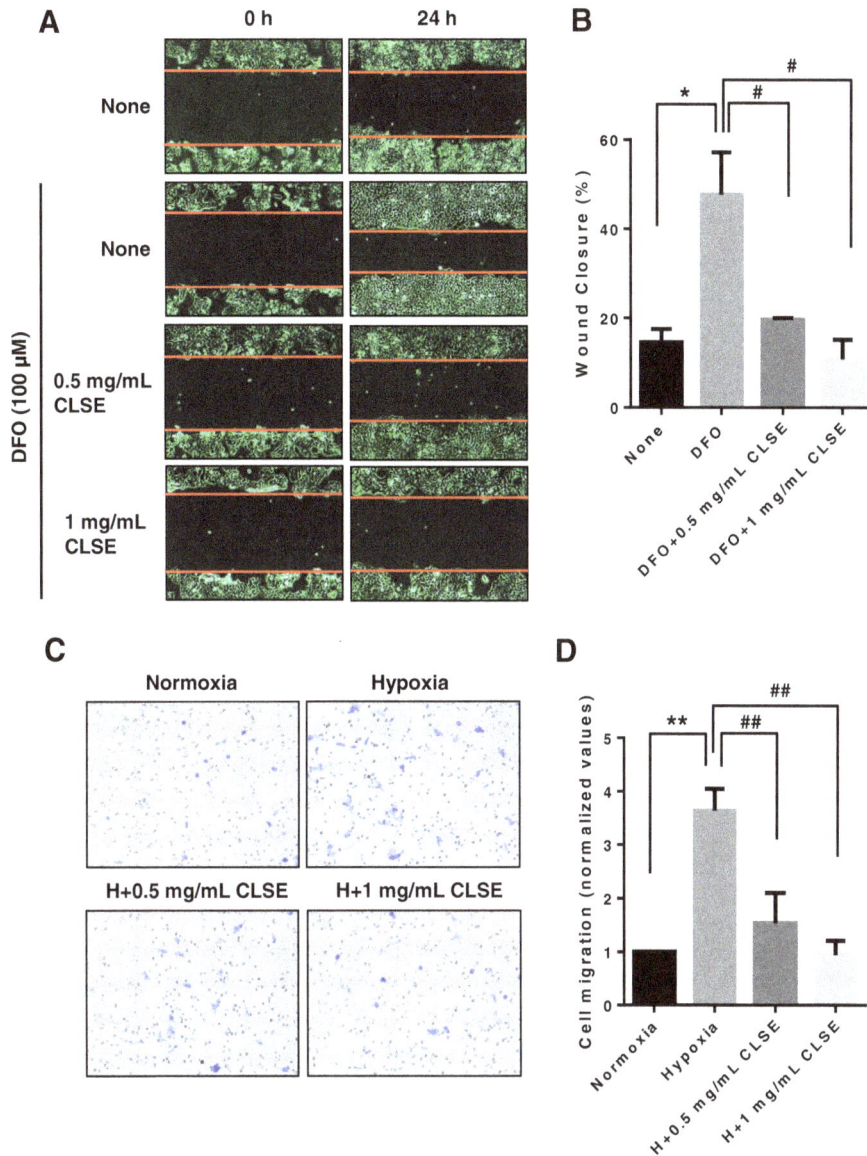

Fig. 2 Effect of CLSE on the migratory ability of HCT116 cells under hypoxic conditions. **a**. Representative scratch-wound images showing the effect of CLSE on the healing ability of HCT116 cells (magnification: ×40). After with treatment DFO (100 μM) and CLSE (0.5, 1 mg/mL) for 24 h, the migratory ability was analyzed by scratch-wound healing assay. **b**. Percentage of HCT116 cells that migrated into the wound following CLSE treatment relative to untreated control cells. * $p < 0.05$ versus untreated control group. #$p < 0.05$ versus DFO-only group. **c**. Representative images showing the effect of CLSE on HCT116 cell migration through a Transwell® chamber membrane (magnification: ×200). After treatment with CLSE (0.5, 1 mg/mL) for 24 h, the migration cells in transwells were stained by crystal violet solution. **d**. Percentage of HCT116 cells that migrated following CLSE treatment relative to control cells (normoxia). ** $p < 0.01$ versus normoxia control group. ##$p < 0.01$ versus hypoxia-only group. Data are mean ± SD (n = 3). CLSE, *Coix lacryma-jobi var. ma-yuen* Strapt sprout extract; H, hypoxia; SD, Standard Deviation

HCT116 cells given PMA or SC79. However, activation of other signaling proteins (p38, p65, STAT3, JNK) was not affected by CLSE treatment at an earlier stage (Fig. 4c). In addition, in the scratch-wound healing assay, PMA and SC79 could compromise the inhibitory effect of CLSE on the migration of HCT116 cells under hypoxic conditions by 57–71% and 64–77%, respectively ($p < 0.05$, $p < 0.01$) (Fig. 4d, e). Therefore,

our results suggest that CLSE represses HCT116 cell migration through inactivation of the ERK1/2 and AKT pathways under hypoxic conditions.

CLSE inhibits HUVEC tube formation under hypoxia

The formation of new blood vessels (angiogenesis) is crucial for invasive tumor growth and metastasis. To demonstrate that CLSE affects angiogenesis, conditioned

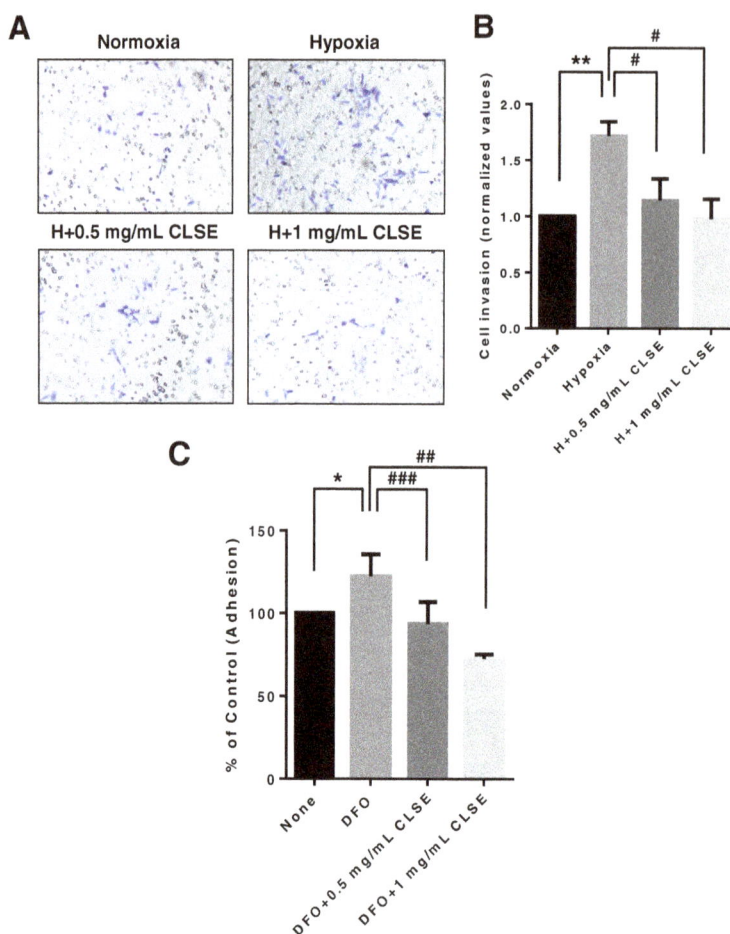

Fig. 3 Effect of CLSE on HCT116 cell invasion and migration under hypoxic conditions. **a**. Representative images showing the effect of CLSE on HCT116 cell invasion through a Matrigel®-coated Transwell® chamber membrane (magnification: 200×). After treatment with CLSE (0.5, 1 mg/mL) for 48 h under hypoxic conditions, cells that had invaded the transwells were analyzed through crystal violet staining. **b**. Number of HCT116 cells that invaded following CLSE treatment. The values are normalized to the number of invaded control cells (normoxia). ** $p < 0.01$ versus normoxia control group. #$p < 0.05$ versus hypoxia-only group. **c**. After treatment with DFO (100 μM) and/or CLSE (0.5, 1 mg/mL) for 24 h, cells were seeded into Matrigel-coated wells and then analyzed using an MTT assay. Number of HCT116 cells that adhered to the Matrigel®-coated plate following CLSE treatment. The values are normalized to the number of adherent control cells (untreated). * $p < 0.05$ versus untreated control group. ##$p < 0.01$, ###$p < 0.001$ versus DFO-only groups. Data are mean ± SD ($n = 3$). CLSE, *Coix lacryma-jobi var. ma-yuen* Stapf sprout extract; H, hypoxia; SD, standard deviation

media, obtained from growing HCT116 cells in media supplemented with CLSE and/or DFO, was used to treat HUVEC cells. The media obtained from DFO-treated HCT116 cells augmented tube formation by HUVECs ($p < 0.01$), whereas conditioned media, obtained from CLSE and DFO-treated HCT116 cells, decreased tube formation by 55–91% ($p < 0.001$). These results suggest that CLSE may mediate its anti-angiogenic effect by regulating the secretion of angiogenic factors by colon cancer cells (Fig. 5).

Discussion

The hallmarks of cancer are self-sufficiency of growth signals, insensitivity to anti-growth signals, limitless replicative potential, evading cell death (apoptosis), tissue invasion, metastasis, and sustained angiogenesis [2].

To investigate the anti-cancer effects of CLSE, we investigated the physiological effect of CLSE on cancer using human colon cancer cells.

In this study, we showed that CLSE had an anti-metastatic effect in colon cancer cells. Specifically, CLSE inhibited colon cancer cell migration, invasion, wound healing, and adhesion. In addition, conditioned media collected from CLSE-treated HCT116 cells had an inhibitory effect on HUVEC tube formation. On the other hand, in the case of the cervical cancer cell line HeLa, CLSE promoted apoptosis and arrested the cell cycle (in submission). Taken together, these results suggest that the mechanism on the anti-cancer effect of CLSE may be organ-specific.

Recently, many studies have tried to identify the active components of *Coix* and determine their mechanism of

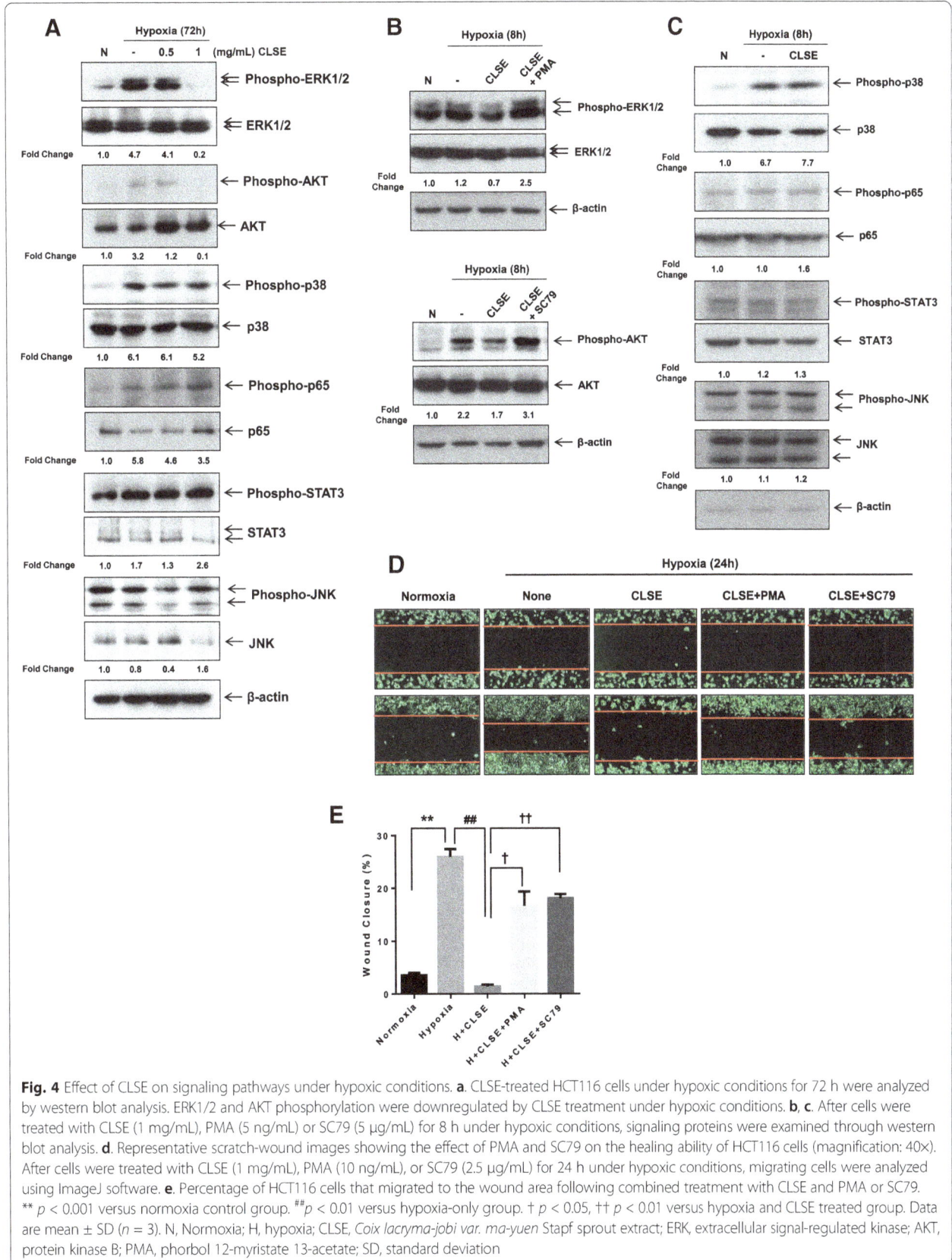

Fig. 4 Effect of CLSE on signaling pathways under hypoxic conditions. **a**. CLSE-treated HCT116 cells under hypoxic conditions for 72 h were analyzed by western blot analysis. ERK1/2 and AKT phosphorylation were downregulated by CLSE treatment under hypoxic conditions. **b**, **c**. After cells were treated with CLSE (1 mg/mL), PMA (5 ng/mL) or SC79 (5 μg/mL) for 8 h under hypoxic conditions, signaling proteins were examined through western blot analysis. **d**. Representative scratch-wound images showing the effect of PMA and SC79 on the healing ability of HCT116 cells (magnification: 40×). After cells were treated with CLSE (1 mg/mL), PMA (10 ng/mL), or SC79 (2.5 μg/mL) for 24 h under hypoxic conditions, migrating cells were analyzed using ImageJ software. **e**. Percentage of HCT116 cells that migrated to the wound area following combined treatment with CLSE and PMA or SC79. ** $p < 0.001$ versus normoxia control group. ## $p < 0.01$ versus hypoxia-only group. † $p < 0.05$, †† $p < 0.01$ versus hypoxia and CLSE treated group. Data are mean ± SD ($n = 3$). N, Normoxia; H, hypoxia; CLSE, *Coix lacryma-jobi var. ma-yuen* Stapf sprout extract; ERK, extracellular signal-regulated kinase; AKT, protein kinase B; PMA, phorbol 12-myristate 13-acetate; SD, standard deviation

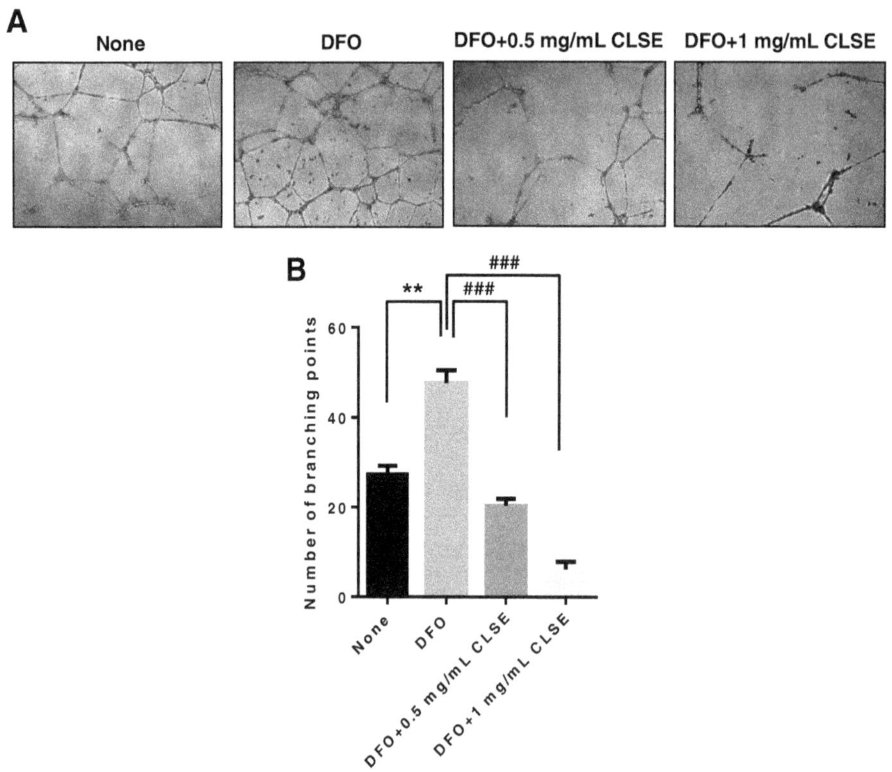

Fig. 5 Effect of CLSE on HUVECs capillary tube formation. **a**. After HUVECs were seeded in matrigel-coated plates and incubated with conditioned media from HCT116 cells treated with DFO (100 µM) and CLSE (0.5, 1 mg/mL) for 24 h. Representative images showing HUVEC tube formation following treatment with conditioned media collected from CLSE-treated HCT116 cells (magnification: ×40). **b**. Number of branching points per unit area following treatment with conditioned media. ** $p < 0.01$ versus untreated control group. ### $p < 0.001$ versus DFO-only group. Data are mean ± SD ($n = 3$). CLSE, *Coix lacryma-jobi var. ma-yuen* Strapt sprout extract; HUVECs, human umbilical vein endothelial cells; SD, standard deviation

action. Specifically, neutral lipid isolated from endosperm of *Coix* inhibits the growth of pancreatic cancer cells [12], and the ethyl acetate fraction from ethanolic extraction of adlay testa has an inhibitory effect on the allergic response [13]. In addition, five compounds (coixspirolactam A, coixspirolactam B, coixspirolactam C, coixlactam, methyl dioxindole-3-acetate) isolated from *Coix* bran exhibit anti-proliferative effect on lung and colon cancer cells [9]. Because CLSE is obtained from a young sprout form *Coix*, we believe it to share a similar chemical composition with the mature plant. As such, it is highly likely that CLSE also contains coixspirolactams and methyl dioxindole-3-acetate, which may contribute to the anti-metastatic effects of CLSE.

Previous reports analyzed the proliferation of cancer cells or the expression of cell cycle regulatory proteins to demonstrate the anti-cancer effects of *Coix* under normal conditions. However, our study focused on the effects of the sprout extract of *Coix* on colon cancer cell metastasis and HUVEC tube formation under hypoxic conditions. Hypoxia, a characteristic feature of locally advanced solid tumors, has emerged as a pivotal factor for the tumor physiome because it can promote tumor

progression and increase tumor resistance to therapy [14]. Migration, invasion, and adhesion of cancer cells result from the loss of epithelial markers and the degradation of basement membrane. Therefore, we expect that CLSE may have anti-metastatic effects via regulation of E-cadherin, vimentin, MMP-2, and MMP-9 in colon cancer cells, and plan to undertake these experiments in the future.

Phosphorylation-mediated activation of AKT and ERK signaling drives tumor invasion [15]. The ERK pathway controls cell migration, invasion, proliferation, and the induction of transcriptional programs [16]. Since AKT contributes to the development or progression of cancer, many consequences of hyperactive AKT signaling are considered hallmarks of cancer [17]. Our data showed that downregulation of ERK1/2 and AKT phosphorylation by CLSE was reversed in the presence of their activators, PMA and SC79 under hypoxic conditions (Fig. 4); therefore, it is likely that CLSE blocked the migration of colon cancer cells via inactivation of ERK1/2 and AKT under hypoxic conditions.

It has been reported in some animal research that *Coix* consumption might cause embryotoxicity and enhance uterine contractility during pregnancy [18]. Furthermore, some herbal medicines are reported to interfere with the efficacy and safety of conventional medicines [19]. Therefore, more research on the stability and efficacy of herbal supplements such as *Coix* is needed. In addition, our primary focus in this research was to explore the overall anti-cancer effects of CLSE, and we have succeeded in this endeavor. Further studies will not only reinforce this research, but will also contribute greatly to the field of oncology through detailed chemical profiling of CLSE and mechanistic studies of each component, as well as in vivo experiments using CLSE.

Conclusions

CLSE can inhibit colon cancer cells migration, invasion, adhesion, and HUVEC tube formation in hypoxic conditions through inhibition of the ERK1/2 and AKT signaling pathways. However, further study is necessary to reveal the possible mechanism of the anti-metastatic effect of CLSE and its active compounds under hypoxic conditions.

Abbreviations
AKT: Protein kinase B; CCK-8: Cell Counting Kit-8; CLSE: *Coix lacryma-jobi var. ma-yuen* Stapf sprout extract; DFO: Deferoxamine; ERK: Extracellular signal-regulated kinase; FBS: Fetal bovine serum; HUVECs: Human umbilical vein endothelial cells; JNK: c-Jun N-terminal kinase; KLT: Kanglaite®; MTT: 3-(4,5-Dimethylthiazol-2-yl)-2,5-diphenyltetrazolium bromide; PBS: Phosphate buffered saline; PMA: Phorbol 12-myristate 13-acetate; SD: Standard deviation; SDS: Sodium dodecyl sulfate; STAT3: Signal transducer and activator of transcription 3; WST-8: 2-(2-methoxy-4-nitrophenyl0-3-(4-nitrophenyl)-5-(2,4-disulfophenyl)-2H–tetrazolium, monosodium salt

Acknowledgements
Not applicable.

Funding
This work was supported by a grant (FRD2014–10-2) funded by Gachon University Gil Medical Center in 2015 to Jeong Woong Park and a grant (PJ0127852017) from the Rural Development Administration to Young Ock Kim.

Authors' contributions
ESS and YOK equally contributed to the research; CGP and KHP provided *Coix lacryma-jobi var. ma-yuen* Stapf sprout extract for this research; SHJ analyzed the data; JWP and S-HK wrote the manuscript and supervised this work. All authors read and approved the final manuscript.

Authors' information
English in this manuscript has been checked by at least two professional editors, both of whom are native speakers of English. For certification, please refer to the following website: http://www.textcheck.com/certificate/YxkEfe

Competing interests
The authors declare that they have no competing interests.

Author details
[1]Department of Internal Medicine, Gachon University Gil Medical Center, 21 Namdong-daero 774 beon-gil, Namdong-gu, Incheon 405-760, Republic of Korea. [2]Department of Herbal Crop Research, National Institute of Horticultural and Herbal Science, RDA, Cheongju, Chungbuk, Republic of Korea. [3]Gachon medical research institute, Gachon University Gil Medical Center, 21 Namdong-daero 774 beon-gil, Namdong-gu, Incheon 405-760, Republic of Korea.

References
1. Weidner N, Semple JP, Welch WR, Folkman J. Tumor angiogenesis and metastasis–correlation in invasive breast carcinoma. N Engl J Med. 1991; 324(1):1–8.
2. Hanahan D, Weinberg RA. The hallmarks of cancer. Cell. 2000;100(1):57–70.
3. Vaupel P, Briest S, Hockel M. Hypoxia in breast cancer: pathogenesis, characterization and biological/therapeutic implications. Wien Med Wochenschr. 2002;152(13–14):334–42.
4. Semenza GL. Hypoxia-inducible factors: mediators of cancer progression and targets for cancer therapy. Trends Pharmacol Sci. 2012;33(4):207–14.
5. Chaudary N, Hill RP. Hypoxia and metastasis. Clin Cancer Res. 2007;13(7): 1947–9.
6. Liu Y, Zhang W, Wang XJ, Liu S. Antitumor effect of Kanglaite(R) injection in human pancreatic cancer xenografts. BMC Complement Altern Med. 2014; 14:228.
7. Chang HC, Huang YC, Hung WC. Antiproliferative and chemopreventive effects of adlay seed on lung cancer in vitro and in vivo. J Agric Food Chem. 2003;51(12):3656–60.
8. Kuo CC, Shih MC, Kuo YH, Chiang W. Antagonism of free-radical-induced damage of adlay seed and its antiproliferative effect in human histolytic lymphoma U937 monocytic cells. J Agric Food Chem. 2001;49(3):1564–70.
9. Lee MY, Lin HY, Cheng F, Chiang W, Kuo YH. Isolation and characterization of new lactam compounds that inhibit lung and colon cancer cells from adlay (Coix Lachryma-Jobi L. Var. ma-Yuen Stapf) bran. Food Chem Toxicol. 2008;46(6):1933–9.
10. Numata M, Yamamoto A, Moribayashi A, Yamada H. Antitumor components isolated from the Chinese herbal medicine Coix Lachryma-Jobi. Planta Med. 1994;60(4):356–9.
11. Kim JH, Hwang YJ, Han SH, Lee YE, Kim S, Kim YJ, Cho JH, Kwon KA, Kim JH, Kim SH. Dexamethasone inhibits hypoxia-induced epithelial-mesenchymal transition in colon cancer. World J Gastroenterol. 2015;21(34):9887–99.
12. Bao Y, Yuan Y, Xia L, Jiang H, Wu W, Zhang X. Neutral lipid isolated from endosperm of Job's tears inhibits the growth of pancreatic cancer cells via apoptosis, G2/M arrest, and regulation of gene expression. J Gastroenterol Hepatol. 2005;20(7):1046–53.
13. Chen HJ, Chung CP, Chiang W, Lin YL. Anti-inflammatory effects and chemical study of a flavonoid-enriched fraction from adlay bran. Food Chem. 2011;126(4):1741–8.
14. Vaupel P, Mayer A. Hypoxia in cancer: significance and impact on clinical outcome. Cancer Metastasis Rev. 2007;26(2):225–39.
15. Huang C, Jacobson K, Schaller MD. MAP kinases and cell migration. J Cell Sci. 2004;117(Pt 20):4619–28.
16. Provenzano PP, Inman DR, Eliceiri KW, Keely PJ. Matrix density-induced mechanoregulation of breast cell phenotype, signaling and gene expression through a FAK-ERK linkage. Oncogene. 2009;28(49):4326–43.
17. Altomare DA, Testa JR. Perturbations of the AKT signaling pathway in human cancer. Oncogene. 2005;24(50):7455–64.
18. Tzeng HP, Chiang W, Ueng TH, Liu SH. The abortifacient effects from the seeds of Coix Lachryma-Jobi L. Var. ma-Yuen Stapf. J Toxicol Environ Health A. 2005;68(17–18):1557–65.
19. Alsanad SM, Howard RL, Williamson EM. An assessment of the impact of herb-drug combinations used by cancer patients. BMC Complement Altern Med. 2016;16(1):393.

12

The prevention of 2,4-dinitrochlorobenzene-induced inflammation in atopic dermatitis-like skin lesions in BALB/c mice by Jawoongo

Jin Mo Ku[1], Se Hyang Hong[1], Soon Re Kim[1], Han-Seok Choi[1], Hyo In Kim[1], Dong Uk Kim[1], So Mi Oh[1], Hye Sook Seo[2], Tai Young Kim[2], Yong Cheol Shin[2], Chunhoo Cheon[2*] and Seong-Gyu Ko[2*] (iD)

Abstract

Background: Jawoongo is an herbal mixture used in traditional medicine to treat skin diseases. This study aimed to investigate whether Jawoongo ameliorates Atopic dermatitis (AD)-like pathology in mice and to understand its underlying cellular mechanisms.

Methods: AD was induced by 2, 4-Dinitrocholrlbenzene (DNCB) in BALB/c mice. Treatment with Jawoongo was assessed to study the effect of Jawoongo on AD in mice. Histological Analysis, blood analysis, RT-PCR, western blot analysis, ELISA assay and cell viability assay were performed to verify the inhibitory effect of Jawoongo on AD in mice.

Results: We found that application of Jawoongo in an ointment form on AD-like skin lesions on DNCB-exposed BALB/c mice reduced skin thickness and ameliorated skin infiltration with inflammatory cells, mast cells and CD4+ cells. The ointment also reduced the mRNA levels of IL-2, IL-4, IL-13 and TNF-α in the sensitized skin. Leukocyte counts and the levels of IgE, IL-6, IL-10 and IL-12 were decreased in the blood of the DNCB-treated mice. Furthermore, studies on cultured cells demonstrated that Jawoongo exhibits anti-inflammatory activities, including the suppression of proinflammatory cytokine expression, nitric oxide (NO) production, and inflammation-associated molecule levels in numerous types of agonist-stimulated innate immune cell, including human mast cells (HMC-1), murine macrophage RAW264.7 cells, and splenocytes isolated from mice.

Conclusion: These findings indicate that Jawoongo alleviates DNCB-induced AD-like symptoms via the modulation of several inflammatory responses, indicating that Jawoongo might be a useful drug for the treatment of AD.

Keywords: Atopic dermatitis, Jawoongo, 2,4-dinitrochlorobenzene, Cytokine, Inflammation

Background

Atopic dermatitis (AD) is the most common chronic inflammatory and chronically relapsing skin disease. The prevalence of AD has increased continuously, and approximately 10 million people worldwide are currently affected. The disease leads to a significantly reduced quality of life [1, 2]. The pathogenesis of AD is not well understood but appears to be associated with the activation of innate immune responses, including inflammation.

Common features of AD include excessive infiltration of inflammatory cells and granulated mast cells into AD skin lesions and high immunoglobulin E (IgE) levels and leukocyte counts in blood [3]. Notably, CD4+ T cells are critical for the development of allergic inflammatory diseases. CD4+ T cell activation induces the secretion of cytokines and chemokines and drives inflammation and allergic sensitization [4]. Furthermore, the development of AD has been attributed to the activation of mast cells [5, 6] and T-helper 2 (Th2)-dependent cells [7, 8]. Mast

---

* Correspondence: pm.thehoo@gmail.com; epiko@khu.ac.kr
[2]Department of Preventive Medicine, College of Korean Medicine, Kyung Hee University, Kyungheedae-ro 26, Dongdaemun-gu, Seoul 02447, South Korea
Full list of author information is available at the end of the article

cells are activated by IgE through the high-affinity IgE receptor (Fc R) [9, 10]. These cells are then recruited into AD skin lesions, where they promote skin hypersensitivity reactions by releasing histamine; prostaglandin D2 (PGD2); AD-related Th2 cytokines, including IL-4, IL-5, and IL-13; and proinflammatory cytokines, including IL-4 and IL-6.

Tacrolimus is an effective immunosuppressant that inhibits the production of various cytokines, such as IL-2, IL-4 and IL-5. Many studies have demonstrated that tacrolimus suppresses allergic cytokine production by T cells [11, 12] and is effective against AD in animal models [13–15]. Tacrolimus ointment is used for the treatment of AD in adults and children [16–18]. However, previous studies have shown that treatment with tacrolimus elevated total and specific IgE levels and caused transient burning and erythema in ~ 60% of patients [19, 20]. Consequently, the development of alternative remedies is necessary to reduce these side effects.

Jawoongo is a traditional herbal medicine composed of Lithospermum root and Angelica gigas Nakai (AGN). AGN contains numerous active ingredients, including decursin. In previous studies, decursin exhibited anti-allergic effects in an asthma model and anti-metastatic effects in colon cancer [21–23]. Decursin has also been used for the treatment of various dermatitis-associated skin diseases, including eczema and chilblain. Recent studies have indicated that decursin is effective in driving artificial wound healing and ameliorating skin inflammation [24–26]. As known as, DNCB allergens elicited a systemic immune response, because increased cytokine levels in the serum of mice [27].

We investigated effect of jawoongo in DNCB induced AD model in Balb/c mice. The goal of this study was to explore the effects of Jawoongo on 2,4-dinitrochlorobenzene (DNCB)-induced AD-like symptoms in BALB/c mice and several types of immune cell.

Methods
Preparation of Jawoongo ointment and tacrolimus ointment
Jawoongo ointment was supplied by Han-poong Pharm Co., Ltd. (Jeonjoo, Republic of Korea). Jawoongo is made from Lithospermum root and *Angelica gigas Nakai* (AGN). The main compound in Lithospermum root is shikonin. Shikonin inhibits inflammation and imflammasomes [28, 29]. The main compounds in AGN are decursin and Nodakenin. Decursin and Nodakenin are known to inhibit inflammation. Additionally, decursin is known to inhibit the proliferation of ovarian cancer cells [30–32]. A 0.1% protopic tacrolimus ointment was also utilized (Astellas Pharma Tech, Japan). Tacrolimus is made from FK506, which has been used to treat dermatitis, as it suppresses the development of Th2 cells [33, 34].

Animals
Six-week-old male BALB/c mice were obtained from Orient Bio, Inc. (Seoul, Korea). The mice were maintained for 1 week under a controlled temperature (23 ± 3 °C) and humidity (55 ± 15%) with a 12 h light/12 h dark cycle before initiating the experiment. The body weights and food intake of the animals were measured once every 2 days. All procedures performed on the mice were approved by the animal care center of Kyung-Hee University (Kyung Hee University Study Proposal (SEOUL) – 12-014; Approval No. KHUASP(SE)-12–014). Upon completion of the experiment, the mice were anesthetized with a 1.2% avertin solution (0.5 g 2,2,2-tribromoethanol powder dissolved into 1 ml 2-methyl-2-butanol and 39 ml phosphate-buffered saline (PBS) at 55 °C) that was filtered through a Nalgene 0.22-μm filter (Thermo Fisher Scientific, Inc., Waltham, MA, USA) and sacrificed via exsanguination [35, 36].

Induction of AD-like lesions and drug treatment
The procedures used for the induction of AD-like lesions and the drug treatment are shown in Fig. 1. The mice were divided into four groups, with eight mice in each group: group 1, normal; group 2, DNCB; group 3, DNCB + tacrolimus; group 4, DNCB + Jawoongo. After shaving, the back skin of the mice was painted with 200 μL of a 2% DNCB solution over 1 × 1 cm patches for one week and challenged again with 200 μL of a 0.2% DNCB solution twice a week. Tacrolimus or Jawoongo was then applied to the sensitized skin for two weeks.

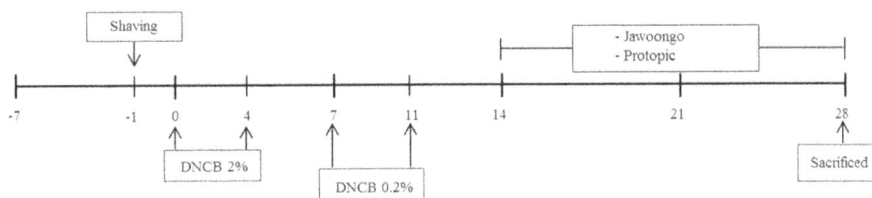

Fig. 1 General schematic diagram for the study protocol

Following the last application of Tacrolimus or Jawoongo, the mice were sacrificed to perform immunological and histological assessments. The method was performed as described previously [37].

Histological analysis

Skin samples (20 μm thick) were embedded in Tissue-Tek optical cutting temperature (OCT) compound (Leica, CA, Richmond, USA). The skin samples were stained with hematoxylin and eosin (H&E) to visualize inflammatory cells and with toluidine blue (TB) to visualize mast cells and then examined under a light microscope (Olympus). The mast cells and inflammatory cells were counted in 10 sections of high-power fields (HPFs) at 40×, 400× and 1000× magnification.

Immunohistochemistry [38]

CD4+ lymphocytes were detected by immunohistochemical analysis using anti-CD4+ antibodies (Santa cruz biotechnology, Dallas, Texas, USA). After deparaffinization, the slides were rehydrated and antigen retrieval done by microwave treatment, they were treated with 3% hydrogen peroxide in PBS for 15 min to inhibit the endogenous peroxidase activity of blood cells. Following the hydrogen peroxide treatment, the sections were incubated with 5% bovine serum albumin (BSA) in PBS as a blocking reagent for 1 h at room temperature. The sections were then incubated with mouse monoclonal CD4+ antibodies (1:100 dilution) overnight at 4 °C. After washing with PBS, subsequently incubated with secondary biotinylated anti-rabbit IgG for 1 h at room temperature. The sections were treated with an avidin-biotin HRP complex (Vectastain ABC kit, Vector Labs, CA, USA) for 30 min at 4 °C and stained with diaminobenzidine (DAB) tetrachloride as a substrate. The slides were mounted in an aqueous mounting solution (DAKO, Glostrup, Denmark) and cover-slipped. All of the sections were analyzed using an Olympus microscope, and images were captured using a digital video camera.

Analysis of mouse blood

Whole blood samples were collected by cardiac puncture and placed in Vacutainer TM tubes containing EDTA (BD Biosciences, USA) to prevent clotting. Anti-coagulated blood was processed to determine leukocyte counts, including lymphocytes, monocytes, eosinophils, basophils and neutrophils, using a HEMAVET 950 hematological analyzer (Drew Scientific, Inc., Oxford, USA).

RT-PCR

RNA was isolated using an Easy-blue RNA Extraction Kit (iNtRON biotech, Republic of Korea). In brief, we harvested cells (HMC-1, RAW264.7 and Splenocyte cells) and mouse tissue and 1 ml of R&A-BLUE solution was added to each. Following this, 200 μl of chloroform was added to the lysate and then vigorously vortexed for 15 s. Then, the lysate was centrifuged at 13,000 rpm for 10 min at 4 °C. We then transferred the appropriate volume of the aqueous phase into a clean tube, added 400 μl of isopropanol and mixed the solution thoroughly by inverting the tube 6–7 times. After centrifuging the tube at 13,000 rpm for 10 min, the supernatant was carefully removed without disturbing the pellet. Then, 1 ml of 75% ethanol was added, and the solution was thoroughly mixed by inverting the tube 4–5 times. The mixture was then centrifuged for 1 min at room temperature, and the supernatant was carefully discarded without disturbing the pellet. Finally, the remaining RNA pellet was dried and then dissolved in 20–50 μl of RNase-free water. The concentration of the isolated RNA was determined using a NanoDrop ND-1000 spectrophotometer (NanoDrop Technologies Inc., Wilmington, USA). We treated DNase to each sample. Two micrograms of total cellular RNA from each sample was reverse-transcribed using a cDNA synthesis kit (TaKaRa, Otsu, Shinga, Japan). PCR was conducted in a 20 μL reaction mixture consisting of a DNA template, 10 pM of each gene-specific primer, 10× Taq buffer, 2.5 mM dNTP mixture, and 1 unit of Taq DNA polymerase (Takara, Otsu, Shinga, Japan). PCR was performed using the specific primers listed in Table 1.

Enzyme-linked immunosorbent assay

Levels of IgE, IL-4, IL-6, IL-10, IL-12 and IL-13 were assessed using a Duoset enzyme-linked immunosorbent assay (ELISA) system (BD Biosciences, USA) according to the manufacturer's instructions. In brief, to assess the level of IgE, IL-4, IL-6, IL-10, IL-12 and IL-13 in the mice serum treated with Tacrolimus and Jawoongo, 96-well plates were coated with capture antibody in ELISA coating buffer and incubated overnight at 4 °C. The plates were then washed with PBS with 0.05% Tween 20 (PBS-T) and subsequently blocked with 10% FBS in PBS for 1 h at 20 °C. Serial dilutions of standard antigen or sample in dilution buffer (10% FBS in PBS) were added to the plates, and the plates were incubated for 2 h at 20 °C. After the plates were washed, biotin-conjugated anti-mouse IgE and streptavidin-conjugated horseradish peroxidase (SAv-HRP) were added to the plates, and the plates were incubated for 1 h at 20 °C. Finally, the tetramethylbenzidine (TMB) substrate was added to the plates, and after 15 min of incubation in the dark, 2 N H_2SO_4 was added to stop the reaction. The optical

Table 1 PCR primer sequences

Primer Type	Primer name	Primer Sequence
Mouse	IL-2	F: 5'-GCA GCT GTT GAT GGA CCT AC-3'
		R: 5'-TCC ACC ACA GTT GCT GAC TC-3'
	IL-4	F: 5'-TCG GCA TTT TGA ACG AGG TC-3'
		R: 5'-GAA AAG CCC GAA AGA GTC TC-3'
	IL-13	F: 5'-CGG CAG CAT GGT ATG GAG TG-3'
		R: 5'-ATT GCA ATT GGA GAT GTT GGT CAG-3'
	iNOS	F: 5'-AAT GGC AAC ATC AGG TCG GCC ATC ACT-3'
		R: 5'-GCT GTG TGT CAC AGA AGT CTC GAA CTC-3'
	TNF-α	F: 5'-ATG AGC ACA GAA AGC ATG ATC-3'
		R: 5'-TAC AGG CTT GTC ACT GGA ATT-3'
	GAPDH	F: 5'-GAG GGG CCA TCC ACA GTC TTC-3'
		R: 5'-CAT CAC CAT CTT CCA GGA GCG-3'
Human	IL-4	F: 5'-TGC CTC CAA GAA CAC AAC TG-3'
		R: 5'-CTC TGG TTG GCT TCC TTC AC-3'
	IL-6	F: 5'-AAC CTT CCA AAG ATG GCT GAA-3'
		R: 5'-CAG GAA CTG GAT CAG GAC TTT-3'
	IL-13	F: 5'-GGT CAA CAT CAC CCA GAA CC-3'
		R: 5'-TTT ACA AAC TGG GCC ACC TC-3'
	TSLP	F: 5'-TAT GAG TGG GAC CAA AAG TAC CG-3'
		R: 5'-GGG ATT GAA GGT TAG GCT CTG G-3'
	GAPDH	F: 5'-CGT CTT CAC CAC CAT GGA GA-3'
		R: 5'-CGG CCA TCA CGC CAC AGT TT-3'

density was measured at 450 nm on an automated ELISA reader. (Versa Max, Molecular Devices, CA, USA).

Detection of nitric oxide

Nitric oxide (NO) production from RAW264.7 cells in culture was measured using Griess reagent (Welgene, Korea). Briefly, 150 μL of cell culture supernatant was mixed with 150 μL of Griess solution and incubated for 30 min at room temperature. The optical density was determined at 570 nm using a microplate reader.

Cell viability assay

An MTS assay was performed to determine cell viability. To accomplish this, cells (HMC-1, RAW264.7 and Splenocyte cells) were seeded into a 96-well plate at a density of 3×10^3 cells per well and treated 24 h later with varying concentrations of Jawoongo (5–500 μg/mL) for an additional 24 h. Ten microliters of WST solution was added to each well of the plate, which was incubated in the dark at 37 °C for another 2 h. Optical density was measured at 450 nm using an ELISA plate reader.

Western blot analysis

Cells (HMC-1, RAW264.7 and Splenocyte cells) were lysed with cell lysis buffer (50 mM Tris-Cl pH 7.4, 1% NP-40, 0.25% sodium deoxycholate, 0.1% SDS, 150 mM NaCl, 1 mM EDTA, and protease inhibitor). Twenty micrograms of protein was separated by SDS-polyacrylamide gel electrophoresis and transferred to a nitrocellulose membrane (Protran nitrocellulose membrane, Whatman, UK). The membrane was blocked with 5% nonfat milk, probed with specific primary antibodies, incubated with HRP-conjugated secondary IgG antibodies (Calbiochem, San Diego, CA, USA), and visualized using an enhanced chemiluminescence detection system (Amersham ECL kit, Amersham Pharmacia Biotech Inc., Piscataway, NJ, USA). The antibodies against COX-2, p-JNK, total JNK and iNos were obtained from Cell Signaling (Danvers, MA, USA). The antibodies against p-Erk, total Erk, phospho-NF-κB p65 (Ser536), total NF-κB and Actin were obtained from Santa Cruz Biotechnology (Dallas, Texas, USA). Tubulin antibody was obtained from Sigma-Aldrich (St. Louis, MO, USA).

Isolation of Splenocytes

Spleen suspensions from normal mice were prepared under aseptic conditions by homogenization in RPMI-1640 medium (containing 10% FBS, 1% antibiotics, and 0.05 mM β-mercaptoethanol). Red blood cell (RBC) lysis buffer (Sigma, St. Louis, MO, USA) was added to the cell suspension to remove RBCs. The spleen cells were centrifuged, suspended in complete RPMI-1640, and maintained at 37 °C in a humidified incubator with 5% CO_2.

Liquid chromatography-mass spectrometry analysis.

An Agilent 1100 series liquid chromatography-mass spectroscopy (LC-MS) with an atmospheric pressure chemical ionization interface was used in negative and positive ionization modes. Data were collected using Chemstation software version A.09.03. A Shiseido capcell-pak C18 column (4.6 mm × 150 mm, 5 μm) was used with an injection volume of 10 μL for the HPLC separation. The mobile phases consisted of (A) Acetonitrile, (B) 0.1% Acetic acid and (C) Methanol at a flow rate of 1.0 mL/min. The gradient of the mobile phases (A: B: C) for separation was 0–90 min (35: 65: 0 to 0: 0: 100). Decursin was used as standard. Mass spectrometry was operated with an electrospray ionization source and positive mode.

Statistical analysis

All experiment results were expressed as the means ± SEM of at least three separate tests. Statistical significance at $P < 0.05 < 0.01$ and < 0.001 has been given respective symbols in the figures. Statistical analyses (ANOVA) were performed using PRISM software (GraphPad Software Inc., La Jolla, CA, USA,).

Results

Effects of Jawoongo on a DNCB-induced mouse model of AD

We investigated the effects of Jawoongo on DNCB-induced AD-like symptoms. We found that skin thickness increased following application of DNCB (2.06 ± 0.12 mm) compared to no treatment (0.57 ± 0.03 mm), and this increase was inhibited by both Jawoongo (1.56 ± 0.21 mm) and tacrolimus (1.25 ± 0.18 mm) treatment (Fig. 2a). In addition, we monitored the body weights and food intake of the mice throughout the study and observed no significant changes, suggesting that Jawoongo did not produce any toxic effects on the mice (Additional file 1: Figure S1A and B). H & E

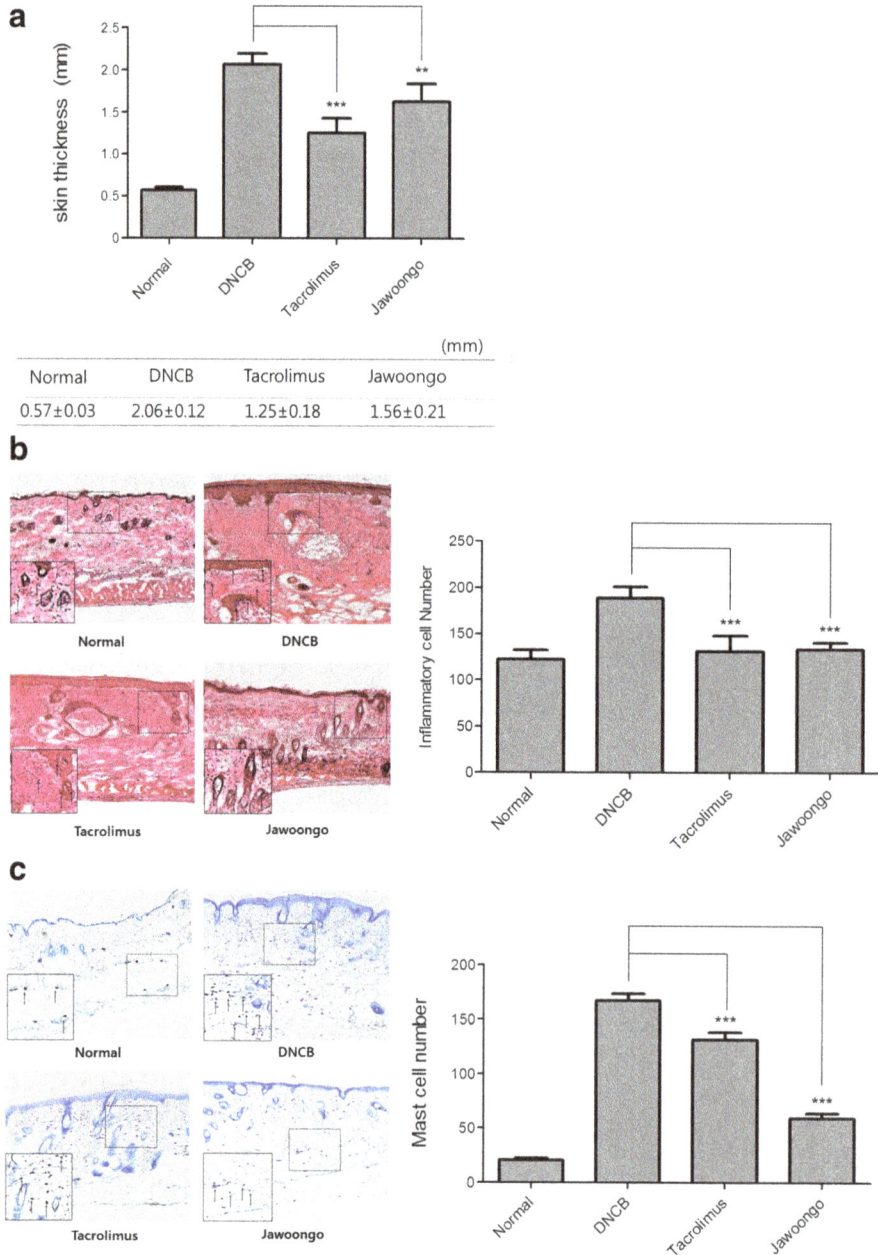

| | | | (mm) |
Normal	DNCB	Tacrolimus	Jawoongo
0.57±0.03	2.06±0.12	1.25±0.18	1.56±0.21

Fig. 2 Effects of Jawoongo on the skin of mice with DNCB-induced AD. Skin thickness in mice with DNCB-induced AD that were treated with Jawoongo (**a**). Jawoongo reduced the infiltration of inflammatory cells into the skin. Skin sections were stained with hematoxylin and eosin (**b**). Arrows indicate inflammatory cells. Jawoongo reduced the infiltration of mast cells into the skin. Skin sections were stained with toluidine blue (**c**). Arrows indicate inflammatory cells. The sections were evaluated under a microscope at an original magnification of 200×. The data were presented as mean ± SEMs (n = 8 mice/group). *P < 0.05, **P < 0.01 and ***P < 0.001 as compared to DNCB-stimulated group, respectively

staining was performed to examine whether Jawoongo reduces the infiltration of inflammatory cells into the skin. The number of inflammatory cells in the mice with DNCB-induced AD lesions was higher than that in the normal mice and decreased following treatment with Jawoongo or tacrolimus (Fig. 2b, left panel). The bar graph indicates the average number of cells counted from a random field of view (Fig. 3b, right panel). Moreover, toluidine blue staining was used to examine whether Jawoongo reduces mast cell infiltration into the skin. There was greater mast cell infiltration in the skin of the mice with DNCB-induced AD lesions than that of the normal mice. Treatment with Jawoongo or tacrolimus decreased the infiltration of mast cells into the skin (Fig. 2c, left panel). The bar graph indicates

the average number of cells counted from a random field of view (Fig. 2c, right panel).

Jawoongo treatment lowered the number of WBCs in the blood of mice

Application of DNCB increased both the total number of white blood cells (WBCs) and the number of each WBC subtype, including neutrophils, basophils, eosinophils, monocytes, and lymphocytes, in the serum of the mice. Importantly, treatment with Jawoongo or tacrolimus lowered the increased number of WBCs, indicating that Jawoongo and tacrolimus suppress inflammation by decreasing the number of WBCs in the blood (Fig. 3a, b, c, d, e and f).

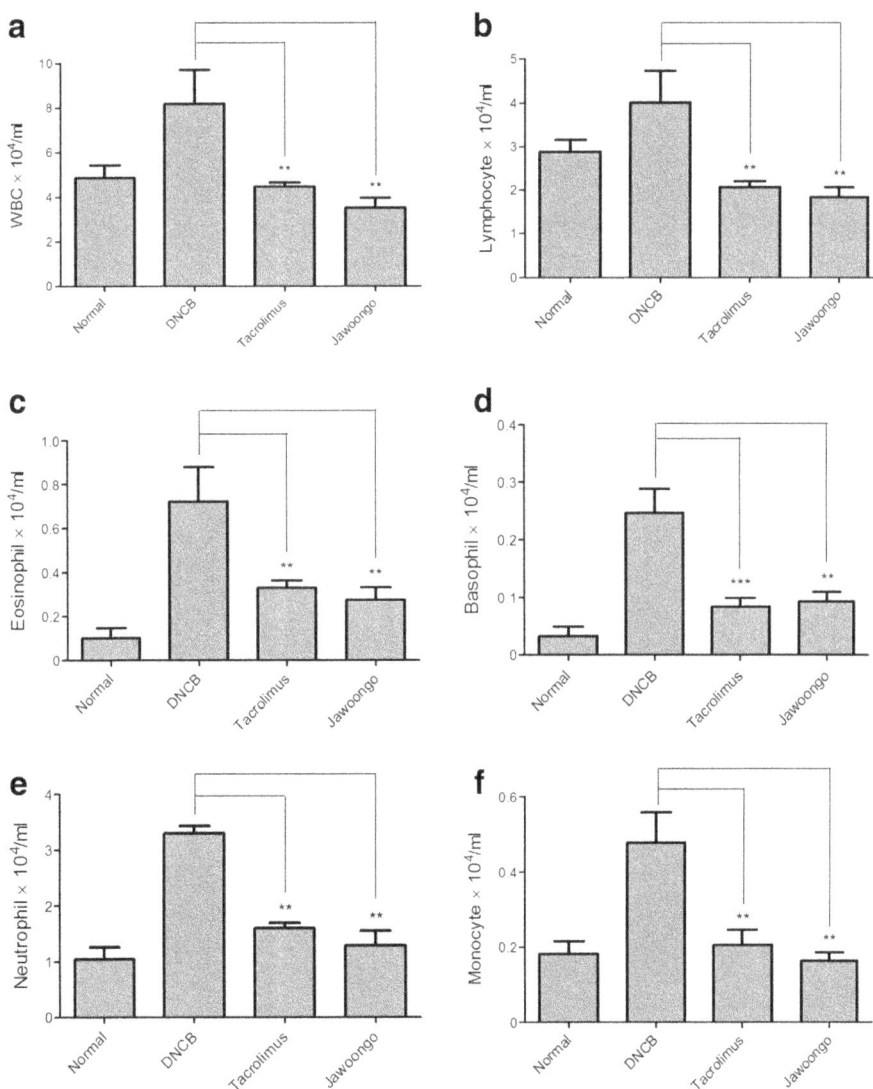

Fig. 3 Jawoongo reduced leukocyte numbers in the blood. Blood samples were analyzed using a HEMAVET 950 hematological analyzer. The data were presented as mean ± SEMs ($n = 8$ mice/group). *$P < 0.05$, **$P < 0.01$ and ***$P < 0.001$ as compared to DNCB-stimulated group, respectively

Jawoongo treatment reduced the serum levels of IgE, IL-6, IL-10 and IL-12 in mice

We next measured proinflammatory cytokine levels by ELISA. We found that Jawoongo treatment reduced the serum levels of IgE, IL-6, IL-10 and IL-12 whose expression was induced after DNCB application. Tacrolimus treatment increased the serum levels of IgE (Fig. 4a, b, c and d).

Jawoongo treatment down-regulated mRNA expression of IL-2, IL-4, IL-13, and TNF-α in mouse skin

RT-PCR analysis of RNA extracted from mouse skin revealed that DNCB increased the levels of AD-associated cytokines such as IL-2, IL-4, IL-13 and TNF-α when applied to skin, and subsequent treatment with Jawoongo or tacrolimus suppressed the increased cytokine levels (Fig. 5a, b, c and d).

Jawoongo treatment reduced the number of CD4+ cells in skin

We performed immunocytochemistry to examine whether Jawoongo treatment can reduce the level of CD4+ in skin. The level of CD4+ in the mice with DNCB-induced AD lesions was higher than that in the normal mice.

Additional treatment with Jawoongo or tacrolimus decreased the number of CD4+ cells (Fig. 6).

Jawoongo inhibited agonist-induced cytokine production in HMC-1 cells

Based on the observation that Jawoongo inhibited AD-associated cytokine production in mice, we next investigated whether Jawoongo affects cytokine expression in human mast cell line 1 (HMC-1) cells. To accomplish this, HMC-1 cells were stimulated with ionomycin and PMA before treatment with varying concentrations of Jawoongo. RT-PCR analysis showed that Jawoongo dose-dependently suppressed the IL-4, IL-13 and TSLP mRNA expression that was induced by treatment with ionomycin and PMA (Fig. 7a). Moreover, Western blot analysis indicated that Jawoongo significantly reduced agonist-stimulated Erk, JNK, NF-κB and COX-2 protein expression in a dose-dependent manner (Fig. 7b). We also demonstrated that Jawoongo inhibited agonist-stimulated IL-4, IL-6, and IL-13 secretion, as determined by ELISA (Fig. 7c). No significant effect on cell viability was observed in HMC-1 cells treated with Jawoongo alone or in combination with ionomycin and PMA (Additional file 2: Figure S2A).

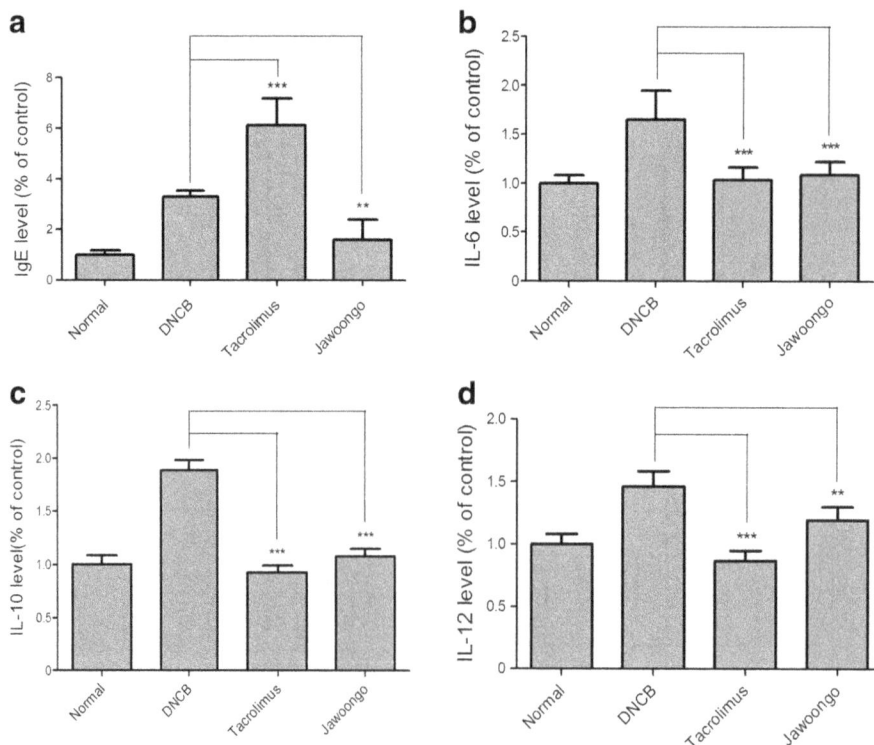

Fig. 4 Jawoongo reduced cytokine levels in serum. Cytokine levels were measured by ELISA. The data were presented as mean ± SEMs ($n = 8$ mice/group). *$P < 0.05$, **$P < 0.01$ and ***$P < 0.001$ as compared to DNCB-stimulated group, respectively

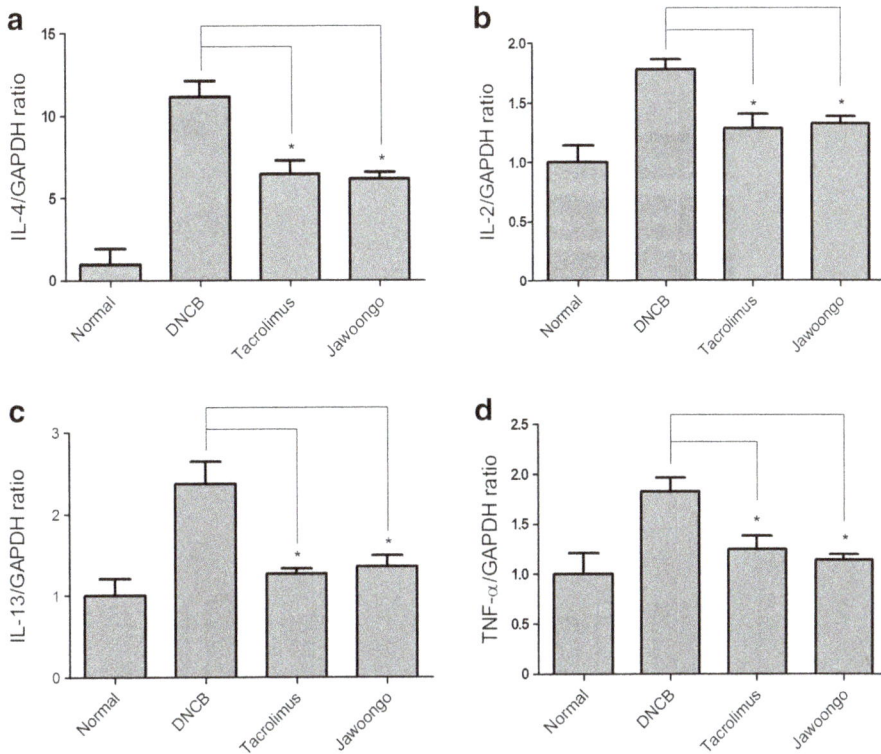

Fig. 5 Effects of Jawoongo on cytokine mRNA expression in mouse skin tissue. IL-2, IL-4, IL-13 and TNF-α mRNA expression was measured by RT-PCR, shown in (**a**), (**b**), (**c**), and (**d**), respectively, in mouse skin tissue. The data were presented as mean ± SEMs ($n = 8$ mice/group). *$P < 0.05$, **$P < 0.01$ and ***$P < 0.001$ as compared to DNCB-stimulated group, respectively

Jawoongo inhibited LPS-induced inflammatory responses in RAW264.7 cells

Because NO plays an important role in allergic responses, we next examined the effects of Jawoongo on NO production and inducible nitric oxide synthase (iNOS) mRNA expression in the murine RAW264.7 macrophage cell line. As shown in Fig. 8a and b, Jawoongo reduced LPS-induced NO production and iNOS mRNA expression in a dose-dependent manner. Jawoongo also decreased LPS-induced increases in mRNA and protein expression of inflammation-related genes, such as tumor necrosis factor-α (TNF-α) and COX-2. Moreover, Jawoongo had an inhibitory effect on ERK and JNK activation in relation to various inflammatory responses (Fig. 8c). When using a low concentration of Jawoongo (~ 100 g/ml), no significant effect on RAW264.7 cell viability was observed (Additional file 2: Figure S2B).

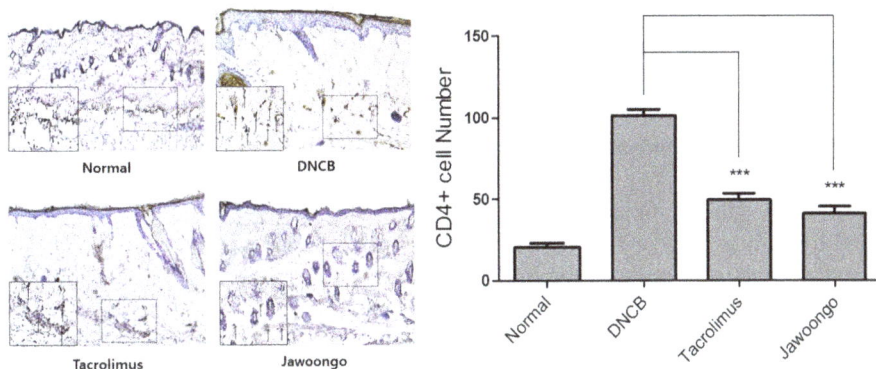

Fig. 6 Distribution of CD4+ cells in the skin of mice with DNCB-induced AD. Skin sections were immunostained with CD4+ antibodies. CD4+ cells display a brown color. The sections were evaluated under a microscope at an original magnification of 200×

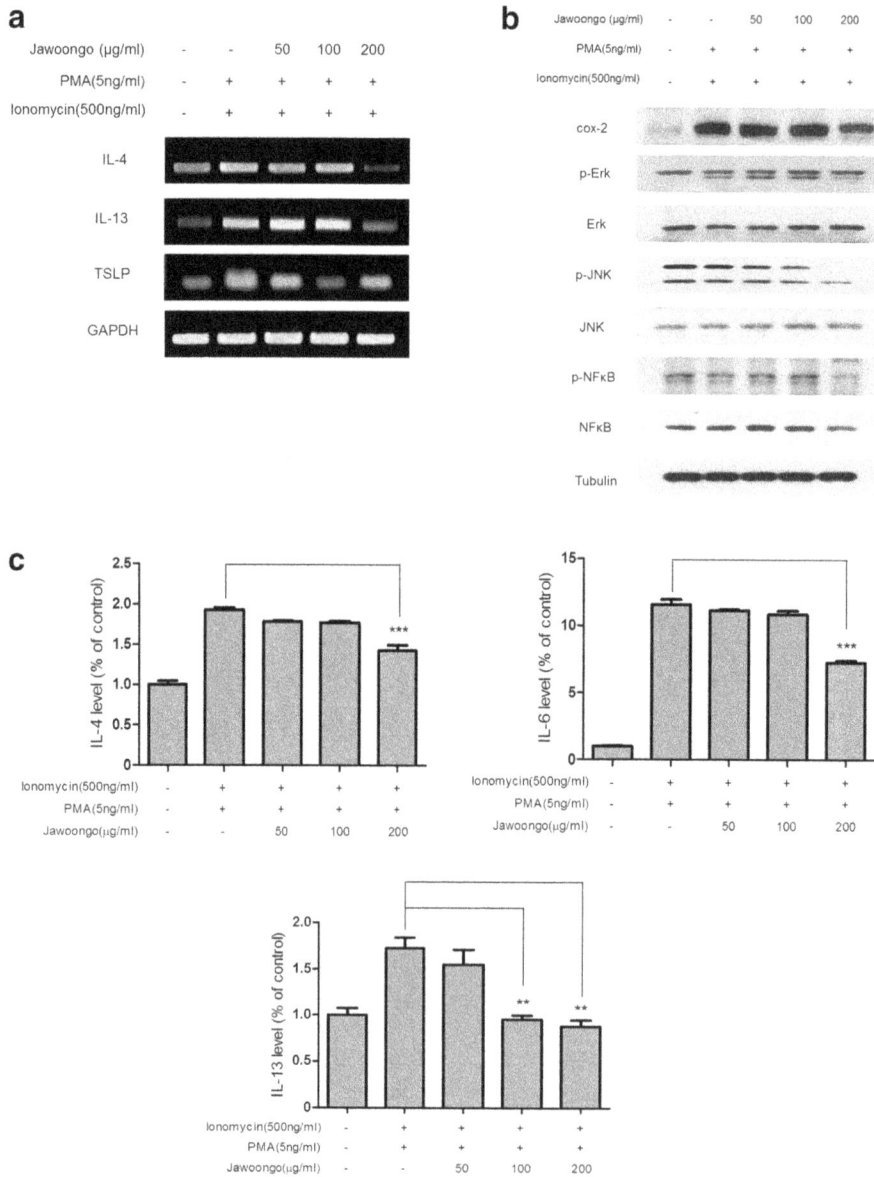

Fig. 7 Effects of Jawoongo on cytokine expression in HMC-1 cells. HMC-1 cells were stimulated with ionomycin (500 ng/ml) and PMA (5 ng/ml) and then treated with different concentrations of Jawoongo (50–200 μg/ml) for 24 h. IL-4, IL-13 and TSLP mRNA expression was measured by RT-PCR (**a**). Whole cell lysates were analyzed by Western blotting (**b**). The culture medium of the cells was harvested, and IL-4, IL-6 and IL-13 cytokine levels were measured by ELISA (**c**). The data were presented as mean ± SEMs (*n* = 8 mice/group). *$P < 0.05$, **$P < 0.01$ and ***$P < 0.001$ as compared to Ionomycin and PMA-stimulated group, respectively

Jawoongo inhibited LPS-induced inflammatory responses in isolated Splenocytes

We further tested Jawoongo's anti-inflammatory activities in splenocytes isolated from mice. Similar to HMC-1 and RAW264.7 cells, Jawoongo treatment reduced the mRNA levels of proinflammatory cytokines, including IL-4, IL-6, and TNF-α in LPS-stimulated splenocytes (Fig. 9a). Dose-dependent inhibition of IL-6 and TNF-α secretion by Jawoongo was also observed (Fig. 9b). Finally, Western blot analysis demonstrated that treatment with a high

dose of Jawoongo decreased COX-2 and iNOS levels and NF-κB activity in LPS-induced splenocytes (Fig. 9c). At a concentration of ~ 200 g/ml, as was used in these experiments, Jawoongo showed no significant toxic effects on splenocytes (Additional file 2: Figure S2C).

Decursin is an Indicator molecule for Jawoongo

Liquid chromatography-mass spectrometry was used to measure the retention time of decursin. Chromatograms were acquired at 215 nm on an HPLC by UV detection

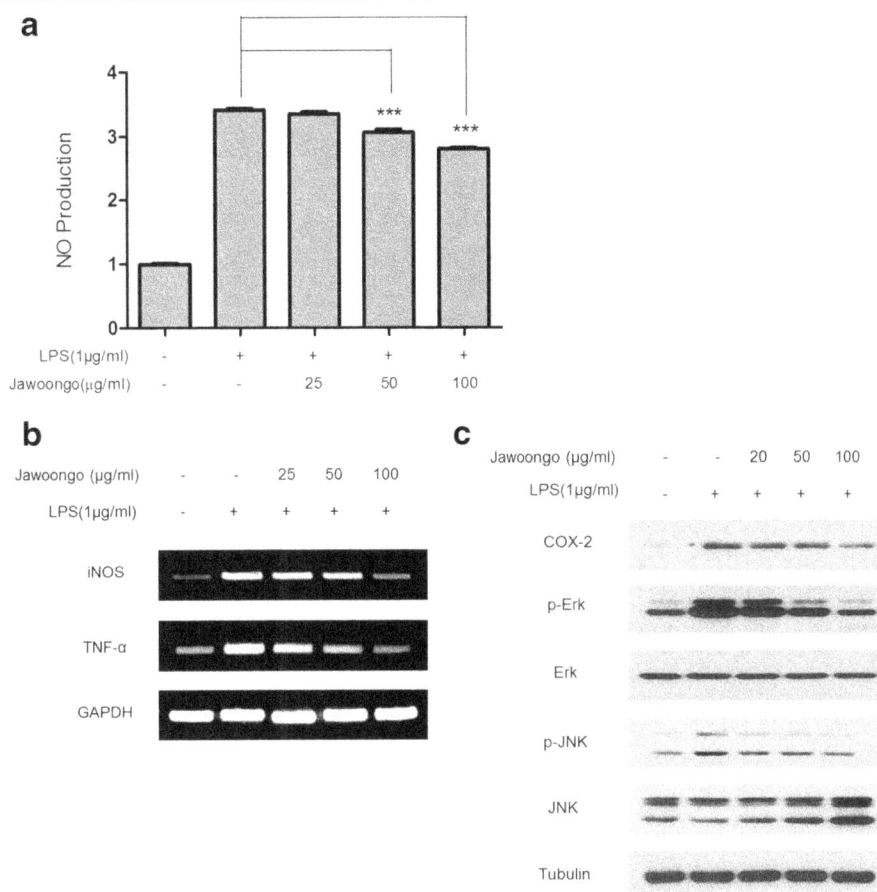

Fig. 8 Effects of Jawoongo on NO production in RAW264.7 cells. RAW264.7 cells were stimulated with LPS (1 mg/ml) and then treated with different concentrations of Jawoongo (25–100 μg/ml) for 24 h. NO production was measured using the Griess reagent system (**a**). iNOS and TNF-α mRNA expression was measured by RT-PCR (**b**). Whole cell lysates were analyzed by Western blotting (**c**). The data were presented as mean ± SEMs ($n = 8$ mice/group). *$P < 0.05$, **$P < 0.01$ and ***$P < 0.001$ as compared to LPS-stimulated group, respectively

(Fig. 10a), and the retention time of decursin was 53.028 min (Fig. 10b).

Discussion

AD is a common pruritic and chronically relapsing inflammatory skin disease. Affecting approximately 10–20% of children and 1–3% of adults worldwide [39], AD is a major global public health problem. Additionally, the incidence of AD has steadily increased every year [40].

Several mouse models have been developed to evaluate drugs for the treatment of AD. A DNCB-patch model using BALB/c mice has been proposed as a suitable representative of human AD because mice treated with DNCB show symptoms similar to human AD, including epidermal hyperplasia, dermal mast cell infiltration, and elevated serum IgE levels [41]. Activated mast cells release inflammatory mediators such as histamines, cytokines and chemokines [42, 43]. In this study, we investigated the anti-AD effects of Jawoongo using DNCB-treated BALB/c mice. We found that topical application of Jawoongo strongly suppressed DNCB-induced AD-like lesions and reduced skin thickness, CD4 levels and mast cell infiltration in sensitized skin. We observed that Jawoongo suppresses skin inflammation by inhibiting various DNCB-stimulated inflammatory responses.

Until now, the exact pathogenesis of AD has remained unclear. However, Th1 and Th2 cytokines play an important role in the etiology of AD. In particular, Th2 cytokines are important mediators of AD development [44]. CD4+ T cells are key factors implicated in the pathogenesis of AD, and skin infiltration of CD4+ T cells is known to increase in severe AD cases [45].

Therefore, we investigated cytokines related to Th2 in an in vivo model. Jawoongo treatment reduced the

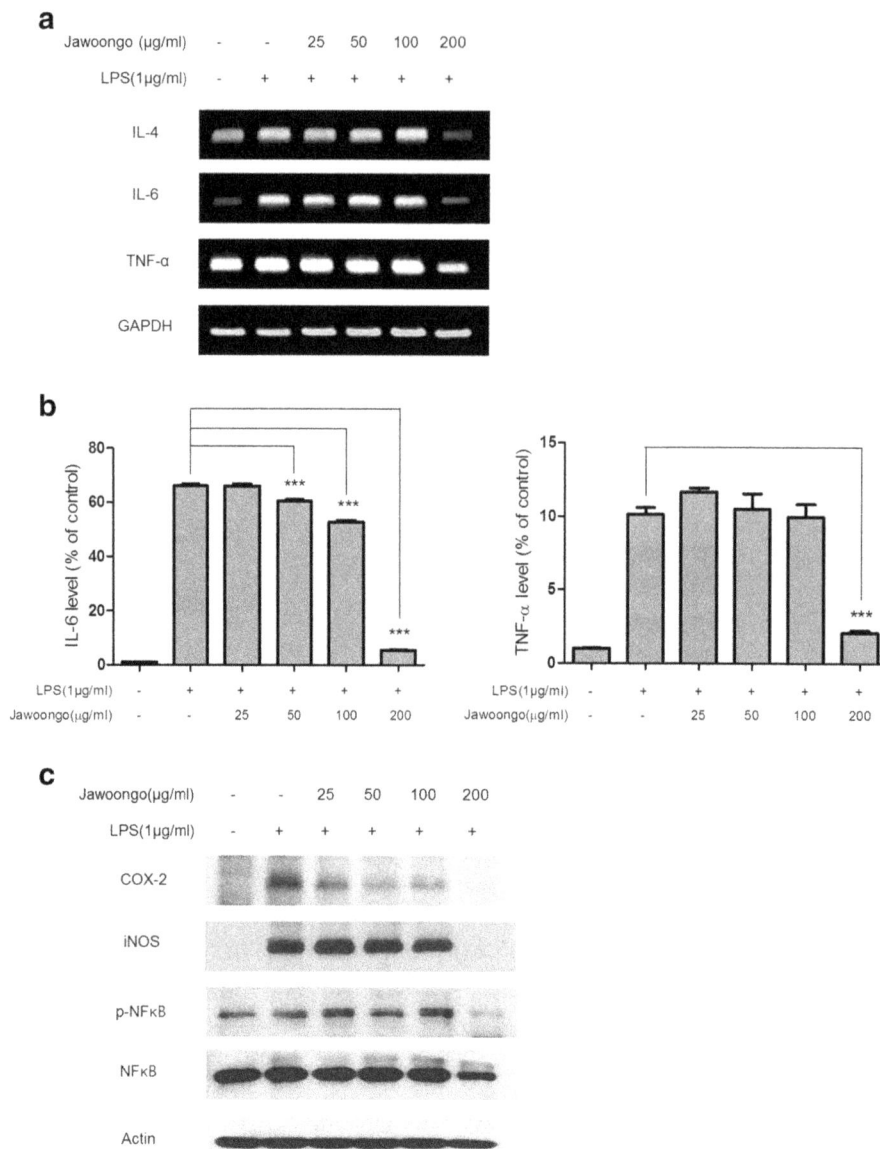

Fig. 9 Effects of Jawoongo on cytokine expression in splenocytes. Splenocytes were stimulated with LPS (1 µg/ml) and then treated with different concentrations of Jawoongo (25–200 µg/ml) for 24 h. IL-4, IL-6 and TNF-α mRNA expression was measured by RT-PCR (**a**). The culture medium of the cells was harvested, and IL-6 and TNF-α cytokine levels were measured by ELISA (**b**). Whole cell lysates were analyzed by Western blotting (**c**). The data were presented as mean ± SEMs ($n = 8$ mice/group). $*P < 0.05$, $**P < 0.01$ and $***P < 0.001$ as compared to LPS-stimulated group, respectively

increased serum levels of IgE, IL-6, IL-10 and IL-12 induced by DNCB treatment In fact, it was reported that IL-12 was increased by DNCB [46, 47], and this increase was suppressed by Jawoongo as expected. We also found that Jawoongo reduced DNCB-stimulated increases in eosinophil, neutrophil, monocyte, basophil, lymphocyte and WBC numbers and in IL-4, IL-13 and TNF-α mRNA expression. These results suggest that Jawoongo decreased the number of CD4+ cells entering the skin. Of note, Jawoongo and tacrolimus, which was used as a positive control in this study, showed similar effects on AD-like skin lesions, but Jawoongo exhibited more favorable effects than tacrolimus in some aspects, such as in decreased mast cell recruitment and serum IgE levels.

To improve our understanding of Jawoongo's actions at the cellular level, we evaluated the effects of Jawoongo on several types of innate immune cell, including human mast cells (HMC-1), murine macrophage RAW264.7 cells, and splenocytes isolated from mice.

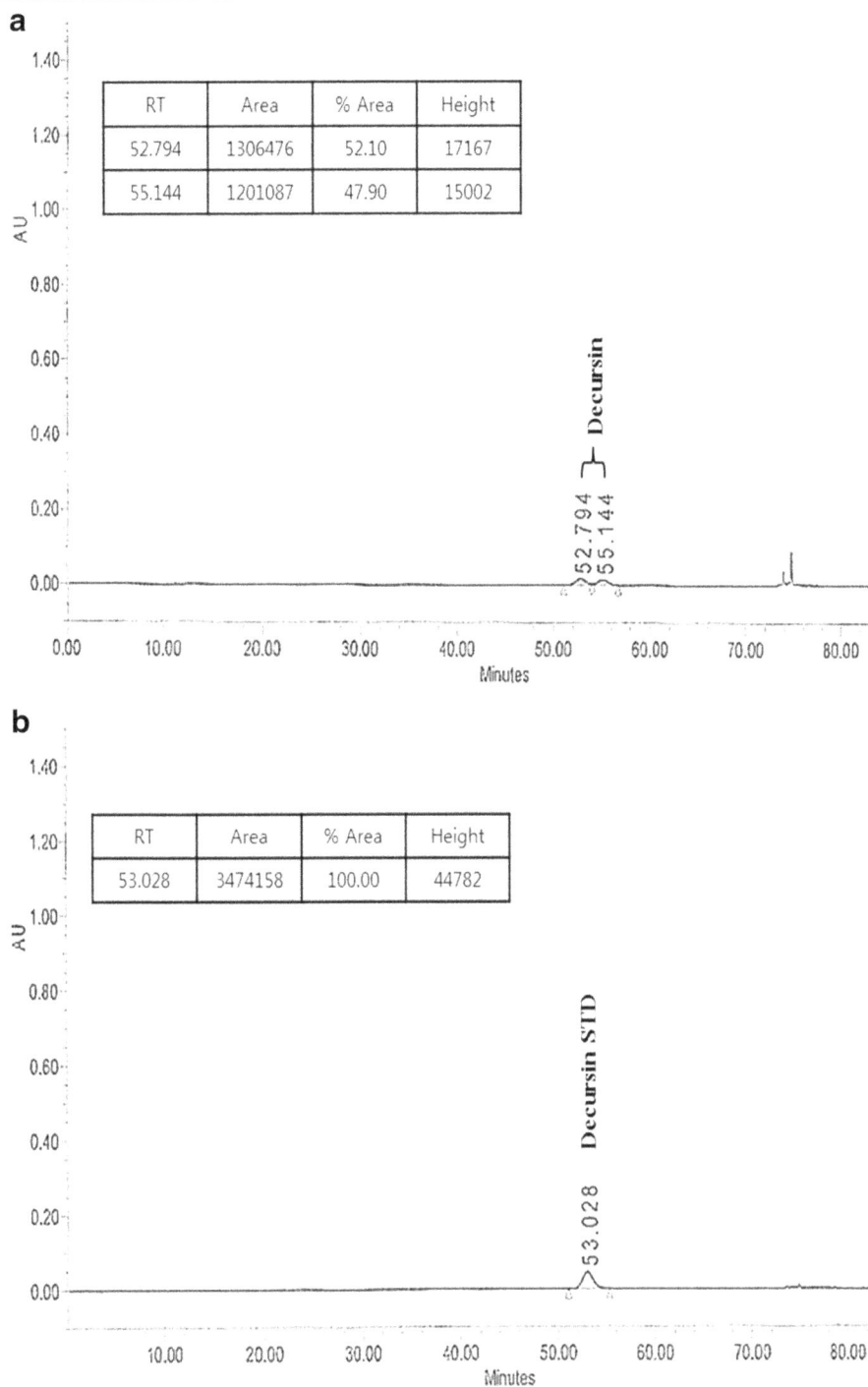

a

RT	Area	% Area	Height
52.794	1306476	52.10	17167
55.144	1201087	47.90	15002

b

RT	Area	% Area	Height
53.028	3474158	100.00	44782

Fig. 10 LC-MS chromatogram. **a** Identification of decursin in Jawoongo. **b** Mass spectrum peak at 53.028 min

Inflammation causes cells to respond to stimulation by releasing various cytokines and by increasing COX-2 expression. Therefore, COX-2 expression can be measured to evaluate anti-inflammatory effects [48, 49]. In the present study, Jawoongo treatment suppressed AD-associated cytokine production, such as IL-4, Erk, JNK, p-NF-κB and COX-2 expression, in HMC-1 cells. iNOS produces NO after it is activated by various cytokines. Inflammatory and immune responses lead to vasodilation, erythema and edema in response to increasing NO levels. Excessive NO aggravates the inflammatory response due to the immune-regulatory

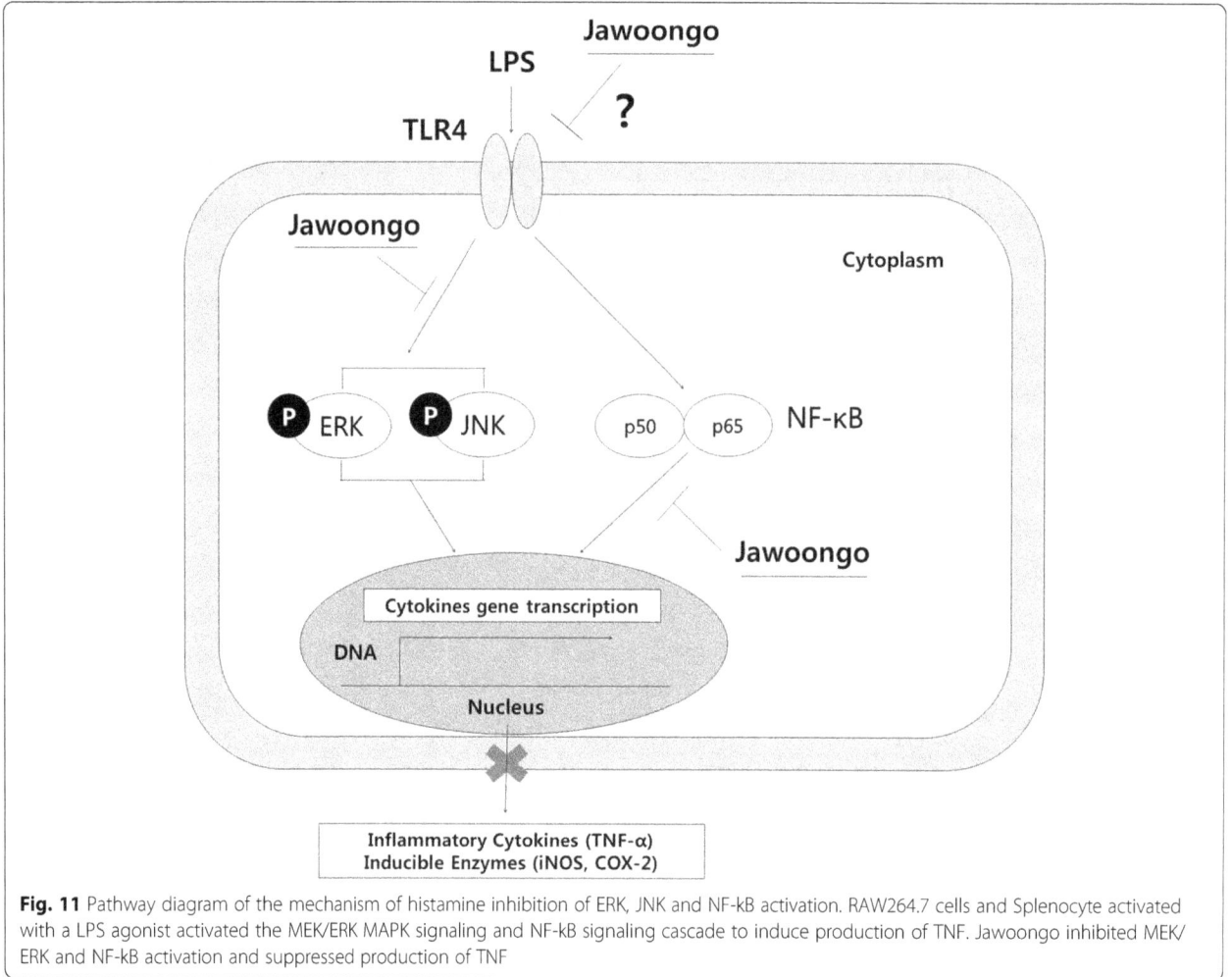

Fig. 11 Pathway diagram of the mechanism of histamine inhibition of ERK, JNK and NF-kB activation. RAW264.7 cells and Splenocyte activated with a LPS agonist activated the MEK/ERK MAPK signaling and NF-kB signaling cascade to induce production of TNF. Jawoongo inhibited MEK/ERK and NF-kB activation and suppressed production of TNF

role of NO [50, 51]. Macrophages contain several factors that regulate cytokine and chemokine secretion in AD. Therefore, macrophages have an important role in both the acute and chronic inflammation associated with AD [52–54]. Macrophages are involved in the initiation and maintenance of acute and chronic inflammatory responses [55]. Treatment of murine macrophage RAW264.7 cells with Jawoongo suppressed LPS-stimulated NO production, reduced iNOS and TNF-α mRNA levels, and decreased ERK and JNK activation. We also found that Jawoongo treatment reduced IL-4, IL-6 and TNF-α mRNA levels; COX-2 and iNOS protein levels; and NFκB activity in LPS-induced splenocytes. It appears that high concentrations of Jawoongo are required to mediate an effect in vitro. Because both MAP kinase and NFκB pathways are implicated in AD, Jawoongo appears to inhibit both pathways (Fig. 11). Taken together, our results suggest that Jawoongo regulates proinflammatory cytokine production in several types of immune cell, thereby suppressing the AD-like symptoms caused by DNCB.

Conclusions

Our present study demonstrates that Jawoongo treatment suppresses DNCB-induced AD symptoms by downregulating serum IgE levels and the production of several inflammatory cytokines. In addition, our data indicate that Jawoongo treatment inhibits cytokine expression and activation of the NF-kB and MAPK pathways in several types of immune cell. Taken together, our results suggest that Jawoongo might be a useful candidate drug for the treatment of AD.

Additional files

Additional file 1: Figure S1. Changes in body weight (A) and food intake (B) in DNCB-induced AD mice during treatment with Jawoongo. Values are expressed as the mean ± SEMs ($n = 8$).

Additional file 2: Figure S2. Effects of Jawoongo on cell viability in various cell lines. HMC-1 cells were treated with the combination of ionomycin (500 ng/ml) and PMA (5 ng/ml) with varying concentrations of DMSO and Jawoongo (5–500 µg/ml) for 24 h (A). RAW264.7 cells (B) and splenocytes (C) were treated with the combination of LPS (1 mg/ml) and varying concentrations of DMSO and Jawoongo (5–500 µg/ml) for 24 h.

Cell viability was measured using an MTS assay. The data were presented as mean ± SEMs of three independent experiments. $*P < 0.05$, $**P < 0.01$ and $***P < 0.001$.

Abbreviations

AD: Atopic dermatitis; AGN: Angelica gigas Nakai; BSA: Bovine serum albumin; DAB: Diaminobenzidine; DNCB: 2,4-dinitrochlorobenzene; HMC-1: Human mast cells; IgE: Immunoglobulin E; iNOS: Inducible nitric oxide synthase; MTS: 3-(4,5-dimethylthiazol-2-yl)-5-(3-carboxymethoxyphenyl)-2-(4-sulfophenyl)-2H-tetrazolium; NO: Nitric oxide; OCT: Optical cutting temperature; PGD2: Prostaglandin D2; PMA: Phorbol-12-Myristate-13-Acetate; TB: Toluidine blue; Th2: T-helper 2; TNF-α: Tumor necrosis factor-α; TSLP: Thymic stromal lymphopoietin; WBCs: White blood cells; WST: Tetrazolium salt

Acknowledgements

We thank our colleagues from the Laboratory of Prevention medicine for technique assistance and useful discussions.

Funding

This research was supported by a grant from the Korean Medicine R&D Project of the Ministry of Health and Welfare (HI12C1889 and HI13C0530).

Authors' contributions

JMK carried out the experiment and drafting of manuscript. SHH, SRK, HC, HIK, DUK and SMO revised the research and manuscript and assisted in the research work. HSS, TYK and YCS guided the research, revised and submitted the manuscript. CC and SGK designed, supervised the experiments and corrected the manuscript. All the authors read and approved the final manuscript.

Competing interests

The authors declare that they have no competing interests.

Author details

[1]Department of Science in Korean Medicine, Graduate School, Kyung Hee University, Kyungheedae-ro 26, Dongdaemun-gu, Seoul 02447, Republic of Korea. [2]Department of Preventive Medicine, College of Korean Medicine, Kyung Hee University, Kyungheedae-ro 26, Dongdaemun-gu, Seoul 02447, South Korea.

References

1. Kaiko GE, Phipps S, Angkasekwinai P, Dong C, Foster PS. NK cell deficiency predisposes to viral-induced Th2-type allergic inflammation via epithelial-derived IL-25. J Immunol. 2010;185(8):4681–90.
2. Yang JQ, Liu H, Diaz-Meco MT, Moscat J. NBR1 is a new PB1 signalling adapter in Th2 differentiation and allergic airway inflammation in vivo. EMBO J. 2010;29(19):3421–33.
3. Shirinbak S, Taher YA, Maazi H, Gras R, van Esch BC, Henricks PA, Samsom JN, Verbeek JS, Lambrecht BN, van Oosterhout AJ, et al. Suppression of Th2-driven airway inflammation by allergen immunotherapy is independent of B cell and Ig responses in mice. J Immunol. 2010;185(7):3857–65.
4. Grewe M, Bruijnzeel-Koomen CA, Schopf E, Thepen T, Langeveld-Wildschut AG, Ruzicka T, Krutmann J. A role for Th1 and Th2 cells in the immunopathogenesis of atopic dermatitis. Immunol Today. 1998; 19(8):359–61.
5. Torii M, Wang L, Ma N, Saito K, Hori T, Sato-Ueshima M, Koyama Y, Nishikawa H, Katayama N, Mizoguchi A, et al. Thioredoxin suppresses airway inflammation independently of systemic Th1/Th2 immune modulation. Eur J Immunol. 2010;40(3):787–96.
6. Mabalirajan U, Agrawal A, Ghosh B. Comment on "Ym1/2 promotes Th2 cytokine expression by inhibiting 12/15(S)-lipoxygenase: identification of a novel pathway for regulating allergic inflammation". J Immunol. 2009; 183(10):6039. author reply 6039-6040
7. Kitajima M, Iwamura C, Miki-Hosokawa T, Shinoda K, Endo Y, Watanabe Y, Shinnakasu R, Hosokawa H, Hashimoto K, Motohashi S, et al. Enhanced Th2 cell differentiation and allergen-induced airway inflammation in Zfp35-deficient mice. J Immunol. 2009;183(8):5388–96.
8. Akitake R, Nakase H, Tamaoki M, Ueno S, Mikami S, Chiba T. Modulation of Th1/Th2 balance by infliximab rescues postoperative occurrence of small-intestinal inflammation associated with ulcerative colitis. Dig Dis Sci. 2010; 55(6):1781–4.
9. Dubois A, Deruytter N, Adams B, Kanda A, Delbauve S, Fleury S, Torres D, Francois A, Petein M, Goldman M, et al. Regulation of Th2 responses and allergic inflammation through bystander activation of CD8+ T lymphocytes in early life. J Immunol. 2010;185(2):884–91.
10. Girtsman T, Jaffar Z, Ferrini M, Shaw P, Roberts K. Natural Foxp3(+) regulatory T cells inhibit Th2 polarization but are biased toward suppression of Th17-driven lung inflammation. J Leukoc Biol. 2010;88(3):537–46.
11. Jie Z, Jin M, Cai Y, Bai C, Shen Y, Yuan Z, Hu Y, Holgate S. The effects of Th2 cytokines on the expression of ADAM33 in allergen-induced chronic airway inflammation. Respir Physiol Neurobiol. 2009;168(3):289–94.
12. Perros F, Hoogsteden HC, Coyle AJ, Lambrecht BN, Hammad H. Blockade of CCR4 in a humanized model of asthma reveals a critical role for DC-derived CCL17 and CCL22 in attracting Th2 cells and inducing airway inflammation. Allergy. 2009;64(7):995–1002.
13. Singh SP, Mishra NC, Rir-Sima-Ah J, Campen M, Kurup V, Razani-Boroujerdi S, Sopori ML. Maternal exposure to secondhand cigarette smoke primes the lung for induction of phosphodiesterase-4D5 isozyme and exacerbated Th2 responses: rolipram attenuates the airway hyperreactivity and muscarinic receptor expression but not lung inflammation and atopy. J Immunol. 2009; 183(3):2115–21.
14. Niu N, Laufer T, Homer RJ, Cohn L. Cutting edge: limiting MHC class II expression to dendritic cells alters the ability to develop Th2- dependent allergic airway inflammation. J Immunol. 2009;183(3):1523–7.
15. Park SK, Cho MK, Park HK, Lee KH, Lee SJ, Choi SH, Ock MS, Jeong HJ, Lee MH, Yu HS. Macrophage migration inhibitory factor homologs of anisakis simplex suppress Th2 response in allergic airway inflammation model via CD4+CD25+Foxp3+ T cell recruitment. J Immunol. 2009;182(11):6907–14.
16. Min HJ, Won HY, Kim YC, Sung SH, Byun MR, Hwang JH, Hong JH, Hwang ES. Suppression of Th2-driven, allergen-induced airway inflammation by sauchinone. Biochem Biophys Res Commun. 2009;385(2):204–9.
17. Xia H, Cai SX, Tong WC, Luo LM, Yu HP. respiratory syncytial virus infection promotes the production of thymic stromal lymphopoietin and accelerates Th2 inflammation in mouse airway. Nan Fang Yi Ke Da Xue Xue Bao. 2009; 29(4):724–8.
18. Cai Y, Kumar RK, Zhou J, Foster PS, Webb DC. Ym1/2 promotes Th2 cytokine expression by inhibiting 12/15(S)-lipoxygenase: identification of a novel pathway for regulating allergic inflammation. J Immunol. 2009; 182(9):5393–9.
19. Granot E, Yakobovich E, Bardenstein R. Tacrolimus immunosuppression - an association with asymptomatic eosinophilia and elevated total and specific IgE levels. Pediatr Transplant. 2006;10(6):690–3.
20. Tomi NS, Luger TA. The treatment of atopic dermatitis with topical immunomodulators. Clin Dermatol. 2003;21(3):215–24.
21. Kim IS, Kim DH, Yun CY, Lee JS. A (S)-(+)-decursin derivative, (S)-(+)-3-(3,4-dihydroxy-phenyl)-acrylic acid 2,2-dimethyl-8-oxo-3,4-dihydro-2H,8H-pyrano[3,2-g]-chromen-3-yl-ester, attenuates the development of atopic dermatitis-like lesions in NC/Nga mice. Mol Biol Rep. 2013;40(3):2541–8.
22. Li L, Li W, Jung SW, Lee YW, Kim YH. Protective effects of decursin and decursinol angelate against amyloid beta-protein-induced oxidative stress in the PC12 cell line: the role of Nrf2 and antioxidant enzymes. Biosci Biotechnol Biochem. 2011;75(3):434–42.
23. Son SH, Park KK, Park SK, Kim YC, Kim YS, Lee SK, Chung WY. Decursin and decursinol from Angelica gigas inhibit the lung metastasis of murine colon carcinoma. Phytother Res. 2011;25(7):959–64.
24. Watanabe M, Kato J, Inoue I, Yoshimura N, Yoshida T, Mukoubayashi C, Deguchi H, Enomoto S, Ueda K, Maekita T, et al. Development of gastric cancer in nonatrophic stomach with highly active inflammation identified

by serum levels of pepsinogen and helicobacter pylori antibody together with endoscopic rugal hyperplastic gastritis. Int J Cancer. 2012;131(11): 2632–42.

25. Qayyum T, McArdle PA, Lamb GW, Going JJ, Orange C, Seywright M, Horgan PG, Oades G, Aitchison MA, Edwards J. Prospective study of the role of inflammation in renal cancer. Urol Int. 2012;88(3):277–81.

26. Park BK, Park YC, Jung IC, Kim SH, Choi JJ, Do M, Kim SY, Jin M. Gamisasangja-tang suppresses pruritus and atopic skin inflammation in the NC/Nga murine model of atopic dermatitis. J Ethnopharmacol. 2015;165:54–60.

27. Park HJ, Choi WS, Lee WY, Choi Y, Park C, Kim JH, Hong KH, Song H. A novel mouse model of atopic dermatitis that is T helper 2 (Th2)-polarized by an epicutaneous allergen. Environ Toxicol Pharmacol. 2017;58:122–30.

28. Fu D, Shang X, Ni Z, Shi G. Shikonin inhibits inflammation and chondrocyte apoptosis by regulation of the PI3K/Akt signaling pathway in a rat model of osteoarthritis. Exp Ther Med. 2016;12(4):2735–40.

29. Zorman J, Susjan P, Hafner-Bratkovic I. Shikonin Suppresses NLRP3 and AIM2 Inflammasomes by Direct Inhibition of Caspase-1. PLoS One. 2016;11(7): e0159826.

30. Kim JH, Jeong JH, Jeon ST, Kim H, Ock J, Suk K, Kim SI, Song KS, Lee WH. Decursin inhibits induction of inflammatory mediators by blocking nuclear factor-kappaB activation in macrophages. Mol Pharmacol. 2006; 69(6):1783–90.

31. Park SJ, Cha HS, Lee YH, Kim WJ, Kim DH, Kim EC, Lee KH, Kim TJ. Effect of nodakenin on atopic dermatitis-like skin lesions. Biosci Biotechnol Biochem. 2014;78(9):1568–71.

32. Choi HS, Cho SG, Kim MK, Kim MS, Moon SH, Kim IH, Ko SG. Decursin in Angelica gigas Nakai (AGN) enhances doxorubicin Chemosensitivity in NCI/ADR-RES ovarian Cancer cells via inhibition of P-glycoprotein expression. Phytother Res. 2016;30(12):2020–6.

33. Matsui K, Tamai S, Ikeda R. Betamethasone, but not tacrolimus, suppresses the development of Th2 cells mediated by Langerhans cell-like dendritic cells. Biol Pharm Bull. 2016;39(7):1220–3.

34. Kim HO, Yang YS, Ko HC, Kim GM, Cho SH, Seo YJ, Son SW, Lee JR, Lee JS, Chang SE, et al. Maintenance therapy of facial seborrheic dermatitis with 0. 1% tacrolimus ointment. Ann Dermatol. 2015;27(5):523–30.

35. Weiss J, Zimmermann F. Tribromoethanol (Avertin) as an anaesthetic in mice. Lab Anim. 1999;33(2):192–3.

36. Woo SM, Choi YK, Kim AJ, Yun YJ, Shin YC, Cho SG, Ko SG. Sip-jeon-dea-Bo-tang, a traditional herbal medicine, ameliorates cisplatin-induced anorexia via the activation of JAK1/STAT3-mediated leptin and IL-6 production in the fat tissue of mice. Mol Med Rep. 2016;13(4):2967–72.

37. Ku JM, Hong SH, Kim HI, Seo HS, Shin YC, Ko SG. Effects of Angelicae dahuricae Radix on 2, 4-dinitrochlorobenzene-induced atopic dermatitis-like skin lesions in mice model. BMC Complement Altern Med. 2017;17(1):98.

38. d'Ettorre G, Baroncelli S, Micci L, Ceccarelli G, Andreotti M, Sharma P, Fanello G, Fiocca F, Cavallari EN, Giustini N, et al. Reconstitution of intestinal CD4 and Th17 T cells in antiretroviral therapy suppressed HIV-infected subjects: implication for residual immune activation from the results of a clinical trial. PLoS One. 2014;9(10):e109791.

39. Moossavi S, Bishehsari F. Inflammation in sporadic colorectal cancer. Arch Iran Med. 2012;15(3):166–70.

40. Rennert PD, Ichimura T, Sizing ID, Bailly V, Li Z, Rennard R, McCoon P, Pablo L, Miklasz S, Tarilonte L, et al. T cell, Ig domain, mucin domain-2 gene-deficient mice reveal a novel mechanism for the regulation of Th2 immune responses and airway inflammation. J Immunol. 2006;177(7):4311–21.

41. Hamed EA, Zakhary MM, Maximous DW. Apoptosis, angiogenesis, inflammation, and oxidative stress: basic interactions in patients with early and metastatic breast cancer. J Cancer Res Clin Oncol. 2012;138(6): 999–1009.

42. Kryvenko ON, Jankowski M, Chitale DA, Tang D, Rundle A, Trudeau S, Rybicki BA. Inflammation and preneoplastic lesions in benign prostate as risk factors for prostate cancer. Mod Pathol. 2012;25(7):1023–32.

43. Alfano CM, Imayama I, Neuhouser ML, Kiecolt-Glaser JK, Smith AW, Meeske K, McTiernan A, Bernstein L, Baumgartner KB, Ulrich CM, et al. Fatigue,

inflammation, and omega-3 and omega-6 fatty acid intake among breast cancer survivors. J Clin Oncol. 2012;30(12):1280–7.

44. Brandt EB, Sivaprasad U. Th2 cytokines and atopic dermatitis. J Clin Cell Immunol. 2011;2(3):1–25.

45. Oflazoglu E, Simpson EL, Takiguchi R, Grewal IS, Hanifin JM, Gerber HP. CD30 expression on CD1a+ and CD8+ cells in atopic dermatitis and correlation with disease severity. Eur J Dermatol. 2008;18(1):41–9.

46. Kim H, Kim JR, Kang H, Choi J, Yang H, Lee P, Kim J, Lee KW. 7,8,4'-Trihydroxyisoflavone attenuates DNCB-induced atopic dermatitis-like symptoms in NC/Nga mice. PLoS One. 2014;9(8):e104938.

47. Choi WJ, Konkit M, Kim Y, Kim MK, Kim W. Oral administration of Lactococcus chungangensis inhibits 2,4-dinitrochlorobenzene-induced atopic-like dermatitis in NC/Nga mice. J Dairy Sci. 2016;99(9):6889–901.

48. Chae HS, Kang OH, Lee YS, Choi JG, Oh YC, Jang HJ, Kim MS, Kim JH, Jeong SI, Kwon DY. Inhibition of LPS-induced iNOS, COX-2 and inflammatory mediator expression by paeonol through the MAPKs inactivation in RAW 264.7 cells. Am J Chin Med. 2009;37(1):181–94.

49. Huang GJ, Bhaskar Reddy MV, Kuo PC, Huang CH, Shih HC, Lee EJ, Yang ML, Leu YL, Wu TS. A concise synthesis of viscolin, and its anti-inflammatory effects through the suppression of iNOS, COX-2, ERK phosphorylation and proinflammatory cytokines expressions. Eur J Med Chem. 2012;48:371–8.

50. Orita K, Hiramoto K, Kobayashi H, Ishii M, Sekiyama A, Inoue M. Inducible nitric oxide synthase (iNOS) and alpha-melanocyte-stimulating hormones of iNOS origin play important roles in the allergic reactions of atopic dermatitis in mice. Exp Dermatol. 2011;20(11):911–4.

51. Liew FY, Li Y, Severn A, Millott S, Schmidt J, Salter M, Moncada S. A possible novel pathway of regulation by murine T helper type-2 (Th2) cells of a Th1 cell activity via the modulation of the induction of nitric oxide synthase on macrophages. Eur J Immunol. 1991;21(10):2489–94.

52. Triggiani M, Petraroli A, Loffredo S, Frattini A, Granata F, Morabito P, Staiano RI, Secondo A, Annunziato L, Marone G. Differentiation of monocytes into macrophages induces the upregulation of histamine H1 receptor. J Allergy Clin Immunol. 2007;119(2):472–81.

53. Homey B, Meller S, Savinko T, Alenius H, Lauerma A. Modulation of chemokines by staphylococcal superantigen in atopic dermatitis. Chem Immunol Allergy. 2007;93:181–94.

54. Holden CA, Chan SC, Hanifin JM. Monocyte localization of elevated cAMP phosphodiesterase activity in atopic dermatitis. J Invest Dermatol. 1986; 87(3):372–6.

55. Kundu JK, Surh YJ. Emerging avenues linking inflammation and cancer. Free Radic Biol Med. 2012;52(9):2013–37.

13

Extract from *Astragalus membranaceus* inhibit breast cancer cells proliferation via PI3K/AKT/ mTOR signaling pathway

Ruijuan Zhou[1], Hongjiu Chen[1], Junpeng Chen[1], Xuemei Chen[2], Yu Wen[2] and Leqin Xu[3*]

Abstract

Background: *Astragalus membranaceus* (AM) is a commonly used herb in traditional Chinese medicine (TCM), which has been used as an essential tonic to treat various diseases for more than 2000 years. In this study, we aimed to investigate the biological effects of extract from AM on breast cancer cell and its mechanism.

Methods: To prepare the extract, dried AM were ground and extracted with water extraction-ethanol supernatant method. Then the main isoflavones in the extract was detect by HPLC analysis. Furthermore, the anti-proliferative activity of AM extract was examined by MTT assay and morphological observation. Cell apoptosis was evaluated with flow cytometric analysis. The expressions of total and phosphorylated PI3K, GS3Kβ, Akt and mTOR were determined by western blot analysis.

Results: HPLC analysis demonstrated that AM extract contained with four kinds of isoflavones, campanulin, ononin, calycosin and formononetin. The MTT test and morphological observation indicated that cells proliferation of MCF-7, SK-BR-3 and MDA-MB-231were inhibited by AM extract in a dose dependent manner. Furthermore, flow cytometric analysis displayed that after treated with 25 μg/ml and 50 μg/ml AM extract, apoptosis of breast cancer cells was significantly increased as compared with DMSO and blank control group (all $p < 0.05$). Western blot analysis found that the level of p-PI3K, p-GS3Kβ, p-Akt, and p-mTOR were significantly decreased, but the level of total-mTOR was observably increased as compared with DMSO control group.

Conclusions: Taken together, the inhibited cell proliferation and induced cell apoptosis effect of AM extract via PI3K/AKT/mTOR pathway confirmed the anti-tumor potential of AM. Therefore, our findings provide a new insight into anti-cancer effect of AM extract as a promising agent in breast cancer treatment.

Keywords: *Astragalus membranaceus*, Extract, Breast cancer, Apoptosis, PI3K, AKT

Background

Breast cancer is the most threatening health problem for women worldwide in incidence and mortality. In 2012, an estimated more than 1.6 million new cases were diagnosed with breast cancer globally with 521,907 women died due to breast cancer [1]. Surgical resection is the most effective treatment for breast cancer. Chemotherapy, radiotherapy and endocrine therapy are usually used to eliminate remaining tumor cells, inhibit tumor growth, and reduce breast cancer recurrence. These therapies improve long-term survival and quality of life for breast cancer patient [2]. Unfortunately, some patients experience treatment-related adverse effects or become resistant to these reagents. Therefore, finding bioactive natural products may provide an alternative strategy in breast cancer treatment.

Aberrant activation of the PI3K/Akt/mTOR signaling pathway has been shown in numerous cancers, including breast cancers [3]. Accumulating evidence indicates that the PI3K/AKT/mTOR signaling pathway plays a pivotal role in the regulation of breast cancer growth, survival, and motility as well as the acquisition of drug resistance, and there are now extensive data indicating that various components of this pathway as potential molecular

* Correspondence: xuleqin@163.com
[3]Department of Science and Education, Xiamen Hospital of Traditional Chinese Medicine, Fujian University of Traditional Chinese Medicine, 1739 Xianyue Road, Xiamen 361009, People's Republic of China
Full list of author information is available at the end of the article

targets for breast cancer treatment [4]. Therefore, PI3K/ AKT/mTOR signaling pathway is considered as an attractive target for the development of new anticancer agents that could be used alone or in combination with other targeted therapies for treating breast cancer patients.

Over the past few decades, researchers have studied many biological properties of a number of promising plants and herbs. *Astragalus membranaceus* (Radix Astragali or "Huang Qi", AM) has been used for medicinal purposes in traditional Chinese medicine over 2000 years. It is well-known for its vital-energy tonifying, skin reinforcing, diuretic, abscess-draining and tissue generative actions [5]. In practice, AM is often combined with other herbs, such as angelica, poria and ginseng, in various complex prescription formulas [6–8]. In our previous studies, we found that Yiqi formula (AM combined with poria) enhanced the antitumor effects of erlotinib on triple-negative breast cancer xenografts [9]. Although AM is usually combined with other herbs, it can be taken separately by itself. It contains several types of bioactive compounds including ploysaccharides, flavonoids, and saponins [10–15]. In recent years, AM has been investigated in treating various cancers [16–22]. However, the effects of AM extract on breast cancer are still unknown and very limited information is available on the mechanism responsible for the anticancer effects.

The purpose of this present work was to extract AM through the water extraction-ethanol supernatant method and determine its anti-proliferative effect on three distinct breast cancer cell lines, MCF-7 (ER+), SK-BR-3 (HER2+) and MDA-MB-231 (triple-negative). Our results demonstrated that AM extract showed a cytotoxic effect on breast cancer cells, and its mechanism of anticancer action seemed to induce breast cancer cell apoptosis via PI3K/AKT/mTOR signaling pathway.

Methods
Chemicals, reagents, and antibodies
Campanulin, ononin, calycosin and formononetin were purchased from Phytomarker Ltd. (Tianjin, China). Penicillin, streptomycin, phosphate-buffered saline (PBS), trypsin-EDTA, DMEM, RPMI 1640 and fetal bovine serum (FBS) were obtained from Invitrogen (Carlsbad, CA, USA). 3-(4,5-dimethylthiazol-2-yl)-2,5-diphenyltetrazolium bromide (MTT) and Annexin V/propidium iodide (PI) were purchased from Sigma (St. Louis, MO, USA). Fluorescein isothiocyanate (FITC)-labeled secondary antibody was obtained from Invitrogen (Carlsbad, CA, USA). Antibodies against PI3K, p-PI3K, GS3Kβ, p-GS3Kβ, AKT, p-AKT, mTOR, p-mTOR and β-actin were purchased from Cell Signaling Technology (Danvers, MA, USA). Goat anti-

rabbit and goat anti-mouse peroxidase conjugated secondary antibodies were purchased from Bio-Rad (Hercules, CA, USA).

Plant material and extract preparation
Root of AM in dried form of preeminent grade was bought from Luyan pharma Co. Ltd. (Fuzhou, China). The scheme of the extraction procedure was shown in Fig. 1. Briefly, for the water extraction, AM were extracted with 100 °C distilled water for 4 h at a ratio of 1:10 (*w/v*). This procedure was repeated twice. The aqueous extract was centrifuged at 12000×g for 20 min and filtered through a filter paper (GF/A, 47 mm; Whatman, UK). Then the water extraction was added to 1 volumes of 100% ethanol and then stored at 4 °C for 48 h. The precipitate and aqueous supernatant 1 were separated and collected by centrifugation at 18,000×g for 30 min. Then the precipitate was washed with 50% ethanol for twice and filtered to obtain the aqueous supernatant 2. The aqueous supernatant 1 and supernatant 2 were added together, then concentrated in a vacuum evaporator and lyophilized to obtain the water extraction-ethanol supernatant.

High pressure liquid chromatography (HPLC) analysis
Analysis of isoflavones in AM extract were performed using a liquid chromatograph (Series 1100, Agilent Technologies, Palo Alto, CA, USA), consisting of ultraviolet (UV) detector, a dual pump, an autosampler, an ELSD (Alltech Associates, Deer field, IL, USA), a ZORBAX ODS C_{18} column and a guard column using HP Chem Station software (Agilent Technologies). The column temperature was maintained at a constant 40 °C, and the mobile phase flow rate was 1 ml/min. The mobile phase consisted of acetonitrile and H_2O, which were applied in a gradient of acetonitrile as follows: 0–10 min, 25–35%; 10–25 min, 35–45%; 25–35 min, 45–55%; 35–42 min, 55–71%. UV detection was performed at 251 nm, and sample size was 20 μl.

Cell culture and maintenance
MCF-7, SK-BR-3 and MDA-MB-231 (human breast cancer) cells were procured from American Type Culture Collection (ATCC, Manassas, VA, USA) and maintained under the conditions as previously described [9, 23]. MCF-7 cell line (ER+, HER2−) was cultured in Dulbecco's modified Eagle medium (DMEM, Hyclone, UT, USA) supplemented with 10% fetal bovine serum (FBS, Hyclone) and 1% penicillin/streptomycin (Invitrogen, NY, USA). SK-BR-3 cell line (ER−, PR−, HER2+) was maintained in McCoy's 5a medium supplemented with 10% FBS and 1% penicillin/streptomycin. MDA-MB-231 cell line (a triple-negative breast cancer (TNBC) cell line, ER−, PR−, and HER2−) was maintained in DMEM containing 10% FBS

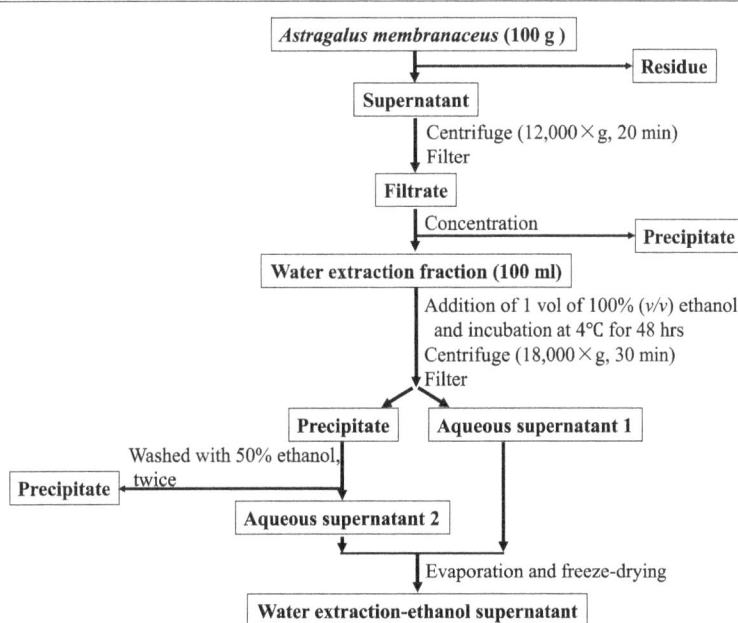

Fig. 1 Schematic depiction of extraction method from AM

with 1% penicillin/streptomycin. All cells were grown as monolayers and were maintained in a humidified CO_2 incubator at 37 °C in 5.0% CO_2 and 95.0% air. The media was changed every two or three days. Cells were detached with 0.25% Trypsin-EDTA in PBS.

Cell proliferation assay
To assess the effects of AM extract on breast cancer cells growth, MTT assay was performed as previously described [23]. MCF-7, SK-BR-3 and MDA-MB-231 cells were seeded into 96-well plates and cultured at a density of 5×10^3 cells per well. After 24 h of incubation, the cells were treated with vehicle (0.1% DMSO) or different concentrations of AM extract (100, 50, 25 µg/ml) for 48 h. Then MTT solution was added to each well (1.2 mg/ml) and incubated at 37 °C for 4 h. The concentration of MTT-formazan product dissolved in DMSO was estimated by measuring absorbance at 490 nm in an absorbance micro-plate reader.

Morphological observation under inverted microscope
In order to investigate the effect of AM extract on cell morphology, breast cells were seeded in 24-well plates (10^5 cells/well). After 24 h of incubation, the cells were treated with different concentrations of AM extract for 48 h. Then breast cancer cells were examined under inverted microscope (OLYMPUS IX70-S8F, Olympus Optical Co., Ltd., Japan) and photographs were taken.

Detection of apoptosis via FITC-Annexin V/PI staining
For Annexin V/propidium iodide (PI) assay, MCF-7, SK-BR-3 and MDA-MB-231 cells were stained with Annexin V-fluorescein isothiocyanate and PI and evaluated for apoptosis by flow cytometry according to the manufacturer's protocol (BD PharMingen, San Diego, CA). In brief, the breast cancer cells were seeded into six-well plates at a density of 2×10^5 cells/well. After 24 h incubation, breast cancer cells were exposed to 50 µg/ml of AM extract for 24 h. Afterward, breast cancer cells were harvested with 0.25% Trypsin–EDTA and washed twice with phosphate-buffered saline (PBS), and then stained with 5 µl of Annexin V-fluorescein isothiocyanate and 10 µl of PI (5 µg/ml) in 1× binding buffer (10 mM HEPES, pH 7.4, 140 mM NaOH, and 2.5 mM $CaCl_2$) for 15 min at room temperature in the dark. Labeled cells were determined using a FACScan Cytometer (BD Biosciences, San Jose, CA). Over 10,000 cells of each sample were counted and there after the percentage of apoptotic cell death was quantitatively analyzed. Three independent experiments were performed.

Western blot analysis
Western blot analysis was performed as previously described by our group [9, 23, 24]. After treatment with various dosages of AM extract for 48 h, the breast cancer cells (MCF-7, SK-BR-3 and MDA-MB-231) were lysed for 15 min with RIPA buffer containing protease and phosphatase inhibitors. The protein concentrations were measured with a BCA kit (Beyotime, China). Equal amounts of protein were separated by sodium dodecyl

sulfate-polyacrylamide gel electrophoresis (SDS-PAGE) and transferred to a polyvinylidene fluoride (PVDF) membrane. The membrane was blocked with a solution containing 5% nonfat dry milk TBST buffer (20 mM Tris–HCl, pH 7.4, 150 mM NaCl and 0.1% Tween 20) for 1 h. The indicated primary antibodies were incubated overnight at 4 °C, washed, and monitored by immunoblotting using a DyLight 800-conjugated secondary antibody. The membrane was scanned using a LI-COR Infrared Imaged Odyssey (Gene Company Limited).

Statistical analysis
All data were presented as the means ± standard deviation (S.D.) of three independent experiments. Statistical analysis was performed by Student's t-test or one-way analysis of variance (ANOVA). In all cases, $p < 0.05$ was considered statistically significant.

Results
Identification of crude isoflavones in AM extract with HPLC analysis
For detecting the isoflavones in AM extract, HPLC analysis was used to compare AM extract with standard components, campanulin, ononin, calycosin, and formononetin (Fig. 2a). Campanulin, ononin, calycosin, and formononetin were detected in AM extract by HPLC analysis at wavelengths of 251 nm. The retention times were 22.245 min, 36.779 min, 42.79 min, and 52.748 min, respectively (Fig. 2b).

AM extract suppressed proliferation of breast cancer cell
The cytotoxic effect of AM extract was evaluated by MTT assay. As indicated in Fig. 3a, AM extract markedly inhibited breast cancer cell growth in a dose dependent manner in 48 h. These results were further confirmed by morphological examination (Fig. 3b).

AM extract induced apoptosis in breast cancer cells
Annexin V/PI staining was used to determine whether the action of AM extract was associated with apoptosis or not. As shown in Fig. 4, AM extract was strongly effective on three cell types. Breast cancer cells treated with 25 μg/ml and 50 μg/ml of AM extract for 24 h showed a marked increase in the number of cells apoptosis (Fig. 4).

Effects of AM extract on the PI3K/AKT signaling pathway
To investigate the effect of AM extract on PI3K/AKT signaling pathway in breast cancer cells, we performed western blot analysis of phosphorylated and total- PI3K, GS3Kβ, Akt and mTOR. Our results showed that AM extract could inhibit the expressions of p-PI3K, p-GS3Kβ, p-AKT and p-mTOR in a dose-dependent manner (Fig. 5).

Discussion
In the present study, we demonstrated that extract from AM, with water extraction-ethanol supernatant method, has anti-proliferative activity on breast cancer cell. This extract contented four kinds of isoflavones, campanulin, ononin, calycosin, and formononetin. As part of inhibitory effect on breast cancer cells proliferation, the AM extract decreased the expression of p-PI3K, p-GS3Kβ, p-AKT and p-mTOR, and led to breast cancer cell apoptosis.

Since many bioactive constituents in plants are flavonoids, polysaccharides and saponins [13]. Flavonoids are found in most parts of plants and have been shown to have multiple biological activities such as anti-cancer, anti-inflammation, antibacteria, antivirus, and immune-stimulation [25, 26]. A recent published review by Auyeung K. K. et al. presents that the AM contains flavonoids within the range of 0.5–3.0 mg/g. A total of 12 different flavonoids can be isolated from AM. These flavonoids include isoflavonones, isoflavans, pterocarpans, flavonones, and chalcones, of which isoflavones are the major constituents [5]. It has been reported that some of isoflavones from AM, such as calycosin and formononetin have inhibited cancer cell proliferation and metastasis effect [17, 23, 25, 27, 28]. The most common extraction method in herbal medicine is to boil the herb in hot water, which is called decoction. Decoction has long been used in traditional Chinese medicine, which is suitable for extracting heat-stable compounds, hard plants materials (e.g. roots and barks) and usually used for extracting oil-soluble compounds [29]. It has been reported that flavonoids were stable during heating reflux in water bath for 30 min and they were better extracted in water-alcoholic solution than by pure solvent [30]. So in this study, we used the water extraction-ethanol supernatant method to extract flavonoids from AM. Due to limited experimental conditions, we only detected four isoflavonoids, campanulin, ononin, calycosin, and formononetin in the AM extract (Fig. 2). Except these four compounds, the extract may content other compounds, such as polysaccharides and saponins. Because, there are many unknown chromatographic peaks in the AM extract (Fig. 2b). We will analyze the other compounds in this extract, detect their biology activities in further experiments and compare the content of active components with different extraction methods.

The anti-proliferative effect of AM extract on different breast cancer cell lines was present in Fig. 3. The presented results showed that exposure of breast cancer cells to AM extract for 48 h resulted in growth inhibition in a dose-dependent manner. Moreover, treatment with 50 μg/ml AM extract significantly promoted the apoptosis of breast cancer cells (Fig. 4). Thus, these results suggest that the AM extract inhibits the proliferation of

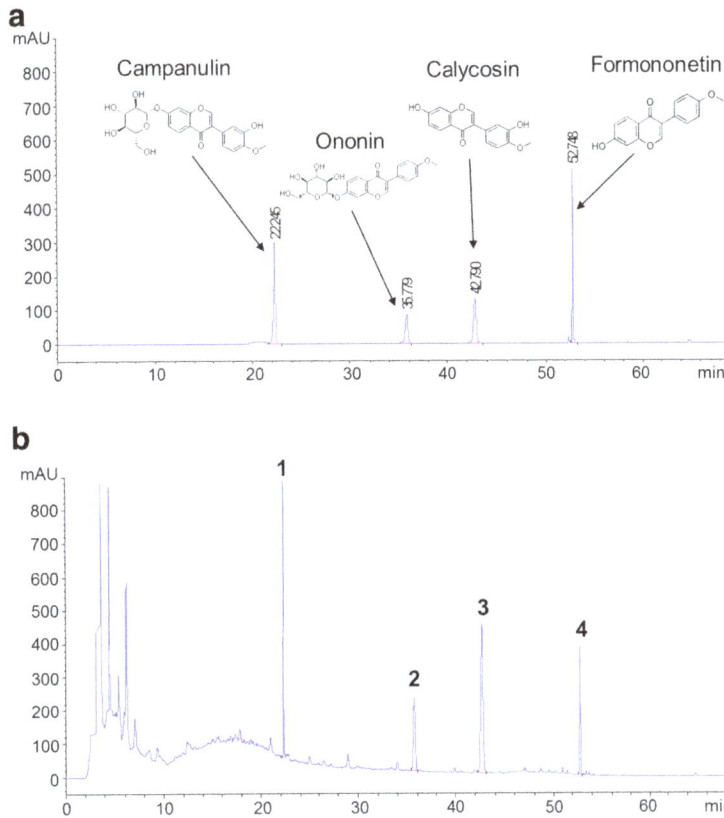

Fig. 2 HPLC profile of AM extract. **a** HPLC chromatogram of mixed standard solutions, campanulin, ononin, calycosin, and formononetin. **b** HPLC chromatogram of AM extract. Campanulin, ononin, calycosin, and formononetin were detected in AM extract. The retention times were 22.245 min (peak 1), 36.779 min (peak 2), 42.79 min (peak 3), and 52.748 min (peak 4), respectively

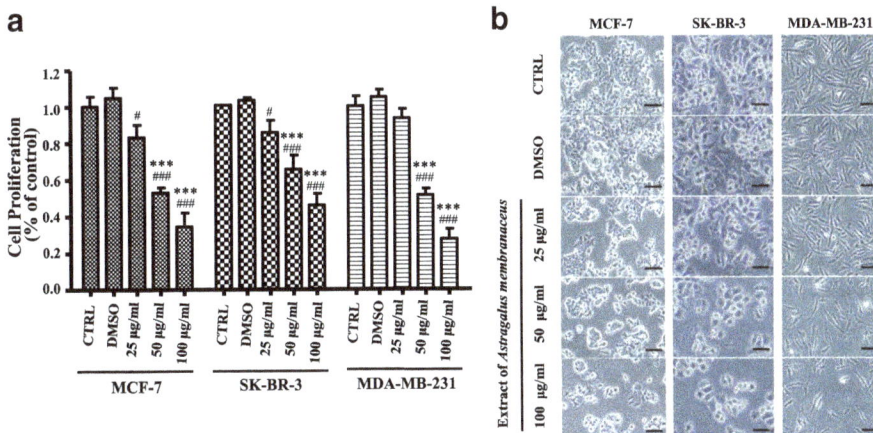

Fig. 3 Cytotoxic effects of AM extract on three distinct breast cancer cell lines. **a** After treated with different concentration of AM extract for 48 h, the cell proliferation was evaluated with MTT assay. Values are the mean ± S.D. of triplicate determinations of three independent experiments. ***$p < 0.001$, compared with blank control group (CTRL); #$p < 0.05$, ###$p < 0.001$, compared with DMSO group. **b** Morphological effect of AM extract on breast cancer cells

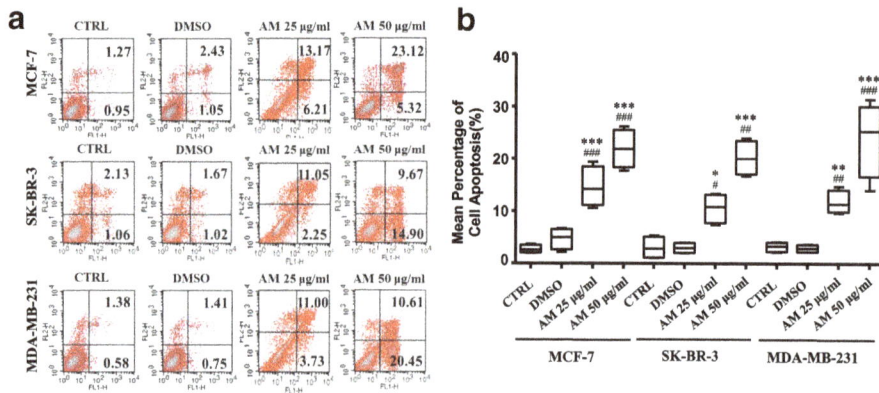

Fig. 4 Analysis of cell apoptosis induced by AM extract in three distinct breast cancer cell lines. Breast cancer cells were treated with 50 μg/ml of AM extract for 24 h, and cell apoptosis was assessed by flow cytometry with FITC-Annexin V/PI Staining. The data are representative of three independent experiments carried out under the same conditions. *$p < 0.05$, **$p < 0.01$, ***$p < 0.001$, compared with blank control group (CTRL); #$p < 0.05$, ##$p < 0.01$, ###$p < 0.001$, compared with DMSO group

breast cancer cells by the induction of apoptosis. Induction of apoptosis is thus considered as a strategy for cancer control. As published data showed that AM extract inhibited the growth of various cancer cells in vitro, such as colon cancer cells [12, 31], hepatocellular carcinoma [18, 21, 32], gastric cancer cell [16] and non-small lung cancer cell [33]. Furthermore, total flavonoids from AM have a significant inhibitory effect on human hepatocellular carcinoma BEL-7402 cell [34] and erythroleukemia K562 cell in vitro [25]. To date, there are two main apoptotic pathways: the extrinsic or death receptor pathway and the intrinsic or mitochondrial pathway [35]. It has

been reported that, AM induced hepatocellular carcinoma cell [18] and gastric cancer cells [16] apoptosis via extrinsic or induced colon cancer cells via intrinsic pathway [31]. However in this study, we only observed the phenomena of AM extract on breast cancer cell proliferation and cell apoptosis. We will analyze the expression of death receptors, such as FasL/FasR, TNF-α/TNFR1, and Bcl-2 family such as Bcl-2, Bcl-x and cytochrome c in our next experiment, to confirm the effect of AM extract on inducing breast cancer cell apoptosis via which pathway.

To investigate the mechanisms by which AM extract inhibit cell growth and promoted apoptosis in breast

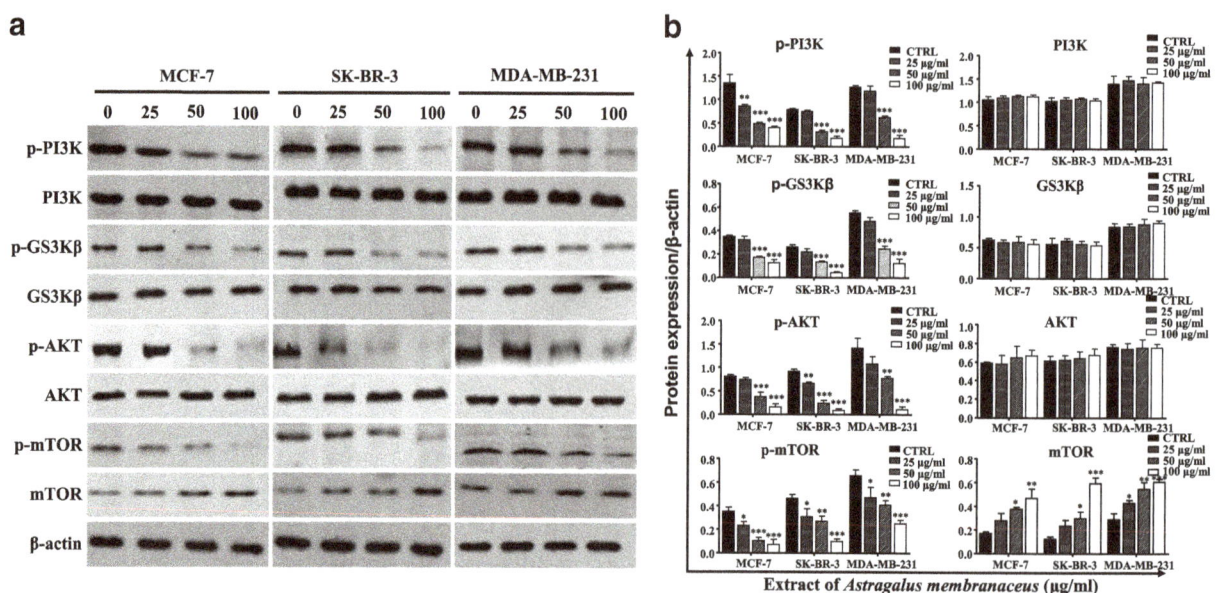

Fig. 5 Protein expressions of PI3K, GS3Kβ, Akt, mTOR, p-PI3K, p-GS3Kβ, p-Akt, and p-mTOR in breast cancer cells by western blot analysis. β-actin was used as a protein loading control. *$p < 0.05$, **$p < 0.01$, ***$p < 0.001$, compared with blank control group (CTRL)

cancer cells, we analyzed PI3K/Akt/mTOR signaling pathways after treatment with the AM extract. The PI3K/Akt/mTOR is a major intracellular signaling pathway, which plays a key role in cell proliferation, growth, migration, metabolism and apoptosis [36]. Aberrant activation of the PI3K/Akt/mTOR pathway is found in many types of cancer including breast cancer [37, 38]. The recent development and clinical testing of PI3K/Akt/mTOR inhibitors have led to the conclusion that targeting the PI3K/Akt/mTOR pathway is a promising approach for the treatment of breast cancer [39]. After treatment with the AM extract, the expression levels of p-PI3K, p-GS3Kβ, p-Akt and p-mTOR were effectively suppressed (Fig. 5). In light of the key role of PI3K/Akt/mTOR signaling pathway in governing apoptosis, our study showed that inhibition of PI3K/Akt/mTOR pathway by the AM extract increase the apoptosis of breast cancer cells. This results indicated that breast cancer cells apoptosis induced AM extract were related to the inhibition of PI3K signaling pathway. However, it is uncertain whether AM extract induces breast cancer cells apoptosis only through the PI3K/Akt/mTOR signaling pathway or by other pathways. We will use siRNA experiments or PI3K/Akt inhibitor in our further study.

Conclusions

In conclusion, in this study, we demonstrate that the extract from AM with water extraction-ethanol supernatant method inhibit cell growth and induce apoptosis in cultured breast cancer cells. The effect of AM extract to suppress breast cancer cells growth was associated with its ability to inhibit PI3K/Akt/mTOR activity. These results suggest that the AM could provide an alternative strategy for breast cancer patients. Further studies are needed to identify all components in the AM extract and determine in vivo effects of this extract in animal models, in order to better evaluate the therapeutic potential of AM.

Additional files

Additional file 1: Figure S1. Cytotoxic effects of AM extract on three breast cancer cell lines for 24 h. After treated with different concentration of AM extract for 24 h, the cell proliferation was evaluated with MTT assay. Values are the mean ± S.D. of triplicate determinations of three independent experiments. **$p < 0.01$, ***$p < 0.001$, compared with blank control group (CTRL); #$p < 0.05$, ##$p < 0.01$, ###$p < 0.001$, compared with DMSO group.

Additional file 2: Figure S2. Analysis of cell apoptosis induced by AM extract in MCF-7 for 48 h. MFC-7 breast cancer cells were treated with 25 μg/ml and 50 μg/ml of AM extract for 48 h, and cell apoptosis was assessed by flow cytometry with FITC-Annexin V/PI Staining.

Abbreviations
Akt: Protein kinase B; AM: Astragalus membranaceus; ATCC: American Type Culture Collection; DMEM: Dulbecco's modified Eagle medium; ER: Estrogen receptor; FBS: Fetal bovine serum; GS3Kβ: Glycogen synthase kinase-3 beta; HER2: Human epidermal growth factor receptor 2; HPLC: High pressure liquid chromatography; mTOR: Mammalian target of rapamycin; MTT: 3-(4,5-dimethylthiazol-2-yl)-2,5-diphenyltetrazolium bromide; PBS: Phosphate-buffered saline; PI: Propidium iodide; PI3K: Phosphatidylinositol-4,5-bisphosphate 3-kinase; PR: Progesterone receptor; TNBC: Triple-negative breast cancer

Funding
This study was financially supported by the Grants from National Natural Science Foundation of China (No. 81704094 and No. 81603642). This work was supported by the Natural Science Foundation of Fujian Province, China (No. 2014D013) and the Science and Technology Planning Projects of Xiamen Science & Technology Bureau, China (No. 3502Z20154052).

Authors' contributions
ZRJ carried out experiment studies. CXM and WY participated in the extraction of AM and HPLC analysis. XLQ performed the statistical analysis and drafted the manuscript. CHJ and CJP provided conceptual advice and critically revised the manuscript. All authors read and approved the final manuscript.

Competing interests
The authors declare that they have no competing interests.

Author details
[1]Department of Chest and Breast Surgery, Xiamen Hospital of Traditional Chinese Medicine, Fujian University of Traditional Chinese Medicine, 1739 Xianyue Road, Xiamen 361009, People's Republic of China. [2]Department of Pharmacy, Xiamen Hospital of Traditional Chinese Medicine, Fujian University of Traditional Chinese Medicine, 1739 Xianyue Road, Xiamen 361009, People's Republic of China. [3]Department of Science and Education, Xiamen Hospital of Traditional Chinese Medicine, Fujian University of Traditional Chinese Medicine, 1739 Xianyue Road, Xiamen 361009, People's Republic of China.

References
1. Ghoncheh M, Pournamdar Z, Salehiniya H. Incidence and mortality and epidemiology of breast cancer in the world. Asian Pacific journal of cancer prevention : APJCP. 2016;17(S3):43–6.
2. Chew HK. Adjuvant therapy for breast cancer: who should get what? West J Med. 2001;174(4):284–7.
3. Cidado J, Park BH. Targeting the PI3K/Akt/mTOR pathway for breast cancer therapy. J Mammary Gland Biol Neoplasia. 2012;17(3–4):205–16.
4. Guerrero-Zotano A, Mayer IA, Arteaga CL. PI3K/AKT/mTOR: role in breast cancer progression, drug resistance, and treatment. Cancer Metastasis Rev. 2016;35(4):515–24.
5. Auyeung KK, Han QB, Ko JK. Astragalus membranaceus: a review of its protection against inflammation and gastrointestinal cancers. Am J Chin Med. 2016;44(1):1–22.
6. Woo SM, Choi YK, Cho SG, Park S, Ko SG: A new herbal formula, KSG-002, Suppresses Breast Cancer Growth and Metastasis by Targeting NF- kappa B-Dependent TNF alpha Production in Macrophages. Evidence-based complementary and alternative medicine : eCAM 2013, 2013:728258.
7. Choi YK, Cho SG: Herbal extract SH003 suppresses tumor growth and metastasis of MDA-MB-231 breast cancer cells by inhibiting STAT3-IL-6 signaling. 2014, 2014:492173.
8. Choi YY, Kim MH, Hong J, Kim K: Effect of Dangguibohyul-Tang, a Mixed Extract of Astragalus membranaceus and Angelica sinensis, on Allergic and Inflammatory Skin Reaction Compared with Single Extracts of Astragalus membranaceus or Angelica sinensis. 2016, 2016:5936354.

9. Liao MJ, Ye MN, Zhou RJ, Sheng JY, Chen HF. Yiqi formula enhances the antitumor effects of erlotinib for treatment of triple-negative breast cancer xenografts. Evidence-based complementary and alternative medicine : eCAM 2014. 2014:628712.

10. Ma Y, Liu C, Qu D, Chen Y, Huang M, Liu Y. Antibacterial evaluation of sliver nanoparticles synthesized by polysaccharides from Astragalus membranaceus roots. Biomed Pharmacother. 2017;89:351–7.

11. Zhu J, Zhang H, Zhu Z, Zhang Q, Ma X, Cui Z, Yao T. Effects and mechanism of flavonoids from Astragalus complanatus on breast cancer growth. Naunyn Schmiedeberg's Arch Pharmacol. 2015;388(9):965–72.

12. Wang Y, Auyeung KK, Zhang X, Ko JK. Astragalus saponins modulates colon cancer development by regulating calpain-mediated glucose-regulated protein expression. BMC Complement Altern Med. 2014;14:401.

13. Fu J, Wang Z, Huang L, Zheng S, Wang D, Chen S, Zhang H, Yang S. Review of the botanical characteristics, phytochemistry, and pharmacology of Astragalus membranaceus (Huangqi). Phytother Res. 2014;28(9):1275–83.

14. Denzler K, Moore J, Harrington H, Morrill K, Huynh T, Jacobs B, Waters R, Langland J. Characterization of the physiological response following in vivo administration of Astragalus membranaceus. Evidence-based complementary and alternative medicine : eCAM 2016. 2016:6861078.

15. Lian Y, Xie L, Chen M, Chen L. Effects of an astragalus polysaccharide and rhein combination on apoptosis in rats with chronic renal failure. Evidence-based complementary and alternative medicine : eCAM 2014. 2014:271862.

16. Wang Z, Dong L, Zhen Y, Wang Y, Qi D, Xu A, Meng X, Li W. Astragalus extract inhibits proliferation but enhances apoptosis in gastric cancer. BMC Complement Altern Med. 2016;29(5):1473–82.

17. Cheng XD, Gu JF, Yuan JR, Feng L, Jia XB. Suppression of A549 cell proliferation and metastasis by calycosin via inhibition of the PKCalpha/ERK1/2 pathway: an in vitro investigation. Mol Med Rep. 2015;12(6):7992–8002.

18. Huang WH, Liao WR, Sun RX. Astragalus polysaccharide induces the apoptosis of human hepatocellular carcinoma cells by decreasing the expression of Notch1. Int J Mol Med. 2016;38(2):551–7.

19. Tseng A, Yang CH, Chen CH, Chen CH, Hsu SL, Lee MH, Lee HC, Su LJ. An in vivo molecular response analysis of colorectal cancer treated with Astragalus membranaceus extract. Oncol Rep. 2016;35(2):659–68.

20. Wang SF, Wang Q, Jiao LJ, Huang YL, Garfield D, Zhang J, Xu L. Astragalus-containing traditional Chinese medicine, with and without prescription based on syndrome differentiation, combined with chemotherapy for advanced non-small-cell lung cancer: a systemic review and meta-analysis. Current oncology (Toronto Ont). 2016;23(3):e188–95.

21. Lai X, Xia W, Wei J, Ding X. Therapeutic effect of Astragalus polysaccharides on hepatocellular carcinoma H22-bearing mice. Dose-response: a publication of International Hormesis Society. 2017;15(1):1559325816685182.

22. Zhou Z, Meng M, Ni H. Chemosensitizing effect of Astragalus polysaccharides on nasopharyngeal carcinoma cells by inducing apoptosis and modulating expression of Bax/Bcl-2 ratio and caspases. Medical science monitor: international medical journal of experimental and clinical research. 2017;23:462–9.

23. Zhou R, Xu L, Ye M, Liao M, Du H, Chen H. Formononetin inhibits migration and invasion of MDA-MB-231 and 4T1 breast cancer cells by suppressing MMP-2 and MMP-9 through PI3K/AKT signaling pathways. Horm Metab Res. 2014;46(11):753–60.

24. Xu L, Luo J, Jin R, Yue Z, Sun P, Yang Z, Yang X, Wan W, Zhang J, Li S, et al. Bortezomib inhibits Giant cell tumor of bone through induction of cell apoptosis and inhibition of osteoclast recruitment, Giant cell formation, and bone resorption. Mol Cancer Ther. 2016;15(5):854–65.

25. Zhang D, Zhuang Y, Pan J, Wang H, Li H, Yu Y, Wang D. Investigation of effects and mechanisms of total flavonoids of Astragalus and calycosin on human erythroleukemia cells. Oxidative Med Cell Longev. 2012;2012:209843.

26. Kumar S, Pandey AK. Chemistry and biological activities of flavonoids: an overview. ScientificWorldJournal. 2013;2013:162750.

27. Jin YM, Xu TM, Zhao YH, Wang YC, Cui MH. In vitro and in vivo anti-cancer activity of formononetin on human cervical cancer cell line HeLa. Tumour Biol. 2014;35(3):2279–84.

28. Yang Y, Zhao Y, Ai X, Cheng B, Lu S. Formononetin suppresses the proliferation of human non-small cell lung cancer through induction of cell cycle arrest and apoptosis. Int J Clin Exp Pathol. 2014;7(12):8453–61.

29. Azwanida NN, Review A. On the extraction methods use in medicinal plants, principle, strength and limitation. Med Aromat Plants. 2015;4(3):196.

30. Biesaga M. Influence of extraction methods on stability of flavonoids. J Chromatogr A. 2011;1218(18):2505–12.

31. Auyeung KK, Mok NL, Wong CM, Cho CH, Ko JK. Astragalus saponins modulate mTOR and ERK signaling to promote apoptosis through the extrinsic pathway in HT-29 colon cancer cells. Int J Mol Med. 2010;26(3):341–9.

32. Li LK, Kuang WJ, Huang YF, Xie HH, Chen G, Zhou QC, Wang BR, Wan LH. Anti-tumor effects of Astragalus on hepatocellular carcinoma in vivo. Indian journal of pharmacology. 2012;44(1):78–81.

33. He CS, Liu YC, Xu ZP, Dai PC, Chen XW, Jin DH. Astragaloside IV enhances cisplatin Chemosensitivity in non-small cell lung cancer cells through inhibition of B7-H3. Cellular physiology and biochemistry: international journal of experimental cellular physiology, biochemistry, and Pharmacology. 2016;40(5):1221–9.

34. Wang DQ, Li Y, Tian YP, Wang CB. Inhibition effects of total flavonids of Astragalus on BEL-7402 cell in vitro. Academic Journal of PLA Postgraduate Medical School. 2005;26(5):331–3.

35. Fulda S, Debatin KM. Extrinsic versus intrinsic apoptosis pathways in anticancer chemotherapy. Oncogene. 2006;25(34):4798–811.

36. Arcaro A, Guerreiro AS. The phosphoinositide 3-kinase pathway in human cancer: genetic alterations and therapeutic implications. Curr Genomics. 2007;8(5):271–306.

37. Ghayad SE, Cohen PA. Inhibitors of the PI3K/Akt/mTOR pathway: new hope for breast cancer patients. Recent Pat Anticancer Drug Discov. 2010;5(1):29–57.

38. Porta C, Paglino C, Mosca A. Targeting PI3K/Akt/mTOR signaling in cancer. Front Oncol. 2014;4:64.

39. Gonzalez-Angulo AM, Blumenschein GR Jr. Defining biomarkers to predict sensitivity to PI3K/Akt/mTOR pathway inhibitors in breast cancer. Cancer Treat Rev. 2013;39(4):313–20.

14

The inhibitory effects of compound Muniziqi granule against B16 cells and harmine induced autophagy and apoptosis by inhibiting Akt/mTOR pathway

Nan Zou[1,2†], Yue Wei[1†], Fenghua Li[2], Yang Yang[2], Xuemei Cheng[1] and Changhong Wang[1*] ⓘ

Abstract

Background: Compound Muniziqi granule (MNZQ) is a multi-component herbal preparation and a popular traditional Uighur medicine used in China for treating endocrine disorder-induced acne, chloasma, dysmenorrhea, menopausal syndrome, and melanoma. Harmine presented in MNZQ has been confirmed potential anticancer effect on the B16 cells among others. The purpose of this study is to explore the inhibitory effects of MNZQ against B16 cells and mechanism of autophagy and apoptosis induced by harmine in B16 cells.

Methods: The cell viability was calculated by CCK8 assay. The in vitro tyrosinase activity was determined by spectrophotometry. The harmine-induced autophagy was demonstrated by electron microscopy and MDC staining. Flow cytometry was used to measure cell death and cell cycle distribution. All proteins expression was assessed by western blot.

Results: MNZQ and some herb extracts contained in preparation displayed inhibitory effects on B16 cells but without inhibition on mushroom tyrosinase compared with kojic acid. The formation of autophagosome was markedly induced by harmine with the accretion of LC3-II and the degeneration of p62 in B16 cells, which indicated that harmine was an autophagy inducer. Cell death and sub-G2 population suggested that harmine could induce cell death. Particularly, 3-MA, an autophagy inhibitor, was discovered to prevent harmine-induced decrease of the cell viability and cell cycle arrest on G2 phase, indicating that autophagy was vital to the cell death. In addition, the results indicated that harmine could inhibit the phosphorylation of Akt and mTOR, which might mediate autophagy.

Conclusion: Harmine could induce autophagy and apoptosis by inhibiting Akt/mTOR pathway in B16 cells. Harmine might be a promising therapeutic agent for treatment of melanoma in MNZQ.

Keywords: Compound Muniziqi granule, Melanoma, Harmine, Autophagy, Apoptosis, Akt/mTOR pathway

Background

Herbal medicines have gained growing popularity and have been used elsewhere worldwide as alternative and complementary medicine and food supplements [1]. According to the statistics, almost 80% of people use herbs to treat related diseases in the whole world based on their health care needs [1]. In China, mostly 1000 herbs are proven effective and prescribed by TCM practitioners or produced as herbal preparations by pharmaceutical manufacturers [2].

Compound Muniziqi granule (MNZQ), recorded in Pharmaceutical Standards-Uighur Medicine and the Ministry of Health of the People's Republic of China, is a multi-component herbal preparation and a popular traditional Uighur medicine (TUM) used in China [3]. MNZQ consists of 13 species of plants for medicinal uses, including seeds of *Peganum harmala, Cichorium intybus, Dracocephalum moldavica, Ocimum basilicum, Althaea rosea,* and *Nigella*

* Correspondence: wchcxm@shutcm.edu.cn
†Equal contributors
[1]Institute of Chinese Materia Medica, Shanghai University of Traditional Chinese Medicine, The MOE Key Laboratory for Standardization of Chinese Medicines and The SATCM Key Laboratory for New Resources and Quality Evaluation of Chinese Medicine, 1200 Cailun Road, Shanghai 201203, China
Full list of author information is available at the end of the article

glandulifera; fruits of *Pimpinella anisum*; roots of *Apium graveolens*, *Glycyrrhiza uralensis* and *Cichorium intybus*; cortex of *Foeniculum vulgare*; and herbs of *Matricaria chamomilla* and *Cymbopogon caesius*. Previously study has showed that hormone synthesis and metabolism can be effectively regulated by treating with MNZQ. What is more, it can also treat endocrine disorder-induced acne, chloasma, dysmenorrhea, menopausal syndrome, and melanoma [4].

Melanoma has usually evolved from skin diseases such as chloasma [5]. Despite melanoma has been viewed as a complex disease, the inhibition of tyrosinase is the most common pathway to achieve skin whiteness as it is the key enzyme that catalyzes the rate-limiting step of melanin biosynthesis [6]. Therefore, it has become a focus to search for new drugs from folk medicine which could inhibit tyrosinase activity and decrease the proliferation of melanoma cell.

Apoptosis, or type I programmed cell death, is classified as cell membrane blebbing, cell shrinkage, nuclear condensation and fragmentation, and formation of apoptotic bodies [7]. The mechanism of apoptosis includes the extrinsic and intrinsic apoptotic pathway which results from the activation of caspases (cysteine proteases), which is activated by either death receptor ligation or emission of apoptotic mediators from the mitochondria [8–10]. The tumor cell death is involved in killing cell and inhibiting cell division. During the cell cycle, successful proportion of cells in the G2/M is a critical factor to cell proliferation [11]. Cell cycle regulation imbalance is described in the cancer cells, which promotes the occurrence and development of tumor [12].

Autophagy is a process of self-eating that degrades and recycles cytoplasmic supplies to sustain metabolism and survival of the cell [13]. The formation of notable double-membraned vesicles, named autophagosomes, is one of the characterizing features of this procedure employed to transfer cargo proposed for degradation. Some principal methods are presently used to monitor the induction of autophagy, including electron microscopy, monodansylcadaverine (MDC) staining, biochemical detection of protein LC3-II and P62 [14]. To make a distinction between induction of autophagy and suppression of down-stream steps of autophagy, it was necessary to monitor autophagic flux of autophagy inhibitors. Cell growth, propagation, and angiogenesis are highly associated with the Akt/mTOR pathway [15, 16].

Harmine is a naturally occurring β-carboline alkaloid present in a number of medicinal plants such as *P. harmala* L., *Passiflora incarnata* L. and *Banisteriopsis caapi* (Spruce ex Griseb.) Morton [17]. It has been found that harmine is the most important compound which has been demonstrated to exert strong anticancer activities by suppressing proliferation [18, 19], migration [20], invasion [21] and preventing from tumorigenesis. Harmine can down-regulation

the expression of pro-metastatic genes (e.g. MMP-9, ERK and VEGFs) which is related to the foregoing activity, and it was crucial to melanoma cell invasion [22]. Some studies have been reported that harmol (a metabolite of harmine) and β-carboline derivatives could induce autophagy instead of apoptosis [23]. However, harmine has been reported to modulate autophagy and perturb molecular targets of apoptosis, the exact mechanism of harmine-induced autophagy remains unclear.

In the present study, the exciting inhibitory effects of MNZQ and extract from *P. harmala* against B16 cells have been observed. However, MNZQ and extract from *P. harmala* did not exhibit inhibitory effects on tyrosinase activity. MNZQ and the main β-carboline alkaloids harmine among others contained in extract from *P. harmala* showed potential effects on melanoma. The induction of autophagy by harmine in B16 cells was demonstrated by electron microscopy and MDC staining, the expression of LC3-II and p62. In addition, the nuclear morphology was analyzed by hoechst 33,258 assay. Apoptosis rate and cell cycle distribution were detected by annexinV-FITC/PI staining assay and cell cycle analysis. It was identified that 3-MA was found to prevent harmine-induced cell death and cell cycle arrest on G2 phase. Autophagy induced by harmine is mediated by increased autophagy activity and inhibition of the Akt/mTOR signaling pathway.

Methods
Chemicals and drugs
Harmine, harmaline, harmane, and harmol (purity > 98%), methylsulfoxide (DMSO), 3-Methyladenine (3-MA), monodansylcadaverine (MDC), L-dopa, hoechst 33,258 and mushroom tyrosinase were purchased from Sigma-Aldrich. Liquiritin, isoliquiritin and glycyrrhizic acid were purchased from Natural Biological Technology Co., LTD (Shanghai). Cell Counting Kit-8 (CCK8, YEASEN, China), bafilomycin A1 (Calbiochem, US), annexin V- fluorescein isothiocyanate (FITC), and apoptosis detection Kit (BD Bioscience, USA) were used. RPMI Medium Modified, fetal bovine serum (FBS), phosphate buffered saline (PBS) and penicillin-streptomycin were obtained from Gibco (Carlsbad, CA, USA). Primary antibodies of GAPDH, LC3, P62, mTOR, p-mTOR, Akt, p-Akt, ERK1/2, p-ERK1/2 were purchased from Cell Signaling Technology (Danvers, MA). MNZQ was offered by Xinjing Uighur Pharmaceutical Co., Ltd. (Xinjiang, China; Batch No.151144). The information, including plant name, herbal name, Chinese name, medicinal parts, formula dosage, and voucher number of 13 species of medicinal plants comprising MNZQ could be referred to our previous study [4].

Preparation of herbs extracts, MNZQ, and chemicals
The extracts of 13 herbs were prepared according to the preparation process of MNZQ [3]. The 13 dried raw

materials (60 g) in MNZQ were pulverized as powder and decocted with 600 mL of water thrice in reflux, each for 2 h, 1.5 h, and 1 h, respectively. The decoctions were combined, filtrated, and concentrated under reduced pressure at 60 °C to afford concentrated extracts (ca. 60 mL). Due to the different extract yield, the 13 concentrated extracts were converted to equivalent amount of raw material concentrations in formula of MNZQ as follow: *P. harmala* 0.8 g/mL, *F. vulgare* 0.8 g/mL, *P. anisum* 2 g/mL, *N. glandulifera* 0.8 g/mL, *M. chamomilla* 0.8 g/mL, *C. intybus* (seed) 0.8 g/mL, *C. intybus* (root) 2 g/mL, *A. graveolens* 0.8 g/mL, *D. moldavica* 0.2 g/mL, *G. uralensis* 0.8 g/mL, *C. caesius* 0.8 g/mL, *O. basilicum* 1 g/mL, *A. rosea* 2 g/mL, respectively. For cell viability test, the 13 concentrated extracts (5 µL) were diluted to 1 mL with culture medium to give concentrations of *F. vulgare*: 4 mg/mL, *P. anisum*: 10 mg/mL, *M. chamomilla*: 4 mg/mL, *C. intybus* (seed): 10 mg/mL, *C. intybus* (Root): 10 mg/mL, *A. graveolens*: 4 mg/mL, *D. moldavica*: 1 mg/mL, *G. uralensis*: 4 mg/mL, *C. caesius*: 4 mg/mL, *O. basilicum*: 5 mg/mL, *A. rosea*: 10 mg/mL. And two herbs were diluted to *P. harmala*: 1 mg/mL and *N. glandulifera*: 2 mg/mL. MNZQ (60 mg) was dissolved in 1 mL water at a concentration of 60 mg/mL. Harmine, harmaline, harmane, and harmol were dissolved in DMSO at a concentration of 40 mM. All of stock solutions were stored at –20 °C until use.

Cell culture
B16-F-10 melanoma cells (B16 cells) were gained from the Cell Bank of the Chinese Academy of Sciences (Shanghai, China). B16 cells were cultured in RPMI 1640 medium supplemented with 10% fetal bovine serum (FBS) with 100 U/mL penicillin/streptomycin in a dynamic incubation system at 37 °C under an atmosphere of 5% CO_2 (Thermo Fisher Scientific, USA). When the cells were in the logarithmic growth phage, the cells were used for the following experiments.

Chemical analysis of MNZQ
A high performance liquid chromatography (HPLC) fingerprinting of MNZQ has been established previously [4] and eight characteristic peaks were identified as chlorogenic acid, caffeic acid, ferulic acid, liquiritin, harmaline, harmine, apigenin 7-O-glucoside, and isoliquiritin in MNZQ dissolved in 0.05 M hydrochloric acid solution and extracted with ethyl acetate. In order to reducing interference of impurity and accurately determine the contents of targeted markers, including liquiritin, harmaline, harmine, isoliquiritin and glycyrrhizic acid, the separation condition of HPLC and sample preparation of MNZQ have been modified reasonably (unpublished data). The 12 g aliquot of MNZQ sample was directly dissolved in 20 mL water and extracted three times with 30 mL of n-butyl

alcohol saturated by water in a 125 mL separatory funnel. The organic supernatants were combined to evaporate to dryness and then the residue was dissolved in 5 mL of methanol. The solution was filtered through a Millipore filter (0.45 µm) to obtain the sample solution before injection into LC system for analysis. The sample was separated on a C_{18} chromatographic column (4.6 mm × 250 mm, 5 µm, Boston Lunna Clone, Boston Analytics, Inc., USA) maintained at 30 °C. The mobile phase was consisted of acetonitrile (A) and ammonium acetate buffer (B) at a flow rate of 1 mL/min, and eluted with gradient elution: 0–10 min (19% A), 10–20 min (33% A), 20–35 min (33% A). The injection volume was 10 µL and the detection wavelength was set at 254 nm. The typical chromatographic fingerprints of MNZQ and mixture reference standards were deposited in Fig. 1. The contents of targeted markers liquiritin, harmaline, harmine, isoliquiritin and glycyrrhizic acid were determined as 0.11, 0.43, 0.21, 0.03, and 0.14 mg/g respectively.

Anti-melanoma activity of MNZQ and single herb extracts
Cell viability
The effects of MNZQ and herb extracts on cell growth were evaluated by the CCK8 kit. The B16 cells were seeded in a 96-well plate with the density of 5×10^3 cells/well in the incubator. The cells were treated with abovementioned concentrations of herb extracts, MNZQ (60 mg/mL), harmine, harmaline, harmane, and harmol (50, 100, 150, 200 µM) for 24 h. After the addition of 10 µL CCK8 solution/well, they were incubated for 2 h. A microplate reader (BioTek, USA) was used to measure the absorbance at a wavelength of 450 nm.

Tyrosinase assay
Spectrophotometry was used to detect tyrosinase activity with minor modification [24]. The incubation mixture (150 µL) consisted of 50 U/mL mushroom tyrosinase in PBS (50 µL), 5 mM L-dopa solution (50 µL), stock solutions of individual herb extracts (50 µL) or PBS (50 µL). The mixture was incubated at 37 °C for 10 min and then the absorbance was measured at 475 nm with a microplate reader (BioTek Instruments, Inc., USA).

The autophagy and apoptosis of harmine-induced
Cell morphology
The B16 cells were seeded in culture plates and allowed to attach overnight. The morphology of B16 cells, with or without 40 µM harmine treatment, was evaluated by TEM. Briefly, the cells were immediately fixed in 3% osmium tetroxide in 4 °C for 2 h, along a rinse with distilled water. Dehydrate them in different graded ethanol series then cultured in araldite (Fluka, Buchs, Switzerland). The micrometer thick blocks were stained with toluidine blue, taken photos by a microscope for further observation. They

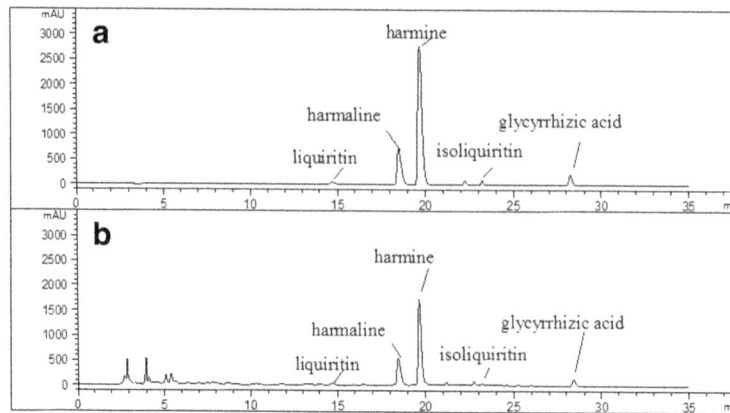

Fig. 1 The typical HPLC fingerprint chromatograms of reference standards of liquiritin, harmaline, harmine, isoliquiritin and glycyrrhizic acid (**a**) and MNZQ sample (**b**)

were then trimmed at interest areas to recognize the morphological changes compatible with autophagy. Cut ultrathin into 60–90 nm thick by a diamond knife for the research of electron microscopic. The steps above were mounted on copper grids, double stained in uranyl acetate as well as lead citrate, checked by electron microscope (FEI Company, USA). Take micrographs for qualitative description. All samples underwent the same fixation and processes.

Autophagosome formation assay
The B16 cells were seeded in 96 well-plates with the density of 5×10^3 cells/well and culture plates in the incubator. The cells were cultured with different concentrations of harmine (40, 50, 60, 80 μM) for 24 h, in order to quantifying the autophagy induction. Cells were cultured in 50 μM MDC for 15 min at 37 °C at last, then washed with PBS (pH 7.4) and the fluorescence measured and photographed by a multimode plate reader (Ex 340 nm and Em 535 nm, Thermo Scientific, USA, OLYMPUS, Japan). All data were performed with three independent, replicate experiments.

Cell viability
In order determining whether the cell death is connected with autophagy, four B16 cells groups were divided, including control group (medium, only), harmine group, 3-MA group, harmine combined with 3-MA group. Among them, the harmine combined with 3-MA group was treated with 3-MA (5 mM) for 1 h previously. The cell viability was evaluated as above.

Hoechst 33,258 staining
The B16 cells were seeded in culture plates and allowed to attach overnight. After being subjected to harmine (80 μM) treatment for 24 h, cells were fixed with 4% paraformaldehyde at room temperature for 30 min, then

washed with PBS and stained with hoechst 33,258 (50 μg/mL) at 37 °C for 20 min in dark. After incubation and washed by PBS, the nuclear morphological changes of the cells were assessed by fluorescence microscopy (OLYMPUS, Japan).

AnnexinV-FITC/PI staining assay
The B16 cells were seeded in 6-well plates and allowed to attach overnight. The cells were cultured with various concentrations of harmine (40, 60, 80 μM). After 48 h incubation, cells were harvested and washed with PBS in cold twice. All cells were re-suspended in 300 μL binding buffer, then added by 5 μL of annexin V-FITC (fluorescein isothiocyanate) (2 mg/mL). Incubated for 15 min in dark, 5 μL of PI (propidium iodide, 20 μg/mL) was added for 5 min. BD FACS Calibur flow cytometer (Becton & Dickinson Company, Franklin Lakes, NJ, USA) was performed to analyze the apoptosis of cells.

Cell cycle analysis
Flow cytometry assay was performed to clarify the distribution of cell period and apoptotic rate. The cells were cultured after treating with harmine (40, 60, 80 μM) for 24 h as described above. After incubation, cells were harvested, washed by phosphate-buffered solution (PBS), and fixed in 70% ice-cold ethanol a night. Then, the cells were incubated with RNase A (100 μg/mL) and PI (40 μg/mL) for 30 min. Use the flow cytometry to determine the DNA content.

In order to investigating whether the cell cycle distribution is connected with autophagy, four B16 cells treatment groups including control group (medium, only), harmine group, 3-MA group, harmine combined with 3-MA group were conducted, in which the harmine combined with 3-MA group was treated with 3-MA (5 mM) for 1 h previously. The evaluation method was as above.

Western blot analysis

Total protein was extracted by incubation of cell pellet with lysis buffer. The protein concentration was determined by using BCA kit (YEASEN, China) according to the instructions of manufacturer. The cell lysate containing 20 μg of protein was fractionated by SDS-PAGE, transferred to a nitrocellulose filter membrane (Millipore, Billerica, MA, USA). Block them with 5% dried skimmed milk, and incubate the membranes for one night at 4 °C with the appropriate primary antibody. Then, it was incubated with HRP-conjugated secondary antibodies at room temperature for an hour. Protein bands were observed by an ECL chemiluminescence reagent and X-ray film (Tanon 5200, China).

Statistical analysis

The results were presented according to the means ± standard deviation. Use the one-way analysis of variance (ANOVA) to conduct statistical comparisons. P value less than 0.05 were used to show a statistically difference. All data were conducted with three independent and replicate tests.

Results

Anti-melanoma activity of MNZQ and herb extracts

The anti-melanoma activities of MNZQ and herb extracts were showed in Fig. 2. It could be seen from Fig. 2a that MNZQ (60 mg/mL), the extracts from *P. harmala* (1 mg/mL), *F. vulgare* (4 mg/mL), *N. glandulifera* (2 mg/mL), *C. intybus* (Seed; 10 mg/mL), *C. intybus* (Root; 10 mg/mL), *A. graveolens* (4 mg/mL), *D. moldavica*

(1 mg/mL) could inhibit the proliferation of B16 cells. It was found that *P. harmala* and *N. glandulifera* have remarkable anti-melanoma effect with IC_{50} values of 0.90 and 1.04 mg/mL at 24 h, respectively. The ingredients of harmine, harmaline, harmane and harmol contained in *P. harmala* inhibited the proliferation of B16 cells in a dose-dependent manner (Fig. 2b). Among these ingredients, harmine was the most notable effective on anti-melanoma activity with the lowest IC_{50} value of 44.92 μM at 24 h. The IC_{50} values of harmol, harmaline, and harmane were 68.50, 107.8, and 149.7 μM, respectively.

The results of tyrosinase inhibition assay indicated that all of 13 herb extracts and MNZQ did not show any inhibitory effects on tyrosinase at treated concentrations compared with kojic acid (data were not showed).

The autophagy and apoptosis of harmine-induced
The autophagy of harmine-induced

Electron microscopy was performed to obtain ultrastructural information regarding the autophagic vacuoles in B16 cells. As showed in Fig. 3a, the electron micrograph of harmine-treated in B16 cell showed cytoplasmic phagolysosomes whereas nucleus was normal after treated with harmine (40 μM). In contrast, few phagolysosomes were observed in the non-treated cells.

As known to all, MDC has been considered as a marker for autophagic vacuoles [25]. As depicted in Fig. 3b and c, the harmine treatment led to the accumulation of MDC-stained autophagic vacuoles. The quantitative analysis of MDC-stained cells confirmed that harmine caused a dose-dependent increase. The qualitative analysis

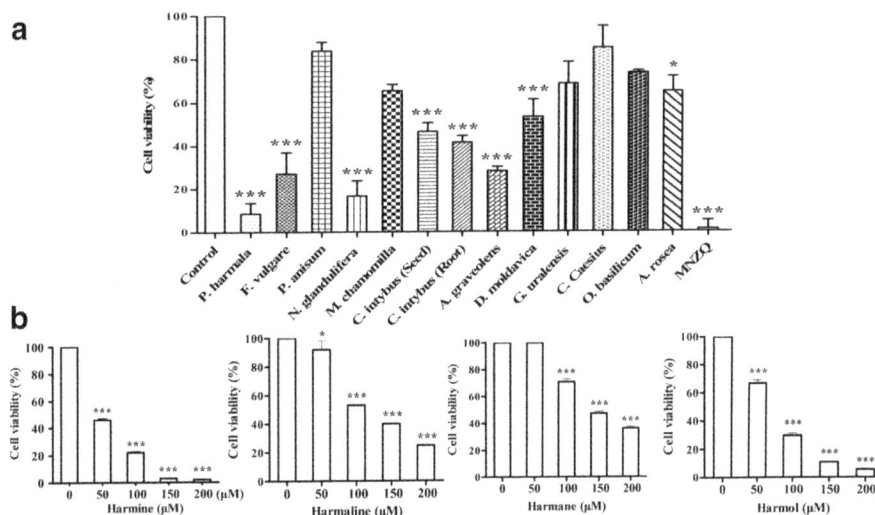

Fig. 2 The anti-melanoma effects of MNZQ, herb extracts and active ingredients on B16 cells assessed by CCK8. **a:** *P. harmala*: 1 mg/mL; *F. vulgare*: 4 mg/mL; *P. anisum*: 10 mg/mL; *N. glandulifera*: 2 mg/mL; *M. chamomilla*: 4 mg/mL; *C. intybus* (seed): 10 mg/mL; *C. intybus* (Root): 10 mg/mL; *A. graveolens*: 4 mg/mL; *D. moldavica*: 1 mg/mL; *G. uralensis*: 4 mg/mL; *C. caesius*: 4 mg/mL; *O. basilicum*: 5 mg/mL; *A. rosea*: 10 mg/mL; MNZQ: 60 mg/mL; **b:** active ingredients of harmine, harmaline, harmane, and harmol with concentration ranging from 50 to 200 μM. Results are expressed as the mean ± SD ($n = 3$). $^*P < 0.05$, $^{***}P < 0.001$ vs. the control group

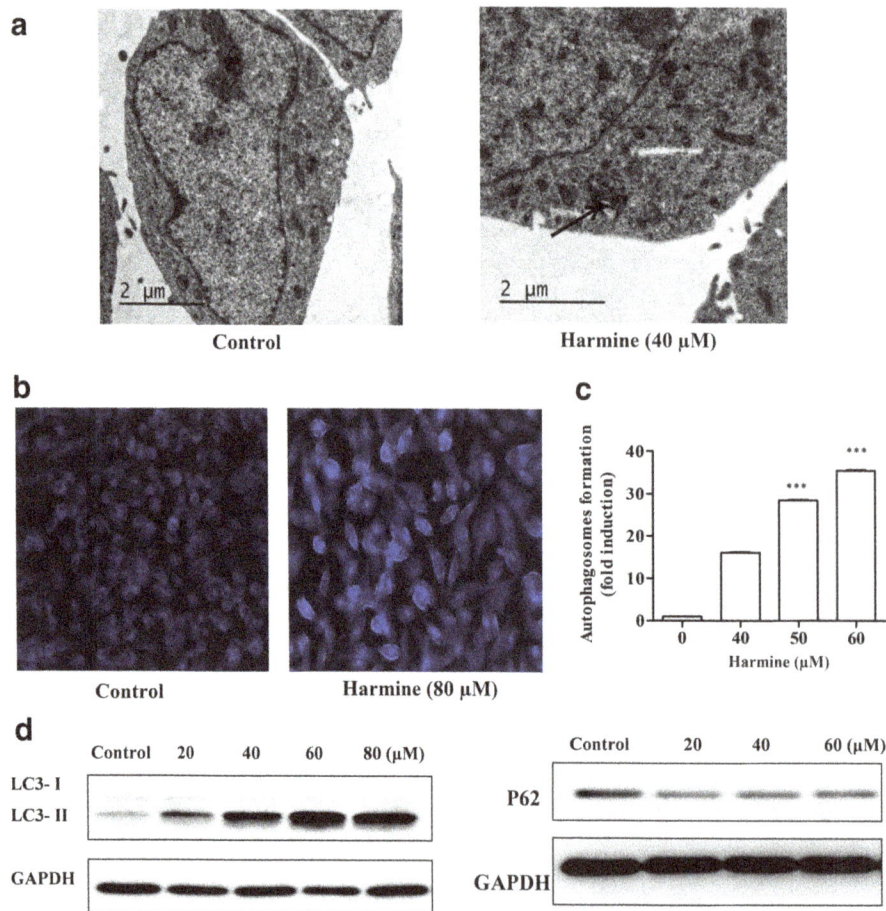

Fig. 3 Harmine induced autophagy in B16 cells. **a:** Electron micrographs of normal B16 cells (Control: magnification × 8200) and harmine-treated (40 μM) B16 cells (magnification × 9900); **b:** Fluorescence microscope (magnification × 200) observation on accumulation of MDC-stained autophagic vacuoles of control and harmine-treated (80 μM) B16 cells; **c:** The quantitative analysis of MDC-stained cells of harmine treated (40, 50 60 μM) expressed as the mean ± SD ($n = 3$). ***$P < 0.001$ vs. the control group; and **d:** the autophagy induction evaluated by western blot analysis for LC3-II treated with harmine (20, 40, 60, 80 μM) for 24 h and P62 proteins treated with harmine (20, 40, 60 μM) for 2 h

confirmed that the control cells showed slight fluorescence, while the cells treated with harmine at 80 μM accumulated MDC into granular structures of high fluorescence intensity.

To measure the occurrence of harmine-induced autophagy, the accumulation of LC3-II and degradation of P62 [26] were assessed by using western blot. The results were followed in Fig. 3d. After treatment of B16 cells with different concentrations of harmine for 24 h, a marked and dose-dependent up-regulation of LC3-II expression was observed compared with the untreated cells. SQSTM1/P62 serves as a link between LC3 and ubiquitinated substrates. After treatment of cells with various concentrations of harmine for 2 h, the levels of p62 presented a declining trend in dose-dependent mode.

The apoptosis of harmine-induced

Apoptotic nuclear morphology was observed after hoechst 33,258 staining. After treatment with 80 μM harmine for 24 h, as shown in Fig. 4a, the morphology of B16 cells changed, such as the volume of nuclear increased. This change was not the characteristics of the nuclear apoptosis. In the control group, the cells were normal in the morphology.

Apoptosis was also detected by annexin V-FITC/PI double staining assay to distinguish and determine the percentage of apoptotic cells. The proportion of apoptotic cells were followed in Fig. 4b. After harmine treatment, the early apoptotic cells increased from 0.84% (40 μM) to 1.87% (60 μM) and 3.85% (80 μM) and the late apoptotic cells increased from 0.82% (40 μM) to 1.83% (60 μM) and 4.80% (80 μM) when incubated with the indicated concentrations of harmine for 48 h.

Flow cytometry with a PI staining assay was assessed to analyze the effects of harmine on the cell cycle distribution. As depicted in Fig. 4c, the results showed that the accumulation of cells in the G2 phase was from 6.18% (40 μM) to 14.94% (60 μM) and 28.62% (80 μM),

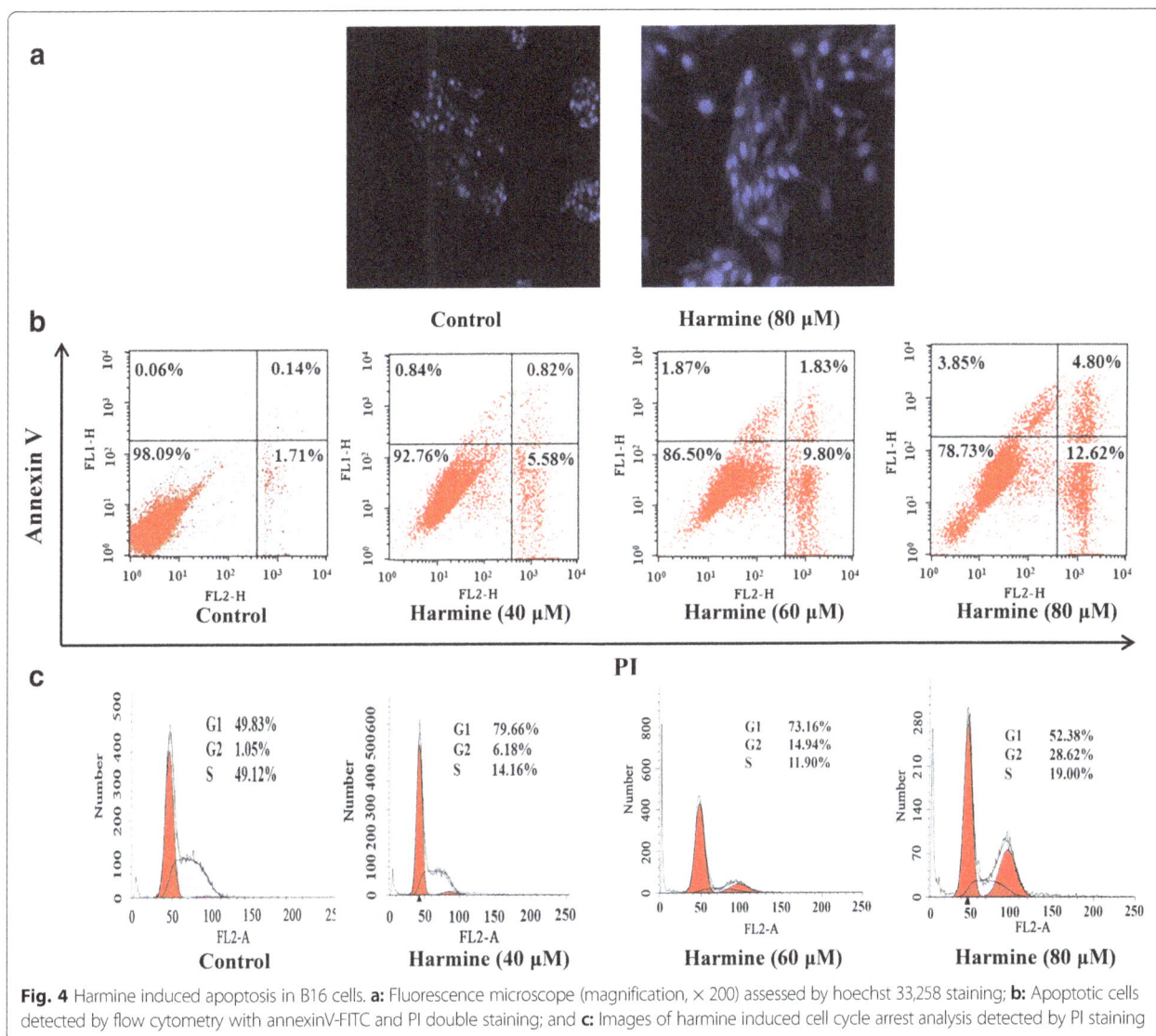

Fig. 4 Harmine induced apoptosis in B16 cells. **a:** Fluorescence microscope (magnification, × 200) assessed by hoechst 33,258 staining; **b:** Apoptotic cells detected by flow cytometry with annexinV-FITC and PI double staining; and **c:** Images of harmine induced cell cycle arrest analysis detected by PI staining

compared to the control group (1.05%). These results indicated that cell cycle distribution was significantly arrested in the G2 phase by harmine treatment.

The relationship between autophagy and apoptosis of harmine-induced

The cell viability of co-administrated harmine and 3-MA was shown in Fig. 5a. Following addition of PI3-kinase inhibitor 3-MA (5 mM), the cell viability was increased compared with corresponding harmine-treated cells.

For the cell cycle of co-administrated harmine and 3-MA, it was observed that 3-MA (5 mM) resulted in an expected reduction in autophagosome formation, which caused a clear decrease in cell cycle arrest of G2 phase compared with the control group as depicted in Fig. 5b. These findings prompted us to explore if the harmine-induced autophagy might has a cytotoxic effect.

In order to identifying the action site of harmine induced autophagy, the protein expression of LC3-II was examined after pretreatment with 3-MA and bafilomycin A1 for 1 h prior to the incubation with B16 cells for 24 h. 3-MA is a PI3-kinase inhibitor that can intervene autophagosome formation [27]. Bafilomycin A1 is a vacuolar H^+-ATPase inhibitor that can avoid endosomal acidification and obstruct autophagosome-lysosome fusion [28]. As shown in Fig. 5c, the expression of LC3-II protein was slightly suppressed by 3-MA in harmine-induced cells, and bafilomycin A1 effectively increased the expression of LC3-II protein in harmine-induced cells.

The effects on the Akt/mTOR signaling pathway

To get some insight into the molecular mechanisms of harmine-mediated autophagy induction in B16 cells, the Akt/mTOR and ERK1/2 signaling pathways were assessed.

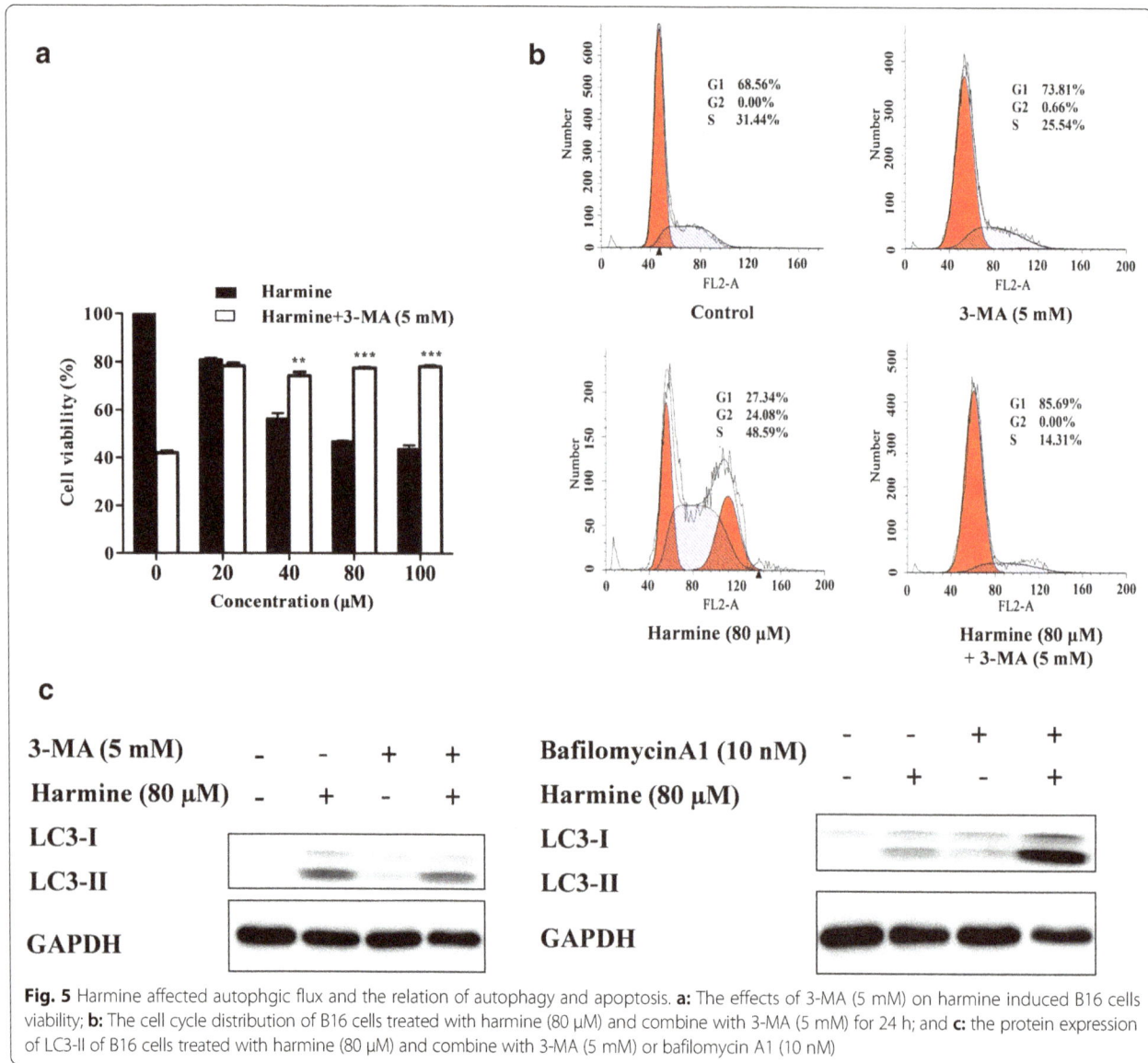

Fig. 5 Harmine affected autophgic flux and the relation of autophagy and apoptosis. **a:** The effects of 3-MA (5 mM) on harmine induced B16 cells viability; **b:** The cell cycle distribution of B16 cells treated with harmine (80 µM) and combine with 3-MA (5 mM) for 24 h; and **c:** the protein expression of LC3-II of B16 cells treated with harmine (80 µM) and combine with 3-MA (5 mM) or bafilomycin A1 (10 nM)

As shown in Fig. 6, treatment with harmine decreased the expression of phosphorylation of Akt and mTOR in a dose-dependent mode without influencing the total protein amount. Meanwhile, the phosphorylation levels of ERK1/2 were also inhibited without affecting the amount of total protein.

Discussion

Although the incidence of melanoma has slowly diminished, it nowadays still is one of widely recognized cancer types in the world [29–31]. It is a highly fatal disease which consists of limited therapeutic options and poor prognosis.

This study showed that MNZQ could display potential inhibitory effects on B16 cells but not affect tyrosinase activity. The target sites of some TCM did not influence the tyrosinase activity, but might play a role on inhibiting

cell proliferation of melanoma by other links of melanin metabolism. The clinical effects of MNZQ were come from the results of the compatibility of the whole 13 medicinal herbs. Alkaloids harmine, harmaline, harmane, and harmol derived from *P. harmala* were the effective ingredients in MNZQ. And harmine was confirmed as the most potent anti-melanoma agent screened from MNZQ. It could provide some evidences for the clinical effect of MNZQ on melanoma. In the previous study, it was found that harmine could significantly inhibit tumor cell proliferation and anticancer mechanism which was related to apoptotic signaling pathways [32, 33].

In harmine-treated cells, it was focused on the formation of autophagic vacuoles, whereas the nucleus remained intact. However, apoptosis is characterized by cell membrane blebbing, cell shrinkage, nuclear fragmentation, chromatin

Harmine (μM)

0   20   40   60   80

mTOR

p-mTOR

AKT

P-AKT

ERK1/2

P-ERK1/2

GAPDH

Fig. 6 The western blot analysis for mTOR, p-mTOR, Akt, p-Akt, ERK1/2 and p-ERK1/2 signaling pathway of B16 cells induced by harmine treated with 20, 40, 60, 80 μM for 1 h

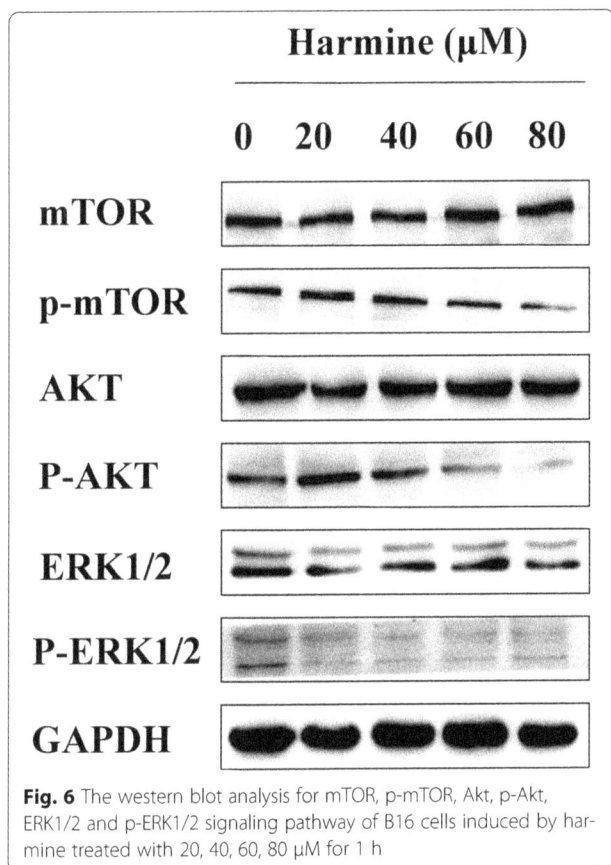

condensation, DNA fragmentation, and formation of apoptotic bodies. These findings indicated that harmine therapy induced autophagy instead of apoptosis in B16 cells. MDC has been regarded as a stalker for autophagic vacuoles. MDC-positive structures contained lysosomal enzymes, but not early/late endosomal marker. Nevertheless, the MDC dots co-localize well with staining for late-endosomal and lysosomal markers. The results of MDC staining showed that the level of autophagy increased in the dose-dependent mode. These two methods from the perspective of different morphology showed harmine induced autophagy.

From the aspects of molecular marker, the results showed that harmine induced the accretion of LC3-II and down-regulated P62 in a dose-dependent mode. The cytoplasmic form LC3-I is treated and recruited to the autophagosomes, in where LC3-II is produced by site-specific proteolysis and lipidation adjacent to the C-terminus. Therefore, there is positive correlation between the number of autophagosomes and the amount of LC3-II. A link between LC3 and ubiquitinated substrates is SQSTM1/P62 [34]. The initiation of autophagy relates with diminished doses of p62. Also, an autophagic flux assay is conducted to differentiate whether autophagosome formation is caused by autophagy induction or obstruction of the down-stream steps. Bafilomycin A1

was reported to inhibit autophagosome-lysosome fusion, expressively elevated the number of LC3-II. The accumulation of LC3-II was markedly changed in the occurrence of bafilomycin A1, suggesting that harmine increased the autophagic flux.

In addition, the rate of early and late apoptotic cells in B16 cells applied with harmine was fundamentally higher than that of control cells. In order to observe the morphological structure of apoptosis, the DNA fragmentation or condensation of the cells was examined by hoechst 33,258 staining [35]. The results revealed that the volume of nuclear enlarged and had no typical characteristic compared with the control group. It could be clearly distinguished from the typical morphologic change of apoptosis. Harmine might change the cell cycle distribution and causes G2 phase arrest. The low apoptosis rate after harmine treatment indicated that apoptosis is not a major mechanism of harmine induced cell death.

The role of autophagy in tumor is complicated and involves several opposite functions, such as promoting cell death or cell survival. As a PI3-kinase specific inhibitor, 3-MA could inhibit cell cycle arrest by blocking autophagosome formation. The data showed that combined treatment with 3-MA increased harmine-induced cell viability. Due to the change of cell cycle distribution in the G2 phase, harmine-induced cell death was not a typical apoptosis and it may be closely related to autophagy. The data provided evidences to explain the tight connection of autophagy, cell cycle distribution, and apoptosis.

Multiple signaling pathways such as AKT/mTOR, and ERK1/2 govern autophagy [36]. Akt/mTOR and ERK1/2 pathways control autophagy-induced nutrient starvation. The Akt/mTOR pathway negatively regulates autophagy [36–38] and the ERK1/2 pathway positively regulates autophagy. These pathways are also usually linked with oncogensis [39]. Some investigations have revealed that the inhibition of phosphorylation of Akt and its downstream mTOR signaling target could induce the initiation of autophagy. In this study, it was found harmine could influence Akt/mTOR and ERK1/2 signals by reducing the expression of p-mTOR, p-Akt, p-ERK1/2 in a dose-dependent manner. The results proved that harmine-induced autophagy was essentially via the Akt/mTOR pathway and in some degree through ERK1/2 pathway. Recently, it has been reported that harmine induced autophagy in MGC-803 and SGC-7901 cells by the inhibition of Akt/mTOR/p70S6K, the activation of AMPK pathway and mitochondrial pathway in human gastric cancer cells [40].

Conclusion

The investigation demonstrated that MNZQ can inhibit cell proliferation of melanoma without inhibiting tyrosinase activity and play a key role in causing autophagy in B16 cells. Harmine could efficiently accelerate cell death and that the cell death is related to autophagy to a great extent. Moreover, harmine could activate multiple autophagy-related signaling pathways, including Akt/mTOR and ERK1/2 pathways. Harmine might be a potential cancer therapy compound for melanoma.

Abbreviations

3-MA: 3-methyladenine; ANOVA: One-way analysis of variance; CCK-8: Cell Counting Kit-8; DMSO: Dimethyl sulfoxide; FITC: Fluorescein isothiocyanate; LC3: Microtubule-associated protein1 light chain 3; MDC: Monodansylcadaverine; MNZQ: Compound Muniziqi granule; mTOR: Mammalian target of rapamycin; PI: Propidium iodide; PI3K: Phosphatidyl inositide 3-kinase

Acknowledgments
The authors also gratefully acknowledge for Dr. Yuanzhi Lao for his kind help in data analysis.

Funding
This study was financially supported by the Key Projects of Joint Funds of the National Natural Science Foundation of China and Xinjiang Uygur Autonomous Region of China (No. U1130303), the Technology Cooperation Projects of Science in Shanghai, China (No. 14495800200) and the Science & Technology Constructing Project (Mandatory) of Xinjiang Uygur Autonomous Region of China (No. 2013911134).

Authors' contributions
CH Wang conceptualized, planned, designed the study and supported the funding. N Zou and Y Wei contributed equally to this work and carried out the experiments and drafted the manuscript. Y Yang, XM Cheng, and FH Li assisted in the analysis of data; N Zou, Y Wei and CH Wang drafted and finalized the manuscript. All authors read and approved the final manuscript.

Competing interests
The authors declare that they have no competing interests.

Author details
[1]Institute of Chinese Materia Medica, Shanghai University of Traditional Chinese Medicine, The MOE Key Laboratory for Standardization of Chinese Medicines and The SATCM Key Laboratory for New Resources and Quality Evaluation of Chinese Medicine, 1200 Cailun Road, Shanghai 201203, China. [2]Institute of Experimental Center for Scientific Technology, Shanghai University of Traditional Chinese Medicine, 1200 Cailun Road, Shanghai, China.

References
1. Lu WI, Lu DP. Impact of Chinese herbal medicine on American society and health care system: perspective and concern. Evid-Based Compl Alt. 2014; https://doi.org/10.1155/2014/251891.
2. Chan K. Chinese medicinal materials and their interface with Western medical concepts. J Ethnopharmacol. 2005;96:1–18.
3. Chinese Pharmacopoeia Committee, Drug Standards of the Ministry of Public Health of the People's Republic of China (Uygur Pharmaceutical Section). Chinese Pharmacopoeia Committee, 1998. China, pp 80.
4. Cheng JJ, Ma TY, Liu W, Wang HX, Jiang JZ, Wei Y, Tian HM, Zou N, Zhu YD, Shi HL, Cheng XM, Wang CH. In in vivo evaluation of the anti-inflammatory and analgesic activities of compound Muniziqi granule in experimental animal models. BMC Complem Altern M. 2016; https://doi.org/10.1186/s12906-016-0999-y.
5. Alqathama A, Prieto JM. Natural products with therapeutic potential in melanoma metastasis. Nat Prod Rep. 2015;32:1170–82.
6. Ye Y, Chou GX, Mu DD, Wang H, Chu JH, Leung AKM, Fong WF, Yu ZP. Screening of chinese herbal medicines for antityrosinase activity in a cell free system and B16 cells. J Ethnopharmacol. 2010;129:387–90.
7. Jeong SY, Seol DW. The role of mitochondria in apoptosis. BMB Rep. 2008; 41:11–22.
8. Li TY, Kon N, Jiang L, Tan MJ, Ludwig T, Zhao YM, Baer R, Gu W. Tumor suppression in the absence of p53-mediated cellcycle arrest, apoptosis, and senescence. Cell. 2012;149:1269–83.
9. Lin CY, Wu HY, Wang PL, Yuan CJ. Mammalian Ste20-like protein kinase 3 induces a caspase-independent apoptotic pathway. Int J Biochem Cell Biol. 2010;42:98–105.
10. Cheng Y, Qiu F, Ye YC, Tashiro S, Onodera S, Ikejima T. Oridonin induces G2/M arrest and apoptosis via activating ERK-p53 apoptotic pathway and inhibiting PTK-Ras-Raf-JNK survival pathway in murine fibrosarcoma L929 cells. Arch Biochem Biophys. 2009;490:70–5.
11. Yun J, Afaq F, Khan N, Mukhtar H. Delphinidin, an anthocyanidin in pigmented fruits and vegetables, induces apoptosis and cell cycle arrest in human colon cancer HCT 116 cells. Mol Carcinog. 2009;48:260–70.
12. Eom HJ, Choi J. P38 MAPK activation, DNA damage, cell cycle arrest and apoptosis as mechanisms of toxicity of silver nanoparticles in jurkat T cells. Environ Sci Technol. 2010;44:8337–42.
13. Mizushima N, Yoshimori T, Levine B. Methods in mammalian autophagy research. Cell. 2010;140:313–26.
14. Kumar D, Shankar S, Srivastava RK. Rottlerin induces autophagy and apoptosis in prostate cancer stem cells via PI3K/Akt/mTOR signaling pathway. Cancer Lett. 2013;343:179–89.
15. Kim J, Kundu M, Viollet B, Guan KL. AMPK and mTOR regulate autophagy through direct phosphorylation of Ulk1. Nat Cell Biol. 2011;13:132–41.
16. Herassandoval D, Pérezrojas JM, Hernándezdamián J, Pedrazachaverri J. The role of PI3K/AKT/mTOR pathway in the modulation of autophagy and the clearance of protein aggregates in neurodegeneration. Cell Signal. 2014;26:2694–701.
17. Li SP, Cheng XM, Wang CH. A review on traditional uses, phytochemistry, pharmacology, pharmacokinetics and toxicology of the genus Peganum. J Ethnopharmacol. 2017;203:127–62.
18. Lamchouri F, Settaf A, Cherrah Y, Zemzami M, Lyoussi B, Zaid A, Atif N, Hassar M. Antitumour principles from Peganum Harmala seeds. Therapie. 1999;54:753–8.
19. Chen Q, Chao RH, Chen HS, Hou XR, Yan HF, Zhou SF, Peng WL, Xu AL. Antitumor and neurotoxic effects of novel harmine derivatives and structure-activity relationship analysis. Int J Cancer. 2004;114:675–82.
20. Zhang H, Sun K, Ding J, Xu H, Zhu L, Zhang K, Li XL, Sun WH. Harmine induces apoptosis and inhibits tumor cell proliferation, migration and invasion through down-regulation of cyclooxygenase-2 expression in gastric cancer. Phytopharmacology. 2014;21:348–55.
21. Dai F, Chen Y, Song Y, Huang L, Zhai D, Dong Y, Lai L, Zhang T, Li DL, Pang XF. A natural small molecule harmine inhibits angiogenesis and suppresses tumour growth through activation of p53 in endothelial cells. PLoS One. 2012; https://doi.org/10.1371/journal.pone.0052162.
22. Hamsa TP, Kuttan G. Harmine inhibits tumour specific neo-vessel formation by regulating VEGF, MMP, TIMP and pro-inflammatory mediators both in vivo and in vitro. Eur J Pharmacol. 2010;649:64–73.
23. Abe A, Yamada H, Moriya S, Miyazawa K. The β-carboline alkaloid harmol induces cell death via autophagy but not apoptosis in human non-small cell lung cancer A549 cells. Biol Pharm Bull. 2011;34:1264–72.
24. Chan YY, Kim KH, Cheah SH. Inhibitory effects of sargassum polycystum on tyrosinase activity and melanin formation in B16F10 murine melanoma cells. J Ethnopharmacol. 2011;137:1183–8.
25. Mizushima N. Methods for monitoring autophagy. Int J Biochem Cell B. 2004;36:2491–502.
26. Lippai M, Lőw P. The role of the selective adaptor p62 and ubiquitin-like proteins in autophagy. Biomed Res Int. 2014; https://doi.org/10.1155/2014/832704
27. Tran AT, Ramalinga M, Kedir H, Clarke R, Kumar D. Autophagy inhibitor 3-methyladenine potentiates apoptosis induced by dietary tocotrienols in breast cancer cells. Eur J Nutr. 2015;54:265–72.
28. Xie ZG, Xie Y, Xu YJ, Zhou HB, Xu W, Dong QR. Bafilomycin A1 inhibits autophagy and induces apoptosis in MG63 osteosarcoma cells. Mol Med Rep. 2014;10:1103–7.
29. Climstein M, Furness J, Hing W, Walsh J. Lifetime prevalence of non-melanoma and melanoma skin cancer in australian recreational and competitive surfers. Photodermatol Photo. 2016;32:207–13.
30. Ivanov VN, Bhoumik A, Ronai Z. Death receptors and melanoma resistance to apoptosis. Oncogene. 2003;22:3152–61.
31. Lomas A, Leonardi-Bee J, Bath-Hextall F. A systematic review of worldwide incidence of nonmelanoma skin cancer. Brit J Dermatol. 2012;166:1069–80.

32. Cao MR, Li Q, Liu ZL, Liu HH, Wang W, Liao XL, Pan YL, Jiang JW. Harmine induces apoptosis in HepG2 cells via mitochondrial signaling pathway. HBPD Int. 2011;10:599–604.

33. Zhang P, Huang CR, Wang W, Zhang XK, Chen JJ, Wang JJ, Lin Jiang JW. Harmine hydrochloride triggers G2 phase arrest and apoptosis in MGC-803 cells and SMMC-7721 cells by upregulating p21, activating caspase-8/bid, and downregulating ERK/bad pathway. Phytother Res. 2015;30:31–40.

34. Wu M, Lao YZ, Xu NH, Wang XY, Tan HS, Fu WW, Lin ZX, Xu HX. Guttiferone k induces autophagy and sensitizes cancer cells to nutrient stress-induced cell death. Phytomedicine. 2015;22:902–10.

35. Fan CD, Su H, Zhao J, Zhao BX, Zhang SL, Mao JT. A novel copper complex of salicylaldehyde pyrazole hydrazone induces apoptosis through up-regulating integrin β4 in H322 lung carcinoma cells. Eur J Med Chem. 2010; 45:1438–46.

36. Shinojima N, Yokoyama T, Kondo Y, Kondo S. Roles of the Akt/mTOR/p70S6K and ERK1/2 signaling pathways in curcumin-induced autophagy. Autophagy. 2007;3:635–7.

37. Vucicevic L, Misirkic M, Janjetovic K, Vilimanovich U, Sudar E, Isenovic E, Prica M, Harhaji-Trajkovic T, Bumbasirevic V, Trajkovic V, Compound C. Induces protective autophagy in cancer cells through ampk inhibition-independent blockade of Akt/mTOR pathway. Autophagy. 2011;7:40–50.

38. Surviladze Z, Sterk RT, Deharo SA, Ozbun MA. Cellular entry of human papillomavirus type 16 involves activation of the phosphatidylinositol 3-kinase/AKT/mTOR pathway and inhibition of autophagy. J Virol. 2013;87:2508–17.

39. Wu YT, Tan HL, Huang Q, Ong CN, Shen HM. Activation of the PI3K-AkT-mTOR signaling pathway promotes necrotic cell death via suppression of autophagy. Autophagy. 2009;5:824–34.

40. Li C, Wang Y, Wang C, Yi X, Li M, He X. Anticancer activities of harmine by inducing a pro-death autophagy and apoptosis in human gastric cancer cells. Phytomedicine. 2017;28:10–8.

15

Acute and chronic toxicity of a polyherbal preparation – Jueyin granules

Yu Chen[1†], Dong-jie Guo[1†], Hui Deng[3], Min-feng Wu[1], Ya-Nan Zhang[1], Su Li[1], Rong Xu[1], Jie Chen[1], Xing-xiu Jin[1], Bin Li, Qi Xu[4*] and Fu-lun Li[1,2*]

Abstract

Background: The potential toxicity of Chinese herbal medicine has attracted more attention in recent years. Jueyin granules (JYG), a polyherbal formula, have been proven to be an effective agent for treating psoriasis in both animal models and clinical research. However, little is known about the possible acute and chronic toxicity of JYG. The objective of this study was to investigate the safety of JYG in ICR mice and Wistar rats.

Methods: To examine the acute toxicity of JYG, ICR mice were randomly divided into an experimental group and a control group, each comprising 20 mice (10 male and 10 female). The experimental group was fed JYG solution at a dose of 21.5 g/kg, equivalent to 143 times the clinical human dosage, for 14 days, whereas control animals were fed distilled water. In the chronic toxicity test, Wistar rats were divided into four groups, each comprising 40 rats (20 male and 20 female). For 6 months, the experimental animals were given JYG at a dose of 7.5, 3.75 and 1.875 g/kg, whereas control animals were given distilled water. The animals' body weight, food and water consumptions were monitored weekly. In addition, their biochemical and hematological parameters, histopathology, and body and organ weights were all measured at specific observation time points.

Results: According to the results of the acute toxicity test, no mortality was found and no abnormal pathological changes in major organs were observed in mice treated with JYG. In the chronic toxicity test, JYG did not cause significant abnormalities in the physiological parameters or pathological changes in the major organs of the rats.

Conclusion: The results indicated that JYG at the given doses did not induce any harmful effects in animals. Thus, it is reasonable to conclude that JYG is safe at the studied dosage levels and causes no acute or chronic toxicity in animal models.

Keywords: Jueyin granules, Acute toxicity, Chronic toxicity

Background

Although traditional medicine provides front-line pharmacotherapy for millions of Chinese, its application is often viewed with skepticism by the Western medicine establishment [1]. There has been wide concern about the toxicity of herbal medicine, and several side effects (such as allergic reactions, hepatotoxicity, nephrotoxicity, and cardiac toxicity) of herbal medicines have been reported in recently years [2].

Psoriasis is a chronic inflammatory skin disease affecting more than 125 million people worldwide [3]. Currently, there is no cure for psoriasis. Patients with psoriasis in China often turn to alternative and complementary treatments, which are considered to be effective and safe [4]. Jueyin granules (JYG), an effective formula consisting of eight Chinese herbs (*Haliotis diversicolor, Flos Lonicerae Japonicae, Radix Rehmanniae* exsiccate, cortex moutan, *Herba Hedyotisdiffusae, Folium isatidis, Smilax china L. and Radix Curcumae*) were discovered in the 1950s by Han Xia (a well-known Chinese surgeon) and have been used to clinically treat psoriasis for over 50 years by Yueyang Hospital of

* Correspondence: isuxuqi@163.com; drlifulun@163.com
†Equal contributors
[4]School of Public Health, Shanghai University of Traditional Chinese Medicine, Shanghai 200433, China
[1]Department of Dermatology, Yueyang Hospital of Integrated Traditional Chinese and Western Medicine, affiliated with Shanghai University of Traditional Chinese Medicine, 110 Ganhe Road, Shanghai 200437, China
Full list of author information is available at the end of the article

Integrated Traditional Chinese and Western Medicine. Our previous study showed that JYG can reduce inflammation and proliferation of keratinocytes and prevent psoriasis in animal models [5]. Moreover, the major ingredients, including *Haliotis diversicolor, Flos Lonicerae Japonicae, Herba Hedyotis diffusae, Folium Isatidis, Smilax china L., Radix Curcumae*, have been demonstrated to have anti-inflammatory effects in vitro and in vivo models [6–12]. The ingredient *Cortex Moutan* has been reported to have an inhibitory effect on proliferation of HaCaT cells in vitro models [13]. However, the toxicity of JYG has not been well studied. The objective of this study was to evaluate the safety of JYG in animal models.

Methods
Testing materials
Jueyin granules(manufactured by Tianyin Pharmaceutical Co. Ltd., Jiangsu Province, China; Certified Number of 20,120,103) were prepared using a water–alcohol extraction method and its quality control was performed using high-performance liquid chromatography (HPLC) by detecting chlorogenic acid and paeonol as shown in a previous publication [5]. The suspension of the drug was prepared by purified water. Its composition is shown in Table 1.

Animals
ICR mice weighing 17.2–19.8 g, purchased from Shanghai Super B & K Laboratory Animal Corp., Ltd., were used for the acute toxicity test. Six-to-seven-week-old SPF grade Wistar rats, purchased from Beijing WeiTongLiHua Experimental Animal Technology Co., Ltd., were used for the chronic toxicity test (Animal certificate no. 11400700011308). All animals were housed in groups of five rats per cage under a schedule of 12 h light/12 h dark and in a controlled temperature of 21 °C–24 °C. Animals had free access to standard laboratory animal feed and water. The experimental protocols were approved by the institutional Animal Ethics Committee of Shanghai University of Traditional Chinese Medicine (No. 14480 and 14,486).

Testing methods
Acute toxicity test
Forty ICR mice were randomly divided into two groups, each comprising 10 males and 10 females. For 18 h before the start of the experiment, the mice had access to water but no food. The mice were fed JYG oral solution, 40 ml/kg, by gavage twice a day for 14 days. The animals' skin, mucous membrane, changes in fur color, eyes, circulation, central nervous system, respiration, and conscious behavior were observed daily. Body weights were also measured once a week. Mice were euthanasized with CO_2 inhaltion on the 14th day.

Chronic toxicity test
A total of 160 Wistar rats were randomly divided into four groups, each group comprising 40 animals of 20 males and 20 females. All rats in the experimental groups were fed JYG oral solution once a day at graded doses of 7.5 (JYG-H), 3.75 (JYG-M), and 1.875 (JYG-L) g/kg for 3 months and 6 months, respectively, followed by a recovery period of 4 weeks. Those in the control group were administered distilled water at 20 ml/kg/d. The rats were observed daily for abnormal behavior and other adverse signs of toxicity. Consumption of food and water as well as body weight were recorded weekly. All animals were euthanasized with CO_2 inhaltion at the end of testing, and blood samples were obtained for the biochemical assays. The liver, kidney, lung, heart, spleen, brain, ovaries, testes and adrenal gland were all collected, weighed, and homogenized. A portion of each organ was removed for histological studies.

Biochemical assay
Hematological assessments
Hematological parameters, such as total white blood cell count, red blood cell count, packed cell volume, hemoglobin, and platelets (PLT), were determined using a fully automated hematology analyzer (Simens, Bayer ADVIA120, Germany).

Table 1 Ingredients of JYG used with English translations

Medicine	English translation	species/ family	dose
Haliotis diversicolor	Concha Haliotidis	Haliotis diversicolor Reeve	15 g
Flos Lonicerae japonicae	Honeysuckle flower	Lonicera japonica Thunb	12 g
Radix Rehmanniae exsiccata	Dried Rehmannia root	Rehmannia glutinosa(Gaertn.)Libosch	15 g
Cortex Moutan	Tree peony bark	Paeonia suffruticosa Andr	12 g
Herba Hedyotisdiffusae	Oldenlandia	Hedyotis diffusa Willd	15 g
Folium isatidis	Dyer's woad leaf	Isatis indigotica Fort	15 g
Smilax china L.	Chinaroot greenbrier rhizome	Smilaz china L	15 g
Radix Curcumae	Turmeric root tuber	Curcuma longa L	9 g

Table 2 Body weight in the control and JYG-treated group in the acute toxicity test

Group	Dose (g/kg)	n	Body weight (X ± S)		
			Day0	Day7	Day14
Control	/	20	18.7 ± 0.8	27.9 ± 1.9	31.0 ± 2.8
JYG	21.5	20	18.5 ± 0.7	26.4 ± 2.6	30.5 ± 3.6

JYG Jueyin granules. Values are expressed as mean ± SEM. JYG-treated groups showed non-significant changes as compared with control mices ($P > 0.05$)

Liver, renal function and serum electrolytes tests

A Hitachi 7020 Automatic Biochemical Analyzer was used to detect aspartate aminotransferase (AST), alanine aminotransferase (ALT), alkaline phosphatase, blood urea nitrogen, total protein, albumin, blood glucose, total bilirubin, creatinine, total cholesterol, triglycerides, creatine kinase, sodium ion concentration, potassium ion concentration, and chloride ion concentration.

Histopathology

The brain, liver, spleen, adrenal gland, epididymis, uterus, heart, kidney, testis, ovary, lung, and thymus were all weighed to calculate organ coefficients. The thyroid, stomach, pancreas, testis, prostate, aorta, bladder and bone marrow were preserved in 10% Faure Marin solution, fixed for 36–48 h, and subjected to conventional histological processes for histopathological examination. The tissue sections were examined under a microscope with a 40× objective to check cell morphology and quantity.

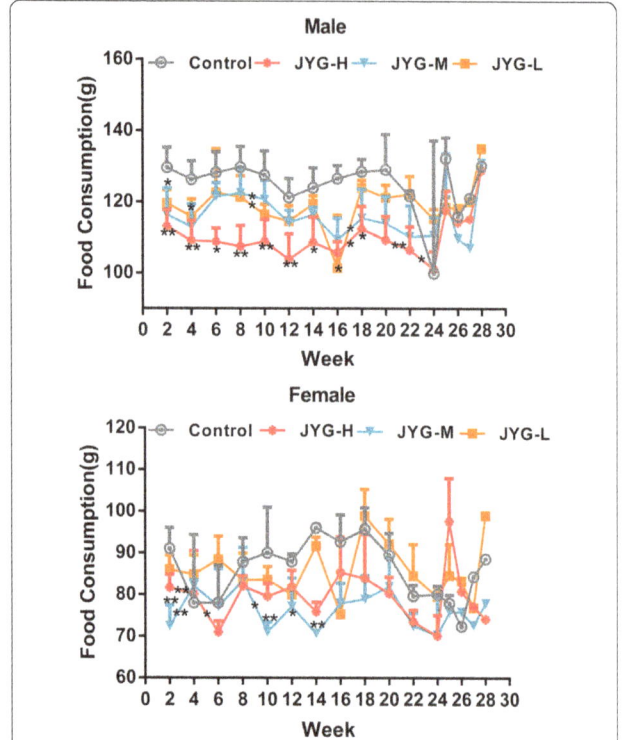

Fig. 2 Food consumption in the control and JYG-treated groups in the chronic toxicity test. Note: JYG-H, JYG-M,JYG-L: Jueyin granules high-dose, medium dose, low-dose group, respectively. The values are expressed as mean ± SEM ($n = 10$ rats for 3 months; $n = 17$–19 rats for 6 months; $n = 10$ rats for 1 month recovery). * $P < 0.05$; ** $P < 0.01$ statistically significant compared to control group

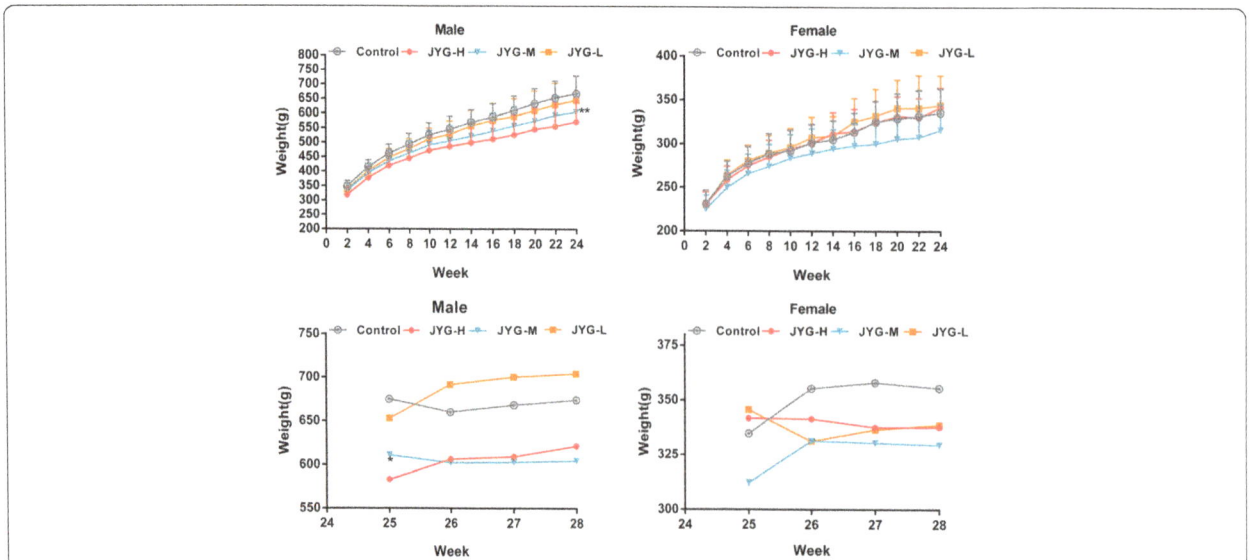

Fig. 1 Body weight in the control and JYG-treated groups in the chronic toxicity test. Note: JYG-H, JYG-M, JYG-L: Jueyin granules high-dose, medium dose, low-dose group, respectively. The values are expressed as mean ± SEM ($n = 10$ rats for 3 months; $n = 17$–19 rats for 6 months; $n = 10$ rats for 1 month recovery). * $P < 0.05$; **$P < 0.01$ statistically significant compared to control group

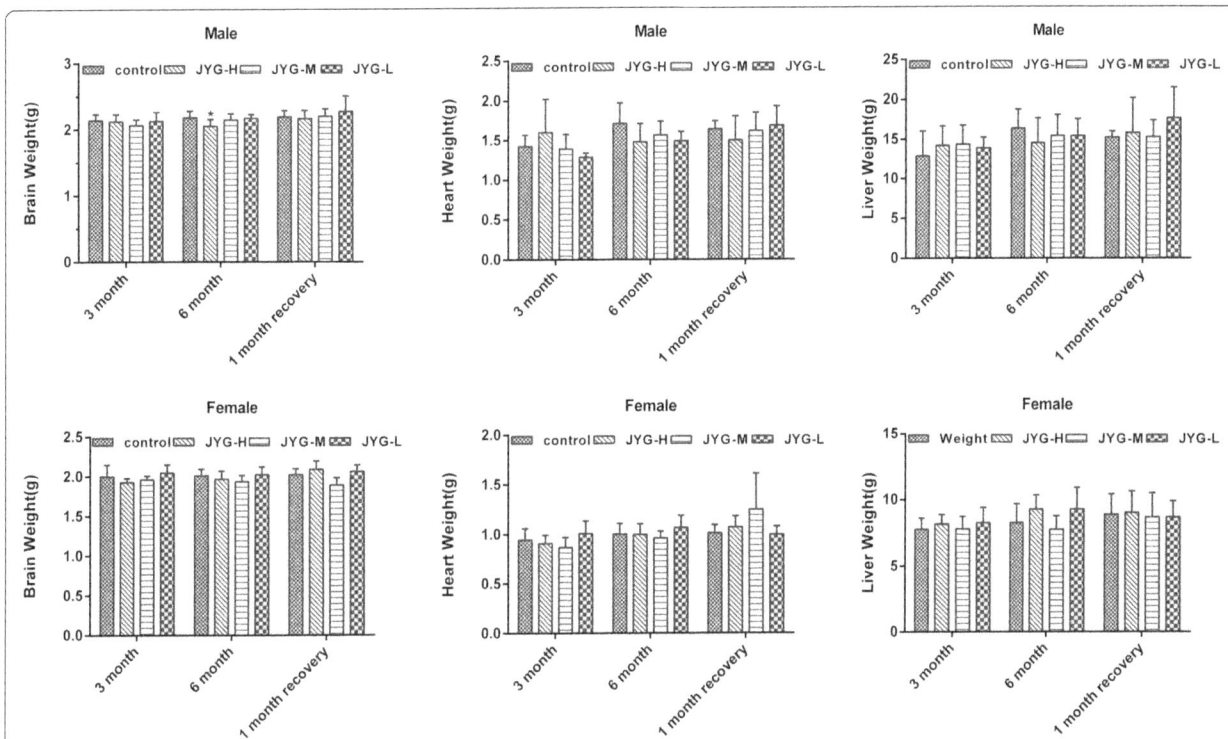

Fig. 3 Organs weight of brain, heart and liver in the control and JYG-treated groups in the chronic toxicity test. Note: JYG-H, JYG-M,JYG-L: Jueyin granules high-dose, medium dose, low-dose group, respectively. The values are expressed as mean ± SEM (*n* = 10 rats for 3 months; *n* = 17–19 rats for 6 months; n = 10 rats for 1 month recovery). * *P* < 0.05 statistically significant compared to control group

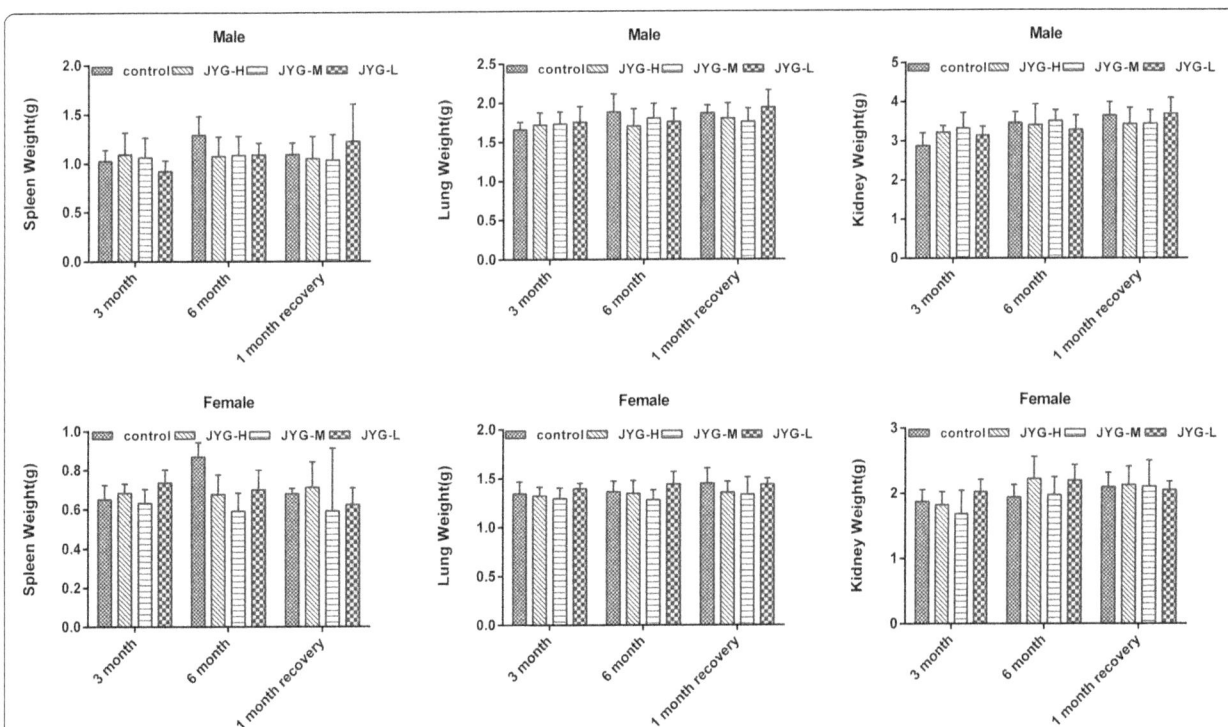

Fig. 4 Organs weight of spleen, lung, and kidney in the control and JYG-treated groups in the chronic toxicity test. Note: JYG-H, JYG-M,JYG-L: Jueyin granules high-dose, medium dose, low-dose group, respectively. The values are expressed as mean ± SEM (n = 10 rats for 3 months; n = 17–19 rats for 6 months; n = 10 rats for 1 month recovery). JYG-treated groups showed non-significant changes as compared with control group (*P* > 0.05)

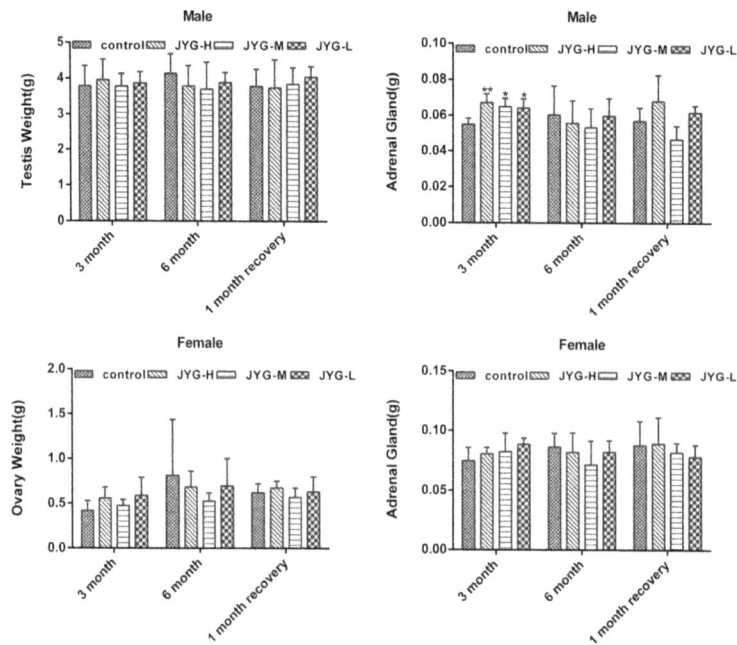

Fig. 5 Organs weight of testis, ovary, and adrenal gland in the control and JYG-treated groups in the chronic toxicity test. Note: JYG-H, JYG-M,JYG-L: Jueyin granules high-dose, medium dose, low-dose group, respectively. The values are expressed as mean ± SEM (n = 10 rats for 3 months; n = 17–19 rats for 6 months; n = 10 rats for 1 month recovery). * $P < 0.05$; ** $P < 0.01$ statistically significant compared to control group

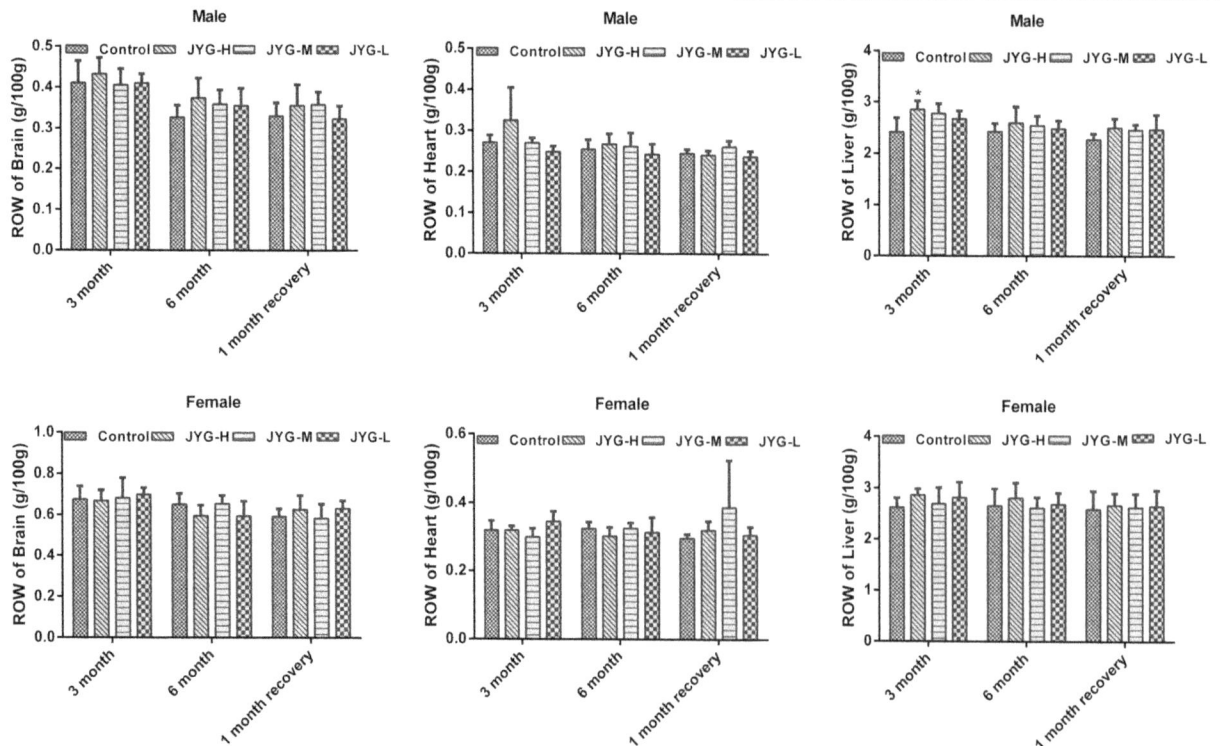

Fig. 6 Relative organs weight of brain, heart and liver in the control and JYG-treated groups in the chronic toxicity test. Note: ROW: relative organs weight; JYG-H, JYG-M, JYG-L: Jueyin granules high-dose, medium dose, low-dose group, respectively. The values are expressed as mean ± SEM (n = 10 rats for 3 months; n = 17–19 rats for 6 months; n = 10 rats for 1 month recovery). * $P < 0.05$ statistically significant compared to control group

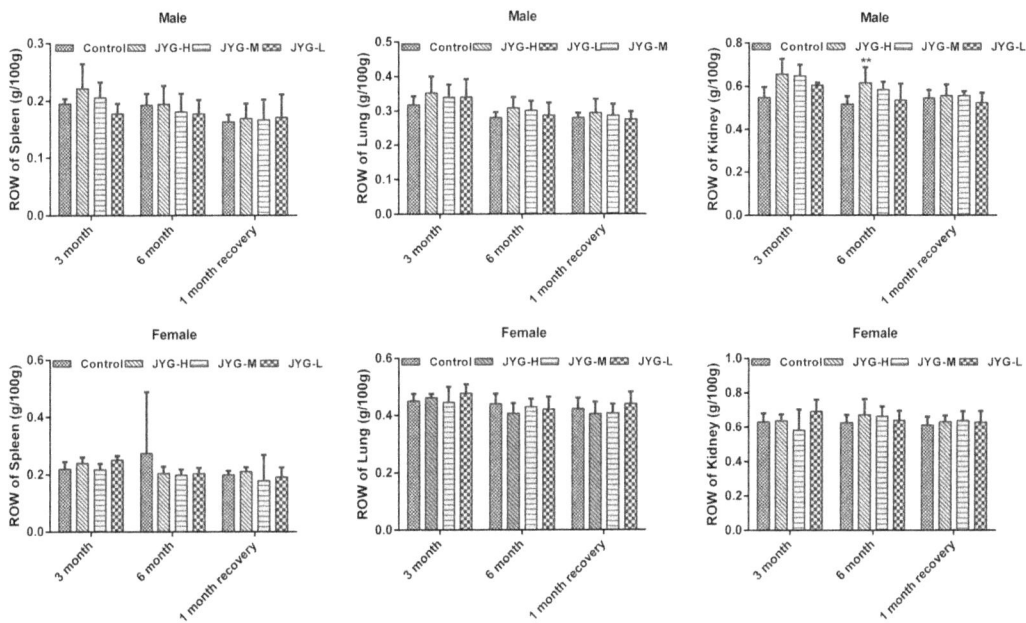

Fig. 7 Relative organs of spleen, lung, and kidney in the control and JYG-treated groups in the chronic toxicity test. Note: ROW: relative organs weight; JYG-H, JYG-M, JYG-L: Jueyin granules high-dose, medium dose, low-dose group, respectively. The values are expressed as mean ± SEM (n = 10 rats for 3 months; n = 17–19 rats for 6 months; n = 10 rats for 1 month recovery). ** $P < 0.01$ statistically significant compared to control group

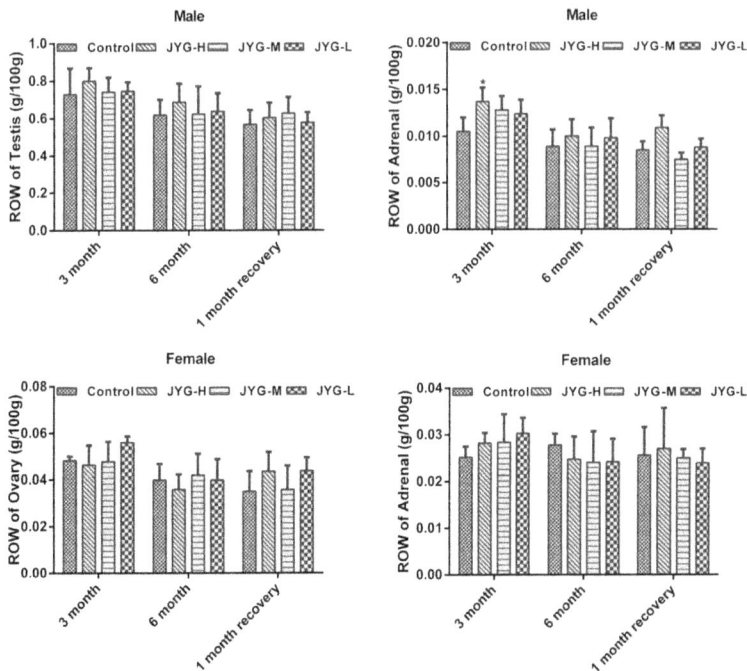

Fig. 8 Relative organs of testis, ovary, and adrenal gland in the control and JYG-treated groups in the chronic toxicity test. Note: ROW: relative organs weight; JYG-H, JYG-M, JYG-L: Jueyin granules high-dose, medium dose, low-dose group, respectively. The values are expressed as mean ± SEM (n = 10 rats for 3 months; n = 17–19 rats for 6 months; n = 10 rats for 1 month recovery). * $P < 0.05$ statistically significant compared to control group

Table 3 Hematological parameters of female rats in chronic toxicity test

Treatments	Time	Control	JYG-H	JYG-M	JYG-L
			7.5 g/kg	3.75 g/kg	1.875 g/kg
WBC	3 month	3.99 ± 1.44	3.46 ± 0.58	3.81 ± 0.49	4.04 ± 2.26
(× 109/L)	6 month	2.41 ± 1.31	1.95 ± 0.42	2.00 ± 0.79	1.90 ± 0.32
	1 month recovery	4.58 ± 1.82	4.86 ± 1.96	4.42 ± 2.22	4.43 ± 0.88
RBC	3 month	7.99 ± 0.42	7.38 ± 0.28*	7.84 ± 0.29	7.91 ± 0.48
(× 1012/L)	6 month	7.55 ± 1.19	7.71 ± 0.25	7.84 ± 0.52	8.03 ± 0.42
	1 month recovery	8.60 ± 0.35	8.35 ± 0.79	8.57 ± 0.44	8.41 ± 0.28
HGB	3 month	15.26 ± 0.61	14.40 ± 0.44*	14.86 ± 0.54	15.24 ± 0.86
(g/L)	6 month	14.30 ± 2.11	14.66 ± 0.89	14.64 ± 0.82	15.00 ± 0.43
	1 month recovery	15.24 ± 0.85	15.24 ± 0.68	15.50 ± 0.88	14.86 ± 0.60
PLT	3 month	1264 ± 54	1254 ± 210	1196 ± 106	1207 ± 172
(× 109/L)	6 month	1209 ± 347	1099 ± 120	1128 ± 110	1109 ± 156
	1 month recovery	1195 ± 140	1210 ± 198	1179 ± 98	1137 ± 121
NEUT	3 month	0.91 ± 0.62	0.98 ± 0.15	0.91 ± 0.13	0.94 ± 0.54
(× 109/L)	6 month	0.84 ± 0.57	0.66 ± 0.24	0.58 ± 0.16	0.58 ± 0.14
	1 month recovery	1.45 ± 0.58	1.65 ± 0.59	1.13 ± 0.65	1.30 ± 0.30
LYMPH	3 month	2.67 ± 1.08	2.15 ± 0.52	2.57 ± 0.40	2.77 ± 1.55
(× 109/L)	6 month	1.14 ± 0.47	1.10 ± 0.25	1.17 ± 0.54	1.11 ± 0.22
	1 month recovery	2.72 ± 1.28	2.75 ± 1.55	2.76 ± 1.57	2.69 ± 0.78
MONO	3 month	0.19 ± 0.10	0.22 ± 0.08	0.18 ± 0.07	0.20 ± 0.13
(× 109/L)	6 month	0.14 ± 0.13	0.09 ± 0.04	0.13 ± 0.13	0.11 ± 0.05
	1 month recovery	0.18 ± 0.12	0.23 ± 0.15	0.19 ± 0.15	0.22 ± 0.14

JYG-H, JYG-M,JYG-L Jueyin granules high-dose, medium dose, low-dose group, respectively. *WBC* total white blood cell count, *RBC* red blood cell, *HGB* hemoglobin, *PLT* blood platelet, *Neut* neutrophil, *Lymph* lymphocyte, *Mono* mononucleosis. The values are expressed as mean ± SEM ($n = 10$ rats for 3 months; $n = 17$–19 rats for 6 months; $n = 10$ rats for 1 month recovery). * Significantly different from control group ($p < 0.05$)

Statistical analysis

The experimental data were analyzed using SPSS 21 statistical software. All data were expressed as the mean ± the standard error of the mean (SEM).Significant differences among the groups were determined by a one-way analysis of variance and post hoc testing was performed for inter-group comparisons for least significant differences (LSDs) using a statistical analysis program for social science (SPSS).

Results

Acute toxicity

The results of acute oral toxicity testing of JYG administered at the dose of 21.5 g/kg are shown in Table 2. No animal mortality occurred at the doses given, and no signs of abnormality were observed throughout the experiment. The weight of the control group and the experimental group were both increased, and the average weight of those groups had no significant difference. In addition, no histopathological changes were observed in either the control or the JYG-treated groups (Additional file 1: Figure S1-S2).

Chronic toxicity

General conditions

Following the oral administration of JYG, rats from the low, medium, and high dose groups as well as those in the control group, were all in good condition. There were no significant abnormalities in fur color, behavior, eating, drinking, or breathing, nor were there any abnormalities in secretions from the eyes, mouths, noses, or other cavities. Eight rats died because of operational errors (Additional file 1: Figure S3-S4).

Effect of JYG on body weight, food consumption, organ weight and relative organ weight

Compared with the control group, JYG-H male rats had lower weight from weeks 2 to 24, although slow appreciable growth was observed at weeks 1, 2, and 18. JYG-M females had lower weight at week 2 (see Fig. 1). In most weeks from week 1 to 23, JYG-H male rats took in less food (except during weeks 3, 15, 16, 18–20, and 22). JYG-M male rats consumed less food during weeks 1, 2, 3, 5, 9, and 17, and JYG-M female rats consumed less food during weeks 1, 2, 3, 9, 10, and 12–14. JYG-L male

Table 4 Hematological parameters of male rats in chronic toxicity test

Treatments	Time	Control	JYG-H 7.5 g/kg	JYG-M 3.75 g/kg	JYG-L 1.875 g/kg
WBC	3 month	5.00 ± 1.01	8.27 ± 3.50	5.82 ± 1.28	6.81 ± 1.10
(× 109/L)	6 month	6.23 ± 2.20	6.06 ± 3.20	5.55 ± 1.23	5.52 ± 1.64
	1 month recovery	2.44 ± 1.30	2.36 ± 1.05	2.78 ± 0.85	2.33 ± 1.21
RBC	3 month	8.42 ± 0.67	8.06 ± 0.23	8.37 ± 0.16	8.58 ± 0.21
(× 1012/L)	6 month	8.80 ± 0.43	8.16 ± 0.51*	8.33 ± 0.47*	8.70 ± 0.39
	1 month recovery	7.05 ± 0.65	7.92 ± 0.76	7.57 ± 0.53	7.06 ± 0.79
HGB	3 month	14.56 ± 0.68	14.76 ± 0.36	15.02 ± 0.23	15.06 ± 0.42
(g/L)	6 month	15.14 ± 0.37	14.51 ± 0.78	14.72 ± 0.76	15.21 ± 0.49
	1 month recovery	13.26 ± 1.14	15.10 ± 1.01*	14.18 ± 1.09	13.14 ± 1.38
PLT	3 month	1214 ± 164	1108 ± 132	1080 ± 79	1186 ± 83
(× 109/L)	6 month	1134 ± 172	1182 ± 202	1102 ± 213	1210 ± 114
	1 month recovery	855 ± 314	897 ± 185	814 ± 238	759 ± 399
NEUT	3 month	1.53 ± 0.65	2.61 ± 1.69	1.51 ± 0.76	1.91 ± 0.70
(× 109/L)	6 month	1.61 ± 0.56	2.01 ± 1.13	1.71 ± 0.47	1.65 ± 0.81
	1 month recovery	0.74 ± 0.31	0.67 ± 0.20	0.93 ± 0.08	1.09 ± 0.86
LYMPH	3 month	2.91 ± 1.42	4.89 ± 1.89	3.78 ± 1.88	4.16 ± 0.62
(×109/L)	6 month	3.84 ± 1.55	3.34 ± 1.86	3.27 ± 0.97	3.36 ± 1.48
	1 month recovery	1.43 ± 0.91	1.39 ± 0.71	1.50 ± 0.71	0.99 ± 0.42
MONO	3 month	0.40 ± 0.24	0.58 ± 0.20	0.38 ± 0.17	0.53 ± 0.16
(×109/L)	6 month	0.49 ± 0.33	0.32 ± 0.24	0.29 ± 0.14	0.26 ± 0.15*
	1 month recovery	0.12 ± 0.07	0.19 ± 0.15	0.24 ± 0.11	0.15 ± 0.09

JYG-H, JYG-M, JYG-L Jueyin granules high-dose, medium dose, low-dose group, respectively, WBC total white blood cell count, RBC red blood cell, HGB hemoglobin, PLT blood platelet, Neut neutrophil, Lymph lymphocyte, Mono mononucleosis. The values are expressed as mean ± SEM (n = 10 rats for 3 months; n = 17–19 rats for 6 months; n = 10 rats for 1 month recovery). *Significantly different from control group ($p < 0.05$).

rats ate less food during weeks 9, 16, and 17 (see Fig. 2). No differences were found in average bodyweight and food intake throughout the six-month experimental period at the other time points. The brain weight of JYG-H male rats was lower and kidney relative weight was heavier at the end of 6 months compared with the control group. The liver relative weight of JYG-H male rats was heavier at the end of 3 months compared with the control group. The adrenal gland weight of male rats in JYG-treated groups was heavier than that of the control group. No significant differences were found in other organ weight values (see Figs. 3, 4, 5, 6, 7 and 8).

Effect of JYG on hematology parameters and biochemistry parameters
In female rats, JYG-H rats had significantly lower RBC and HGB values at the third months. In male rats, JYG-H and JYG-M rats had lower RBC values at the end of 6 months, whereas HGB values were significantly higher in JYG-H rats after 1 month of treatment in comparison to control group. By the sixth month, a significant

decrease in Mono values was noted in low dose compared to the control group (see Tables 3 and 4). At the end of 6 months, JYG-L rats had significantly lower ALT values, whereas AST values was significantly lower in JYG-M and JYG-L rats compared to the control group (see Fig. 9). However, these values were still within the normal range. There was no significant difference in other hematological and biochemistry parameters between the JYG-treated and the control groups.

Effect of JYG on histopathological alterations of visceral organs
No remarkable gross lesions were detected in any organs of the rats in the JYG-treated groups or those in the control groups. Histopathological examination showed no significant differences in the heart, lung, liver, kidney, spleen, pancreas, stomach, jejunum, duodenum, uterus, ovaries. Orchis between JYG-treated groups and the control group (see Figs. 10, 11, 12 and 13).

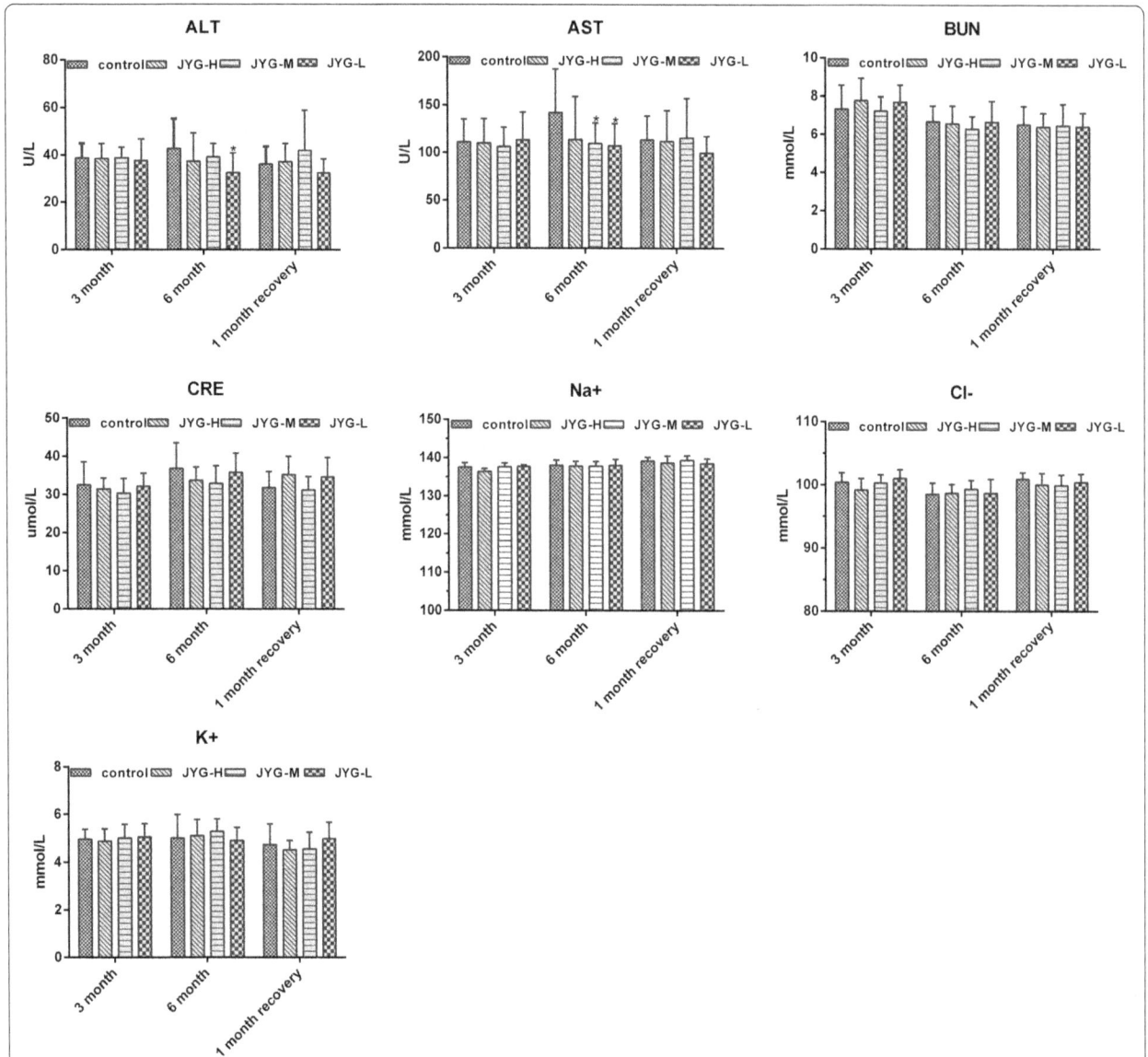

Fig. 9 Biochemical parameters in the control and JYG-treated groups in the chronic toxicity test. Note: JYG-H, JYG-M, JYG-L: Jueyin granules high-dose, medium-dose, low-dose group, respectively; ALT: alanine aminotransferase; AST: aminotransferase; BUN: blood urea nitrogen; CRE: creatinine; Na$^+$: Sodium ion; Cl$^-$: Chloride ion; K$^+$: Potassium ion. The values are expressed as mean ± SEM (n = 10 rats for 3 months; n = 17–19 rats for 6 months; n = 10 rats for 1 month recovery). * $P < 0.05$ statistically significant compared to control group

Discussion

Psoriasis, first defined by Ferdinand von Hebra as a distinct entity in 1841, is a common chronic inflammatory skin disorder. It is characterized by abnormal hyperproliferation of epidermal keratinocytes and infiltration of immunocytes along with angiogenesis [14]. The prevalence of psoriasis has been reported to range from 0.91% to 8.5% in adults and from 0 to 2.1% in children [15]. Despite the advances in what is known about the pathogenesis of psoriasis, modern therapies have had limited effects. People are looking for novel drugs to treat psoriasis, but many patients cannot afford the new therapies because of their high cost [16]. Moreover, patients suffering from

psoriasis are subjected to considerable physical and psychological disorders,which can aggravate the severity of psoriasis. This situation impairs the quality of life of people with psoriasis [17–19].

Recently, more people with psoriasis have turned to complementary and alternative medicine (CAM) because of its low cost and minimal adverse effects [8]. Traditional Chinese medicine is part of such therapies. Deng et al. [20] reported that herbal formulations could significantly improve the modified psoriasis area severity index score. In addition, these herbs and/or their constituents have anti-inflammatory, anti-angiogenic, anti-proliferative, and tissue repair actions. However, some herbal remedies or

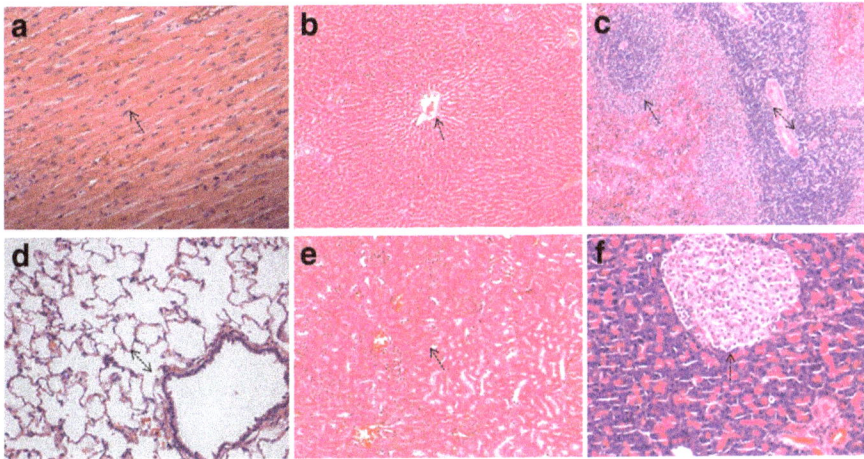

Fig. 10 Histopathological analysis of organs stained with H&E. Histopathology showing normal morphology from rats treated with Jueyin granules at the dose of 7.5 g/kg/day. **a** heart, **b** liver, **c** spleen, **d** lung, **e** kidney, **f** pancreas; scale bar = 100 μm

herbal formulae can produce a wide range of adverse reactions, even death [21–24]. Therefore, in recent years scientific investigation of CAM has been focused mainly on safety and toxicological evaluations [25].

In the present study, we investigated the acute and chronic toxicity of JYG, which was created in the 1950s by a well-known Chinese surgeon named Han Xia. Although clinical experience and animal studies have demonstrated the effectiveness of JYG in treating psoriasis, some patients suffering from weight loss, gastrointestinal symptom and abnormal liver function were reported in a recent publication [26]. Thus an evaluation on the safety of JYG is necessary.

The acute toxicity test results show that JYG cause no abnormalities or mortality with a maximum dose of 21.5 g/kg, equivalent to 143 times the clinical dose (0.15 g/kg) for

a person weighing 60 kg. Therefore JYG could be regarded as a partially nontoxic compound.

In the chronic toxicity test, food consumption and body weight showed a tendency to decrease in the JYG-treated group, especially in male rats. All rats' weight was recovered at 14 days after the withdrawl of the treatment. Although reduced food intake and weight loss were consistent with clinical observations, there was no significant dose response observed among animals in any of the three groups with different doses. In addition, organ weight and histopathological examinations also remained close to or within the normal range suggesting JYG showed no toxic effects on digestive system in JYG-treated rats. Therefore, we speculate that the reason for the differences is that animals could not adapt to the

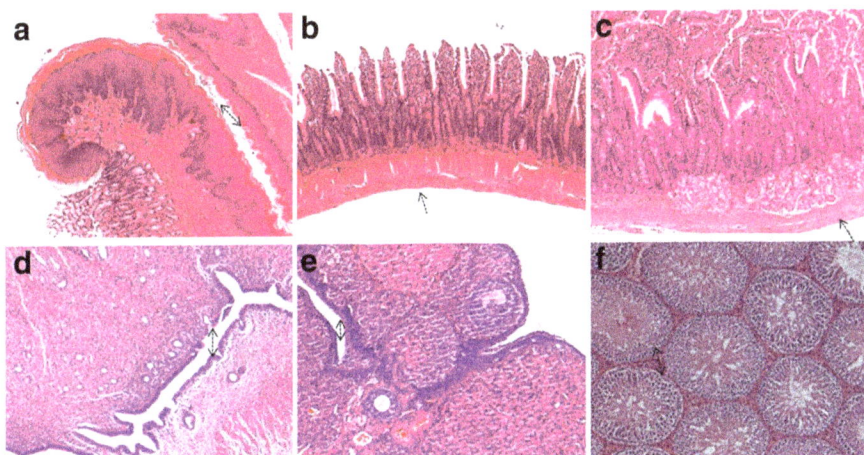

Fig. 11 Histopathological analysis of organs stained with H&E. Histopathology showing normal morphology from rats treated with Jueyin granules at the dose of 7.5 g/kg/day. **a** stomach, **b** jejunum, **c** duodenum, **d** uterus, **e** ovaries, **f** orchis; scale bar = 100 μm

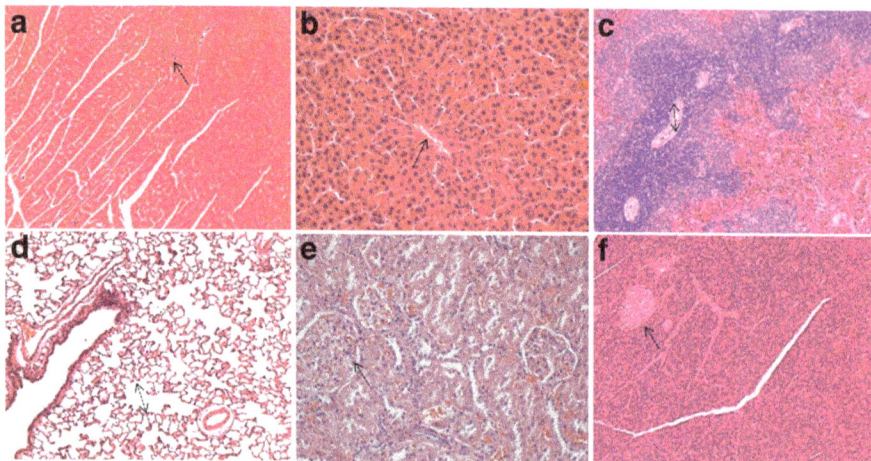

Fig. 12 Histopathological analysis of organs stained with H&E. Histopathology showing normal morphology from control group. **a** heart, **b** liver, **c** spleen, **d** lung, **e** kidney, **f** pancreas; scale bar = 100 μm

solution administered. In addition, we recommend that caution still should be taken in determining the dosage of JYG for children.

The serum enzyme levels, organ weight and histopathological examinations remained close to the control values indicating chronic administration of the drug JYG neither impaired the physiology of the liver nor the cellular structures of the liver, which is inconsistent with the clinical observation. However, we speculated the abnormal liver function in the patient may be caused by other reasons such as alcohol consumption rather than JYG administration, since the patient had an alcohol drinking history [26]. No hematological or other biochemistry alterations, or delayed toxic reactions were found in JYG-treated rats. These results were consistent with the recent clinical study showing that patients treated with JYG formulation twice a day for a continuous four-week period had no adverse effects in hematology or hepatorenal functions [26].

Conclusion

Jueyin granules at the given doses did not produce acute and chronic toxicity in animal models. There were no statistically significant alterations found in behavior, biochemistry, hematological parameters, organ weight, or histopathology. But children, the elderly and those with abnormal digestive function should be used with caution.

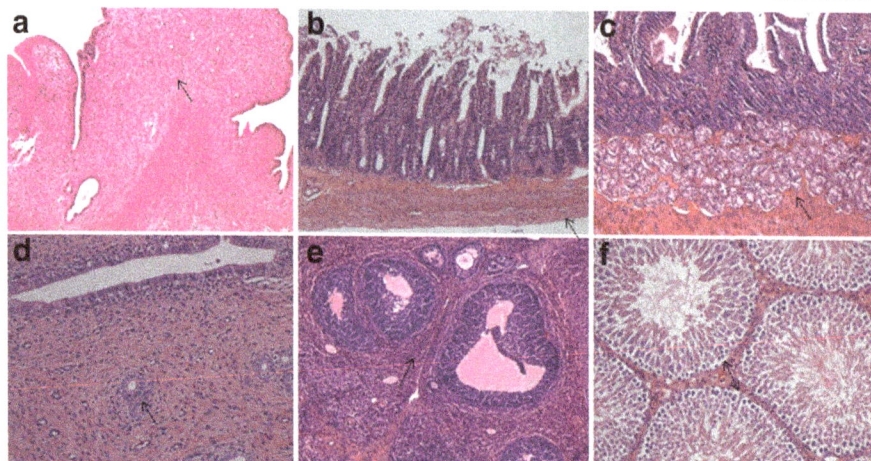

Fig. 13 Histopathological analysis of organs stained with H&E. Histopathology showing normal morphology from control group. **a** stomach, **b** jejunum, **c** duodenum, **d** uterus, **e** ovaries, **f** orchis; scale bar = 100 μm

Additional file

> **Additional file 1: Figure S1** Histopathological analysis of organs stained with H&E. Histopathology showing normal morphology from the acute toxicity test. (A) heart, (B) liver, (C) spleen, (D) lung, (E) kidney, (F) pancreas; scale bar = 100 μm. **Figure S2** Histopathological analysis of organs stained with H&E. Histopathology showing normal morphology from the acute toxicity test. (A) stomach, (B) jejunum, (C) duodenum, (D) uterus, (E) ovaries, (F) orchis; scale bar = 100 μm. **Figure S3** Histopathological analysis of organs stained with H&E. Histopathology showing normal morphology from eight dead rats. (A) heart, (B) liver, (C) spleen, (D) lung, (E) kidney, (F) pancreas; scale bar = 100 μm. **Figure S4** Histopathological analysis of organs stained with H&E. Histopathology showing normal morphology from eight dead rats. (A) stomach, (B) jejunum, (C) duodenum, (D) uterus, (E) ovaries, (F) orchis; scale bar = 100 μm

Abbreviations
ALT: alanine aminotransferase; AST: aspartate aminotransferase; BUN: blood urea nitrogen; CAM: complementary and alternative medicine; Cl⁻: Chloride ion; CRE: creatinine; HGB: hemoglobin; JYG: Jueyin granules; JYG-H: Jueyin granules high-dose group; JYG-L: Jueyin granules low-dose group; JYG-M: Jueyin granules medium-dose group; K⁺: Potassium ion; Lymph: lymphocyte; Mono: mononucleosis; Na⁺: Sodium ion; Neut: neutrophil; PLT: blood platelet; RBC: red blood cell count; ROW: relative organs weight; WBC: total white blood cell count

Acknowledgements
We thank SIFDC for their contribution, especially director Lian Ning, whose work helped us to overcome technical problems.

Funding
This study was supported by grant (No. 81373648, 81673866, 81273764, 81673054) from the National Science Foundation (NSFC) of China, the Shanghai Science and Technology Committee (16411955000,17zr1430500), the "Dawn" Program of Shanghai Education Commission (17SG41) and the Pudong New Area Committee on health and family planning (PWZxq2017–16).

Authors' contributions
YC and DJG made substantial contribution to analysis and interpretation of data and draft the manuscript. HD interpreted the data of acute and chronic toxicity. MFW analysed the data of acute toxicity and drafted manuscript. YNZ and SL analysed the data of JYG on body weight, food consumption, and organ weight. RX and JC analysed the data of the effect of JYG on hematology parameters and biochemistry parameters. XXJ analysed the data of JYG on histopathological alterations of visceral organs. BL critically revised the manuscript. FLL and QX significantly contributed to the designs of all experimental protocols, data analysis and interpretation, revised and finalised the manuscript. All authors read and approved the final manuscript.

Competing interests
The authors declare that they have no competing interests.

Author details
¹Department of Dermatology, Yueyang Hospital of Integrated Traditional Chinese and Western Medicine, affiliated with Shanghai University of Traditional Chinese Medicine, 110 Ganhe Road, Shanghai 200437, China. ²Department of Dermatology, the Seventh People's Hospital of Integrated Traditional Chinese and Western Medicine, affiliated with Shanghai University of Traditional Chinese Medicine, Shanghai 200137, China. ³The Sixth Hospital Affiliated with Shanghai Jiaotong University, Shanghai 200233, China. ⁴School of Public Health, Shanghai University of Traditional Chinese Medicine, Shanghai 200433, China.

References
1. Corson TW, Crews CM. Molecular understanding and modern application of traditional medicines: triumphs and trials. Cell. 2007;130(5):769–74.
2. Ghazanfar K, Dar SA, Akbar S, et al. Safety evaluation of Unani formulation: capsule Shaqeeqa in albino Wistar rats. Scientifica. 2016;2016(5):1–7.
3. Zindancı I, Albayrak O, Kavala M, et al. Prevalence of metabolic syndrome in patients with psoriasis. Indian J Dermatol Venereol Leprol. 2012;76(6):662.
4. Wang G, Liu Y. Traditional Chinese medicine is effective and safe in the treatment of psoriasis. Int J Dermatol. 2004;43(7):552.
5. Ma T, Jiang WC, Li X, et al. Effects of Chinese formula Jueyin granules on psoriasis in an animal model. Evid Based Complement Alternat Med. 2014;(3):1–8.
6. Huang X, Lv B, Zhang S, et al. Effects of radix curcumae-derived diterpenoid C on Helicobacter pylori-induced inflammation and nuclear factor kappa B signal pathways. World J Gastroenterol. 2013;19(31):5085.
7. Jiang L, Lu Y, Jin J, et al. N-butanol extract from folium isatidis inhibits lipopolysaccharide-induced inflammatory cytokine production in macrophages and protects mice against lipopolysaccharide-induced endotoxic shock. Drug Des Devel Ther. 2015;9:5601.
8. Kao ST, Liu CJ, Yeh CC. Protective and immunomodulatory effect of Flos Lonicerae japonicae by augmenting IL-10 expression in a murine model of acute lung inflammation. J Ethnopharmacol. 2015;168:108–15.
9. Jiang M, Han YQ, Zhou MG, et al. The screening research of anti-inflammatory bioactive markers from different flowering phases of Flos Lonicerae Japonicae. PLoS One. 2014;9(5):e96214.
10. Zhu H, Liang QH, Xiong XG, et al. Anti-inflammatory effects of the bioactive compound Ferulic acid contained in Oldenlandia diffusa on collagen-induced arthritis in rats. Evid Based Complement Alternat Med. 2014; 2014(12):573801.
11. Chen ZC, Wu SYS, Su WY, et al. Anti-inflammatory and burn injury wound healing properties of the shell of Haliotis diversicolor. Bmc Complement Altern Med. 2016;16(1):487.
12. Zhong C, Hu D, Hou LB, et al. Phenolic compounds from the rhizomes of Smilax China L. and their anti-inflammatory activity. Molecules. 2017;22(4):515.
13. Lü J, Wang Y, Zhao W, et al. Effects of catalpol, L-shikonin and paeonol extracted from radix rehmanniae, radix arnebiae and cortex moutan on KGF-induced HaCaT cell proliferation. Zhonghua Yi XueZaZhi. 2014;94(16):1265.
14. Nestle FO, Kaplan DH, Barker J. Psoriasis. N Engl J Med. 2009;361(5):496.
15. Parisi R, Symmons DPM, Griffiths CEM, et al. Global epidemiology of psoriasis: a systematic review of incidence and prevalence. J Investig Dermatol. 2013;133(2):377.
16. Pal HC, Chamcheu JC, Adhami VM, et al. Topical application of delphinidin reduces psoriasiform lesions in the flaky skin mouse model by inducing epidermal differentiation and inhibiting inflammation. Br J Dermatol. 2014; 172(2):354.
17. MJ Tribó, SRos, G Castaño, et al. Patients with severe psoriasis have high levels of psychological perceived stress: a pilot study on 300 Spanish individuals with psoriasis[EB/OL].http://xueshu.baidu.com/s?wd=paperuri: (e447ba35f98512a131acc0bd4210bd71)&filter=sc_long_sign&sc_ks_para= q%3DPatients+with+severe+psoriasis+have+high+levels+of+psychological +perceived+stress%3A+a+pilot+study+on+300+Spanish+individuals+with +psoriasis&tn=SE_baiduxueshu_c1gjeupa&ie=utf-8&sc_us= 11636290703603640692.
18. O'Leary CJ, Creamer D, Higgins E, et al. Perceived stress, stress attributions and psychological distress in psoriasis. J Psychosom Res. 2004;57(5):465–71.
19. Fordham B, Griffiths CE, Bundy C. A pilot study examining mindfulness-based cognitive therapy in psoriasis .Psychology. Health Med. 2015;20(1): 121–7.
20. Deng S, May BH, Zhang AL, et al. Topical herbal formulae in the management of psoriasis: systematic review with meta-analysis of clinical studies and investigation of the pharmacological actions of the main herbs. Phytotherapy Research Ptr. 2014;28(4):480–97.
21. Sheng Y, Ma Y, Deng Z, et al. Cytokines as potential biomarkers of liver toxicity induced by Dioscorea bulbifera L. Bioscience Trends. 2014;8(8):32–7.
22. Li H, Wang X, Ying L, et al. Hepatoprotection and hepatotoxicity of Heshouwu, a Chinese medicinal herb: context of the paradoxical effect: Food Chem Toxicol. 2016;108(Pt B):407.
23. Forte JS, Raman A. Regulatory issues relating to herbal products-part 2: safety and toxicity. J Med Food. 2000;3(1):41–57.
24. Martins E. The growing use of herbal medicines: issues relating to adverse reactions and challenges in monitoring safety. Front Pharmacol. 2013;4(4):177.

16

Danshen extract circumvents drug resistance and represses cell growth in human oral cancer cells

Cheng-Yu Yang[1†], Cheng-Chih Hsieh[2†], Chih-Kung Lin[3], Chun-Shu Lin[4,5], Bo Peng[1], Gu-Jiun Lin[6], Huey-Kang Sytwu[7], Wen-Liang Chang[8] and Yuan-Wu Chen[1,9*]

Abstract

Background: Danshen is a common traditional Chinese medicine used to treat neoplastic and chronic inflammatory diseases in China. However, the effects of Danshen on human oral cancer cells remain relatively unknown. This study investigated the antiproliferative effects of a Danshen extract on human oral cancer SAS, SCC25, OEC-M1, and KB drug-resistant cell lines and elucidated the possible underlying mechanism.

Methods: We investigated the anticancer potential of the Danshen extract in human oral cancer cell lines and an in vivo oral cancer xenograft mouse model. The expression of apoptosis-related molecules was evaluated through Western blotting, and the concentration of in vivo apoptotic markers was measured using immunohistochemical staining. The antitumor effects of 5-fluorouracil and the Danshen extract were compared.

Results: Cell proliferation assays revealed that the Danshen extract strongly inhibited oral cancer cell proliferation. Cell morphology studies revealed that the Danshen extract inhibited the growth of SAS, SCC25, and OEC-M1 cells by inducing apoptosis. The Flow cytometric analysis indicated that the Danshen extract induced cell cycle G0/G1 arrest. Immunoblotting analysis for the expression of active caspase-3 and X-linked inhibitor of apoptosis protein indicated that Danshen extract-induced apoptosis in human oral cancer SAS cells was mediated through the caspase pathway. Moreover, the Danshen extract significantly inhibited growth in the SAS xenograft mouse model. Furthermore, the Danshen extract circumvented drug resistance in KB drug-resistant oral cancer cells.

Conclusion: The study results suggest that the Danshen extract could be a potential anticancer agent in oral cancer treatment.

Keywords: Danshen, Oral cancer, Drug resistance, Apoptosis

Background

Oral cancer is one of the most common cancers and the leading cause of cancer deaths worldwide [1]. Recent understanding of oral cancer has led to the development of biological therapies using drugs such as 5-fluorouracil (5-FU) and cisplatin [2]. These drugs have shown remarkable activity against difficult-to-treat oral cancer in early clinical trials; however, prolonged drug exposure may result in the development of de novo drug resistance and unexpected side effects, such as allergic reactions, breathing difficulties, swelling, nausea, fever or chills, and dizziness or weakness [3–5]. Therefore, the identification and validation of novel targeted therapies is urgently required to overcome drug resistance and improve patient outcomes.

Danshen (*Salvia miltiorrhiza*) is a widely used traditional Chinese medicine, which was first described in the Chinese pharmacology book, *Shen Nong's Canon on Materia Medica* [6]. Danshen attenuates inflammatory reactions in cardiovascular, hepatic, and tumoral diseases without appreciable adverse effects [6]. Various Danshen extracts

* Correspondence: h6183@yahoo.com.tw
†Equal contributors
[1]School of Dentistry, National Defense Medical Center, Taipei, Taiwan, Republic of China
[9]Department of Oral and Maxillofacial Surgery, Tri-Service General Hospital, No. 161, Section 6, Min-Chuan East Road, Neihu 114, Taipei 114, Taiwan, Republic of China
Full list of author information is available at the end of the article

contain diterpene quinone and phenolic acid derivatives including tanshinone, cryptotanshinone, isocryptotanshinone, miltirone, tanshinol, salviol, and salvianolic acid B [7–9]. Because of their growth-inhibiting effects on cancer cells [7], Danshen extracts may be suitable as major drug candidates or additional chemotherapeutic agents in oral cancer treatment. In this study, we observed that a Danshen extract (crude) can inhibit human oral cancer SAS, SCC25, OEC-M1, and KB drug-resistant cell lines. It possibly exerts anticancer effects by blocking cell cycle entry into the G1 phase in oral cancer cells.

Methods

Reagents

In this study, 5-FU was purchased from Sigma-Aldrich (F6627); its purity was ≥99%, as determined by high-performance liquid chromatography. The 5-FU was dissolved in saline as a 1.5 mg/mL stock and used as the positive control in an animal model.

Preparation and treatment of the Danshen extract

Danshen (*S. miltiorrhiza*) was obtained from Dr. Wen-Liang Chang of the National Defense Medical Center in Taipei, Taiwan [10, 11]. Danshen roots were obtained from Chien Yuan Herbal Medicinal Co., Taipei, Taiwan, and identified to be Salviae miltiorrhizae Radix. The pulverized roots (4.5 kg) were extracted with 95% ethanol (15 L) exhaustively for five times. The extract was concentrated by evaporation under reduced pressure. The dried extracts were dissolved in dimethylsulfoxide to prepare a 20 mg/mL stock solution and stored at 4 °C. The Danshen extract was diluted with culture media to achieve the indicated final concentration in each experiment.

Cell culture

The human oral squamous cell carcinoma (OSCC) cell line SAS (JCRB0260) was purchased from the Japanese Collection of Research Bioresources Cell Bank. SCC25 (CRL-1628) was obtained from the American Type Culture Collection (ATCC). OEC-M1 cell line was derived from oral cavity epidermal carcinoma [12], which is a generous gift from Prof. Jenn-Han Chen (National Defense Medical Center, Taiwan). KB drug-resistant cancer cells were purchased from the ATCC (CCL-17; Rockville, MA, USA). KB-7D cells were generated through etoposide (VP-16)-driven selection, which demonstrated topoisomerase II downregulation and multidrug resistance-associated protein overexpression. KB-tax cells were generated through taxol-driven selection. These drug-resistant cancer cells were kindly provided by Dr. Jang-Yang Chang (Cancer Research Division of National Health Research Institutes, Taiwan) [13]. Human oral cancer SAS, SCC25, and OEC-M1

cells were cultured in Roswell Park Memorial Institute 1640 medium. The culture medium was supplemented with 10% fetal bovine serum, 1% penicillin/streptomycin, and 2 mmol/L L-glutamine. The cells were grown at 37 °C in a humidified 5% CO_2 incubator.

Cytotoxicity assay

The cells (10,000 cells/well) were cultured in a 24-well plate and then exposed to various concentrations of the Danshen extract for 24 h. The methylene blue dye assay was performed to evaluate the effects of melatonin on cell growth, as described previously [10]. The half-maximal inhibitory concentration (IC50) value resulting from 50% inhibition of cell growth was calculated graphically for comparison with cell growth in controls.

Cell cycle analysis

The cells were harvested with 0.25% trypsin and washed once with phosphate-buffered saline (PBS). After centrifugation, the cells were fixed in 100% ice-cold methanol overnight at −20 °C; next, they were incubated in propidium iodide (50 μg/mL) and RNase (1 mg/mL) for 30 min. Apoptotic cells were identified using a FACScan flow cytometer (Becton Dickinson, Mountain View, CA, USA), and the data were analyzed using CellQuest software. All experiments were performed in triplicate.

Western blot analysis for caspase activity

The cells were lysed directly in an radioimmunoprecipitation assay buffer containing 50 mM Tris (pH 7.8), 0.15 M NaCl, 5 mM ethylenediaminetetraacetic acid, 0.5% Triton X-100, 0.5% NP-40, 0.1% sodium deoxycholate, a protease inhibitor mixture (Calbiochem, Billerica, MA, USA), and a phosphatase inhibitor mixture (Calbiochem, USA). The relative protein concentration in supernatants was determined using a bicinchoninic acid protein assay kit (Thermo Scientific, Rockford, IL, USA). For immunoblotting, in each lane of 10% sodium dodecyl sulfate–polyacrylamide electrophoresis gel, 30 μg protein from cell lysates was loaded, separated, and transferred onto polyvinyldifluoride membranes (GE Healthcare, UK). These membranes were subsequently probed using specific antibodies against caspase-3 (Cell Signaling, #9662), X-linked inhibitor of apoptosis protein (XIAP; Cell Signaling, #2045), and glyceraldehyde-3-phosphate dehydrogenase (Epitomics, #2251-1).

OSCC animal models

To investigate the effects of the Danshen extract on OSCC in vivo, we used oral cancer SAS xenograft animal models. All experiments were approved by the Institutional Animal Use Committee (IACUC) of the National Defense Medical Center, Taiwan (IACUC 16-022). Eight-week-old nonobese diabetic/severe combined immunodeficiency

(NOD/SCID) (NOD.CB17 Prkdc scid/J, National Laboratory Animal Center, Taiwan) mice were maintained in microisolators under specific pathogen-free conditions. These NOD/SCID mice were fed with sterile food and chlorinated sterile water. A total of 12 mice were divided into 3 groups: Danshen extract (10 mg/kg body weight [BW]/d/intraperitoneally [i.p.])-treated; positive control (5-FU, 10 mg/kg BW/d/i.p.); and vehicle control (PBS). Each group of mice was subcutaneously injected with 2×10^6 human oral cancer SAS cells. Drugs were first administered to each group of mice on day 3 prior to tumor palpation, and the treatment was continued until day 32. The size of the transplanted tumors was measured every 3 days using gauged calipers, and the tumor volume was calculated using the following formula: V = 1/2 × (length × width^2). At the end of the treatment, the mice were sacrificed, and the tumors were removed, weighed, and photographed.

Haemotoxylin and eosin and immunohistochemical staining

Mice were sacrificed with CO_2 inhalation and fixed by perfusion with 4% paraformaldehyde in 0.1 M phosphate buffer. Serial 5-μm histologic sections were deparaffinized in xylene and rehydrated. After blocking of endogenous peroxidase by incubation with 3% hydrogen peroxide, the slides were incubated with anticaspase-3 overnight at 4 °C. The expression levels of targeted proteins were examined by using the antimouse and rabbit peroxidase complex, and peroxidase activity was evaluated using 3-amino-9-ethyl-carbazole. The slides were counterstained with hematoxylin (Sigma) and mounted with mounting solution. Scores were obtained by multiplying the immunohistochemical (IHC) intensity with the percentage of cancer cells stained.

Statistical analysis

The experiments were performed in triplicate. The data for cell proliferation and viability assays are expressed as the mean ± standard deviation. Standard deviations for all measured biological parameters are displayed in the appropriate figures. The Student t test was performed to determine the significance of the differences between the control and treated groups for all experimental test conditions. $P < 0.05$ was considered statistically significant. Statistical analysis was performed using GraphPad Prism (GraphPad Software, San Diego, CA, USA).

Results

The growth inhibitory effects of a Danshen extract on human oral cancer SAS, SCC25, and OEC-M1 cells were first demonstrated by conducting microscopic studies. The results showed that the Danshen extract effectively inhibited the growth of both tongue cancer cells (SAS and SCC25) and gingival cancer cells (OEC-M1) (Fig. 1). The antiproliferative effects of the Danshen extract on human oral cancer cells were further confirmed by proliferation assays (Fig. 2). The methylene blue proliferation assay revealed that Danshen treatment (5–10 μg/mL) could result in an approximately 50% reduction in oral cancer cell proliferation (Fig. 2).

To examine whether the Danshen extract inhibited cell proliferation by cell cycle arrest, cell cycle profiling of the SAS cells was performed. The cells were treated with the Danshen extract (20 μg/mL) for 24 h and their cell cycle profiles were analyzed using flow cytometry. The analysis results revealed that the Danshen extract engendered an increase in the G0/G1 phase, with a concomitant reduction in the S phase, in the SAS cells (Fig. 3). In addition, the sub-G1 apoptotic dead cell population increased after Danshen treatment (Fig. 3). These results suggest that the Danshen extract induced oral cancer cell apoptosis and cell cycle G0/G1 arrest.

To gain a clearer understanding of the antioral cancer mechanism in Danshen-extract-treated cancer cells, we investigated the effects of the Danshen extract on the expression levels and activities of intracellular signaling molecules (Fig. 4). Specifically, the expression levels of the apoptotic protein caspase-3 and antiapoptotic protein XIAP were upregulated and downregulated, respectively, in Danshen-extract-treated cancer cells (Fig. 4). To delineate the antiproliferative effects of the Danshen extract, the SAS cells were treated with various concentrations of the extract for different treatment periods. In addition, Western blotting was performed to examine the effects of the Danshen extract on intracellular signaling molecules. The results (Fig. 4) demonstrated that the Danshen extract effectively suppressed XIAP expression and upregulated caspase-3 expression.

The antioral cancer effects of the Danshen extract were further investigated in the SAS solid tumor xenografts of immunodeficient mice. The daily treatments were initiated a day after the SAS cells were transplanted into the NOD/SCID mice. The doses for individual treatments (for 32 d) are outlined as follows: Danshen extract, 10 mg/kg/d/i.p.; 5-FU, 10 mg/kg/d/i.p. During this period, each mouse was manually examined for tumor volume at least four times. The Danshen extract and 5-FU (i.e., the first-line drug for oral cancer treatment) significantly inhibited tumor growth in the NOD/SCID mice, and the bodies weight of the mice were not changed (Fig. 5).

Histologic sections obtained from the SAS xenografts were used to evaluate the antiproliferative effects of the Danshen extract in SAS cells. The expression levels of caspase-3 (apoptotic biomarker) were then analyzed through IHC staining (Fig. 6), which our statistical analysis showed were significantly higher in the Danshen-

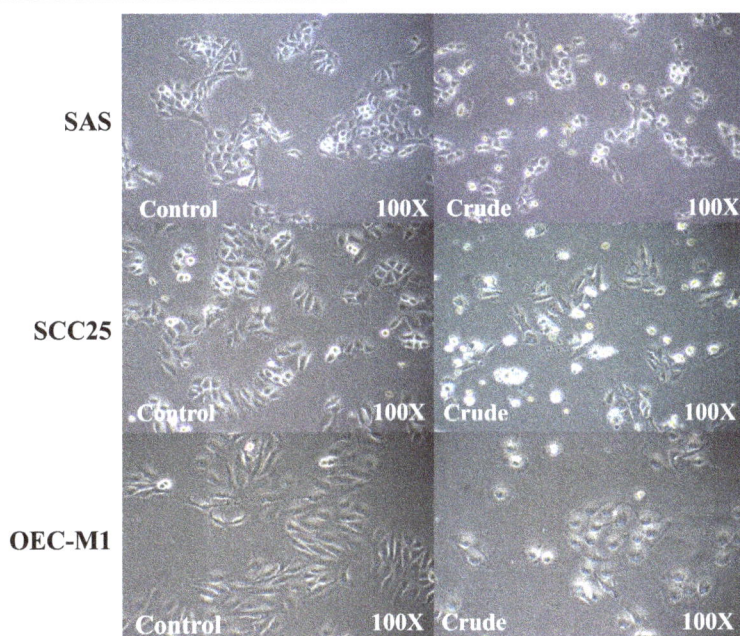

Fig. 1 Danshen crude induced morphological change in oral cancer cells. Effect of the Danshen crude on morphological changes in SAS, SCC25, and OEC-M1 oral cancer cell lines. Original magnification, 100×

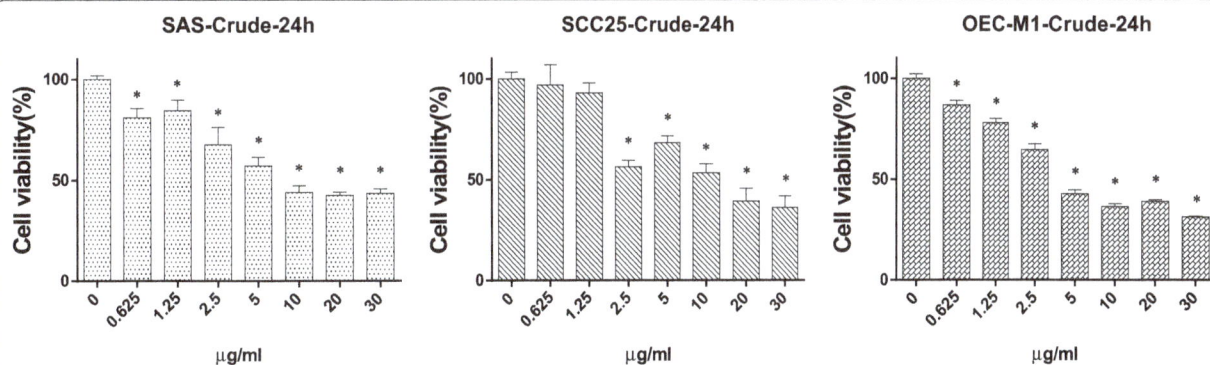

IC50 values of the various oral cancer cells treated with Crude in 24h.

Cell lines	Crude IC$_{50}$ (µg/ml)
SAS	10
SCC25	10
OEC-M1	5

The IC$_{50}$ of Crude on SAS was 10 µg/ml; 10 µg/ml on SCC25 cells; 5 µg/ml on OEC-M1 after a 24 h treatment. These results indicate Extracts of Tanshinone that possesses growth inhibitory effect on these oral cancer cells. (*, $p < 0.05$)

Fig. 2 Inhibition of oral cancer cell (SAS, SCC25, and OEC-M1) growth in vitro via the Danshen crude. The antioral cancer efficacy of the Danshen crude on three oral cancer cell lines (SAS, SCC25, and OEC-M1) treated for 24 h. The extract significantly reduced the cell viability of all three OSCC lines in a dose-dependent manner

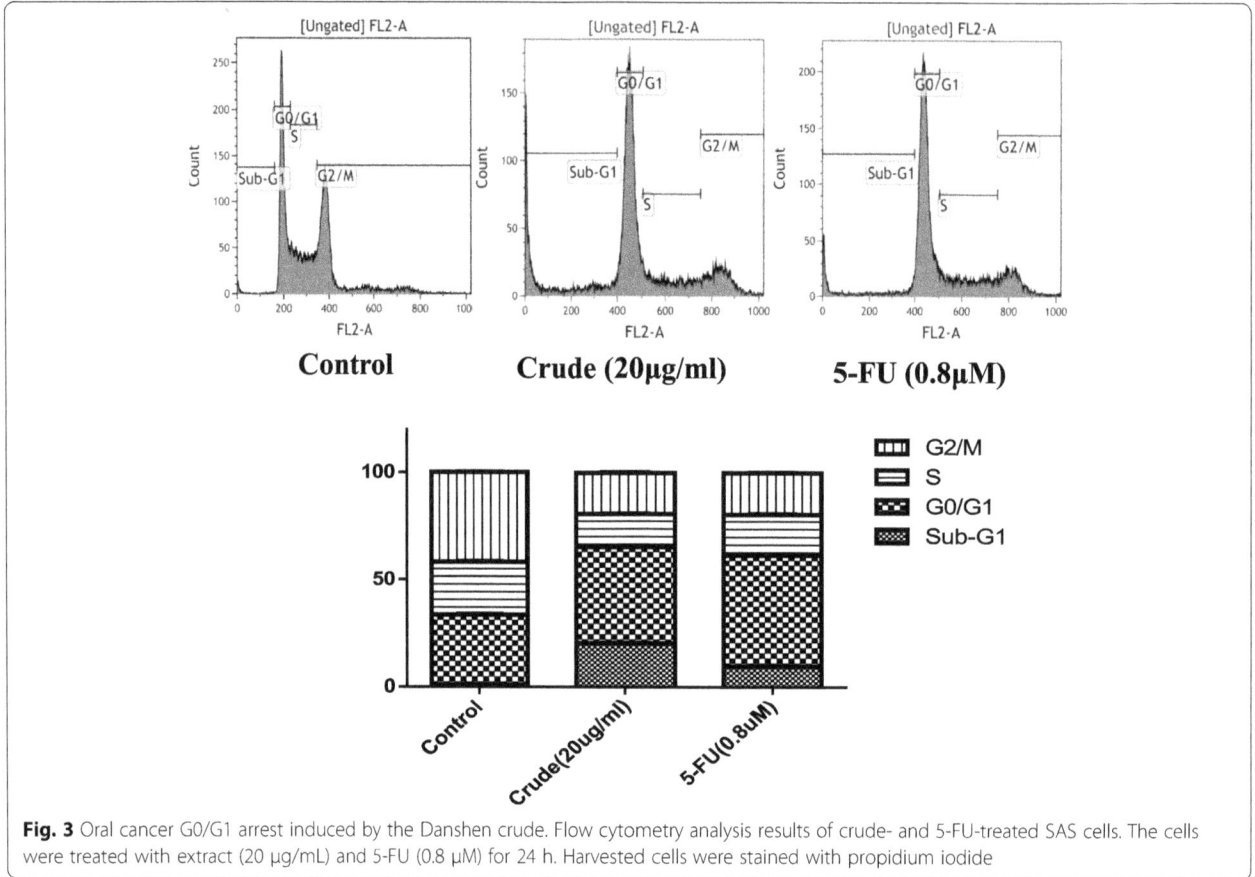

Fig. 3 Oral cancer G0/G1 arrest induced by the Danshen crude. Flow cytometry analysis results of crude- and 5-FU-treated SAS cells. The cells were treated with extract (20 μg/mL) and 5-FU (0.8 μM) for 24 h. Harvested cells were stained with propidium iodide

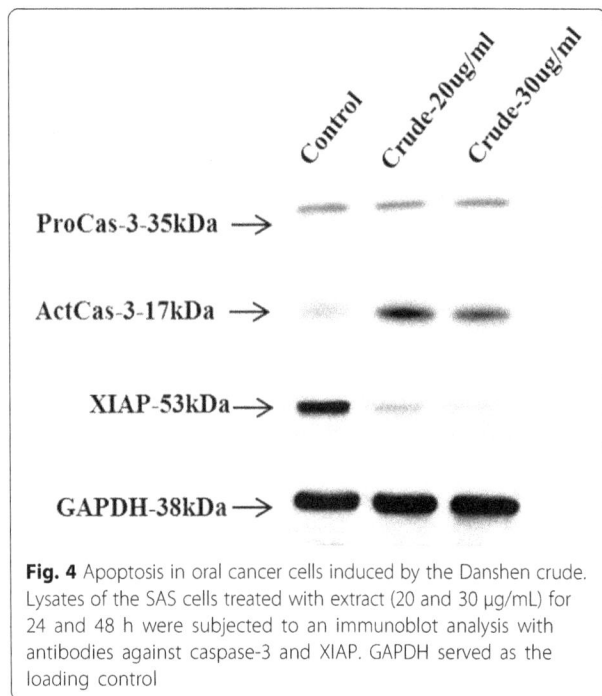

Fig. 4 Apoptosis in oral cancer cells induced by the Danshen crude. Lysates of the SAS cells treated with extract (20 and 30 μg/mL) for 24 and 48 h were subjected to an immunoblot analysis with antibodies against caspase-3 and XIAP. GAPDH served as the loading control

extract-treated group than in the untreated control groups.

The Danshen extract also significantly inhibited the proliferation of KB drug-resistant cells, indicating that the treatment had circumvented drug resistance in these cells (Fig. 7).

Discussion

The prevalence of oral cancer has increased globally in recent years [14], and 5-FU-based chemotherapy has been widely used to reduce the risk of relapse after surgery. The 5-FU plus docetaxel treatment, with the addition of oxaliplatin chemotherapy (which improves survival significantly compared with 5-FU alone [15]), has been widely accepted as the standard adjuvant chemotherapy for OSCC. However, inflammation, neutropenia and lymphopenia, which are common chemotherapy-induced toxicities, may influence the prognosis of adjuvant chemotherapy in cancer treatment [16, 17]. By contrast, Danshen is a natural compound that has anti-inflammation and anticancer effects, which can be effective for the supportive care of cancer patients [18]. Some clinical studies have indicated that bioactive natural compounds play a key role in the treatment of many cancers [6, 19]. In the present study, a

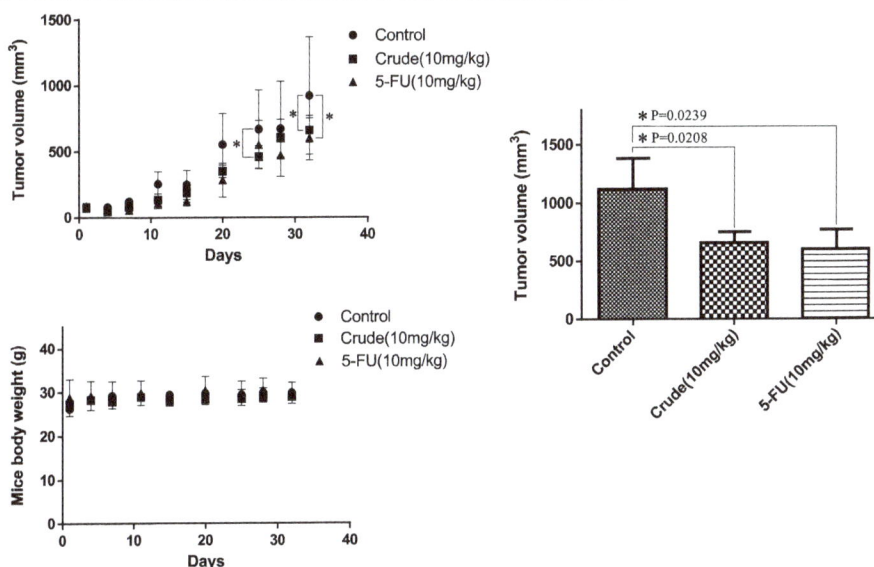

Fig. 5 Repression of tumor cell growth in SAS xenograft mice via the Danshen crude. The Danshen extract inhibited oral cancer cell growth in vivo. The SAS xenograft was exposed to either saline (control) or the Danshen extract (crude, 10 mg/kg), and 5-FU (10 mg/kg) served as the positive control

Danshen extract was observed to inhibit oral cancer cell proliferation (Figs. 1 and 2) through cell cycle G0/G1 arrest (Fig. 3).

Apoptosis is a well-defined self-suicidal process to inhibit tumor growth. Many studies have reported that chemotherapeutic drugs exert antitumor effects by triggering apoptosis through various molecular mechanisms [20]. One previous study revealed that tanshinone IIA induces apoptosis in human oral cancer KB cells through a mitochondria-dependent pathway [8]. Our results demonstrate that the Danshen extract upregulated caspase-3 expression and repressed XIAP expression in SAS cells. In addition, our results confirm the involvement of apoptosis in Danshen-induced in vitro and in vivo growth inhibition in human oral cancer cells (Figs. 4, 5 and 6).

Cell cycle dysregulation results in uncontrolled cell growth, which can lead to cancer development [21]. Therefore, the targeted detection of cell-cycle-related errors in cancer cells is considered a potential strategy for tumor growth control [22]. Research has revealed that the leading bioactive components (salvianolic acid B [23] and tanshinone IIA [8]) of Danshen result in increased G0/G1 and G2/M phases in oral cancer cells, and in head and neck cancer cells, respectively. The present study revealed cell cycle G0/G1 arrest in Danshen-extract-treated SAS

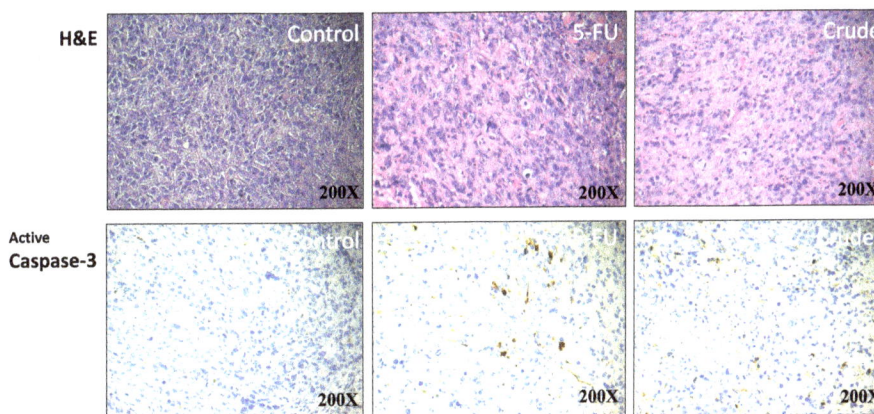

Fig. 6 Active caspase-3 expression induced in oral cancer cells in the SAS xenografts model using the Danshen crude. H&E staining and IHC were performed after administration of the Danshen crude, 5-FU, or PBS (a vehicle control). The SAS xenografts model stained active caspase-3. Immunodetectable proteins are stained brown and the nuclei are counterstained blue. Original magnification, 200×

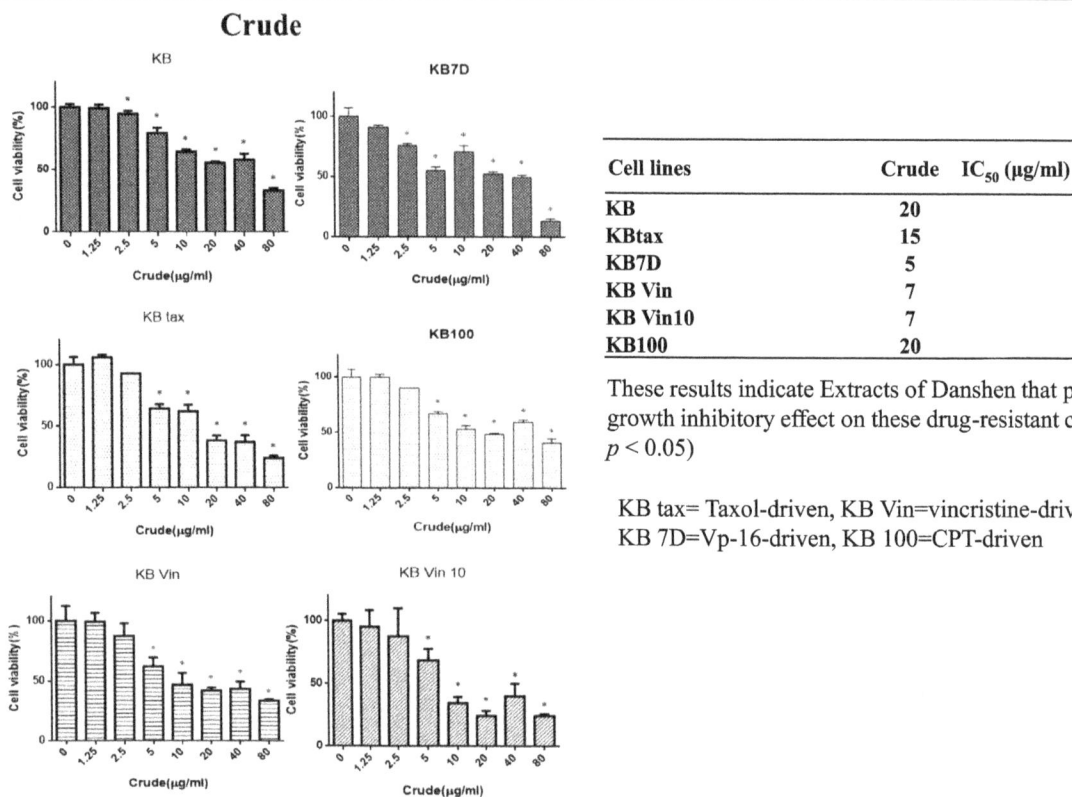

Crude

Cell lines	Crude IC_{50} (µg/ml)
KB	20
KBtax	15
KB7D	5
KB Vin	7
KB Vin10	7
KB100	20

These results indicate Extracts of Danshen that possesses growth inhibitory effect on these drug-resistant cancer cells. (*, $p < 0.05$)

KB tax= Taxol-driven, KB Vin=vincristine-driven, KB 7D=Vp-16-driven, KB 100=CPT-driven

Fig. 7 Inhibition of drug-resistant KB cell growth in vitro via the Danshen crude. An assessment of cell proliferation and viability by using the methylene blue assay in six drug-resistant oral cancer cells treated with varying concentrations of the Danshen crude (0–80 µg/mL) or dimethyl sulfoxide (1 µL/mL) for 24 h

cells and an increased sub-G1 apoptotic dead cell population (Fig. 3). These findings suggest that the Danshen extract induces cell cycle G0/G1 arrest and apoptosis.

Resistance to chemotherapy and molecular-targeted therapies is a major concern in current cancer research. Our results reveal that the Danshen extract suppressed growth in drug-resistant oral cancer cells (including taxol- [24], vincristine- [25], Vp-16- [26], and camptothecin- [27] resistant cells; Fig. 7). These results suggest that the Danshen extract may be a potential novel chemotherapeutic agent in oral cancer treatment.

Conclusions

In conclusion, this in vitro and in vivo study revealed that a Danshen extract exerts antiproliferative effects in human oral cancer cells and KB drug-resistant cells through multiple pathways, such as the induction of apoptosis. Therefore, Danshen treatment should be considered a novel approach for drug-resistant oral cancer prevention and treatment.

Acknowledgements

The authors acknowledge the technical services provided by Instrument Center of National Defense Medical Center and the laboratory animal center of National Defense Medical Center.

Funding

Tri-Service General Hospital, Taiwan, Republic of China (grants No. TSGH-C105-006-008-S05, TSGH-C106-004-006-008-S05, TSGH-C105-190, TSGH-C106-121, Ministry of National Defense, Republic of China (grants No. MAB-106-090) and National Science Council, Taiwan, Republic of China (grants No. MOST 105-2314-B-016-021-MY3) have jointly funded this work.

Authors' contributions

CYY and CCH contributed equally to this work. CYY and CCH performed the biochemical and animal study, analyzed and interpreted the data, designed the study, and drafted the manuscript. CKL and CSL analyzed the IHC data. BP assisted with the animal study. GJL and HKST designed the study and interpreted the data. WLC provided the Danshen extract and reagents. YWC designed the study, interpreted the data, and critically revised the manuscript. All authors read and approved the final manuscript.

Competing interests

The authors declare that they have no competing interests.

Author details

[1]School of Dentistry, National Defense Medical Center, Taipei, Taiwan, Republic of China. [2]Department of Pharmacy Practice, Tri-Service General Hospital, Taipei, Taiwan, Republic of China. [3]Division of Anatomic Pathology, Taipei Tzu Chi Hospital, Taipei, Taiwan, Republic of China. [4]Department of Radiation Oncology, Tri-Service General Hospital, National Defense Medical Centre, Taipei, Taiwan, Republic of China. [5]Graduate Institute of Clinical Medicine, College of Medicine, Taipei Medical University, Taipei, Taiwan, Republic of China. [6]Department of Biology and Anatomy, National Defense Medical Center, Taipei, Taiwan, Republic of China. [7]Graduate Institute of Microbiology and Immunology, National Defense Medical Center, Taipei, Taiwan, Republic of China. [8]School of Pharmacy, National Defense Medical

Center, Taipei, Taiwan, Republic of China. [9]Department of Oral and Maxillofacial Surgery, Tri-Service General Hospital, No. 161, Section 6, Min-Chuan East Road, Neihu 114, Taipei 114, Taiwan, Republic of China.

References

1. Ferlay J, Soerjomataram I, Dikshit R, Eser S, Mathers C, Rebelo M, Parkin DM, Forman D, Bray F. Cancer incidence and mortality worldwide: sources, methods and major patterns in GLOBOCAN 2012. Int J Cancer. 2015;136(5):E359–86.
2. Sankaranarayanan R, Ramadas K, Amarasinghe H, Subramanian S, Johnson N. Oral cancer: prevention, early detection, and treatment. In: Gelband H, Jha P, Sankaranarayanan R, Horton S, editors. Cancer: disease control priorities, third edition (Volume 3). Washington (DC): The International Bank for Reconstruction and Development / The World Bank; 2015 Nov. Chapter 5.
3. Cooley ME, Davis L, Abrahm J. Cisplatin: a clinical review. Part II–nursing assessment and management of side effects of cisplatin. Cancer Nurs. 1994; 17(4):283–93.
4. Xu R, Wang Q. Large-scale automatic extraction of side effects associated with targeted anticancer drugs from full-text oncological articles. J Biomed Inform. 2015;55:64–72.
5. Moschovi M, Critselis E, Cen O, Adamaki M, Lambrou GI, Chrousos GP, Vlahopoulos S. Drugs acting on homeostasis: challenging cancer cell adaptation. Expert Rev Anticancer Ther. 2015;15(12):1405–17.
6. Chen X, Guo J, Bao J, Lu J, Wang Y. The anticancer properties of salvia miltiorrhiza Bunge (Danshen): a systematic review. Med Res Rev. 2014; 34(4):768–94.
7. Yang Y, Ge PJ, Jiang L, Li FL, Zhu QY. Modulation of growth and angiogenic potential of oral squamous carcinoma cells in vitro using salvianolic acid B. BMC Complement Altern Med. 2011;11:54.
8. Tseng PY, Lu WC, Hsieh MJ, Chien SY, Chen MK. Tanshinone IIA induces apoptosis in human oral cancer KB cells through a mitochondria-dependent pathway. Biomed Res Int. 2014;2014:540516.
9. Zhao Y, Guo Y, Gu X. Salvianolic acid B, a potential chemopreventive agent, for head and neck squamous cell cancer. J Oncol. 2011;2011:534548.
10. Wu WL, Chang WL, Chen CF. Cytotoxic activities of tanshinones against human carcinoma cell lines. Am J Chin Med. 1991;19(3–4):207–16.
11. Tsai H-T, Chang W-L, Tu H-P, Fu E, Hsieh Y-D, Chiang C-Y. Effects of salvia miltiorrhiza ethanolic extract on lipopolysaccharide-induced dental alveolar bone resorption in rats. J Dent Sci. 2016;11(1):35–40.
12. Yang CY, Meng CL. Regulation of PG synthase by EGF and PDGF in human oral, breast, stomach, and fibrosarcoma cancer cell lines. J Dent Res. 1994; 73(8):1407–15.
13. Kuo CC, Hsieh HP, Pan WY, Chen CP, Liou JP, Lee SJ, Chang YL, Chen LT, Chen CT, Chang JY. BPR0L075, a novel synthetic indole compound with antimitotic activity in human cancer cells, exerts effective antitumoral activity in vivo. Cancer Res. 2004;64(13):4621–8.
14. Siegel RL, Miller KD, Jemal A. Cancer statistics, 2016. CA Cancer J Clin. 2016; 66(1):7–30.
15. Tamatani T, Ferdous T, Takamaru N, Hara K, Kinouchi M, Kuribayashi N, Ohe G, Uchida D, Nagai H, Fujisawa K, et al. Antitumor efficacy of sequential treatment with docetaxel and 5-fluorouracil against human oral cancer cells. Int J Oncol. 2012;41(3):1148–56.
16. El-Sayyad HI, Ismail MF, Shalaby FM, Abou-El-Magd RF, Gaur RL, Fernando A, Raj MH, Ouhtit A. Histopathological effects of cisplatin, doxorubicin and 5-flurouracil (5-FU) on the liver of male albino rats. Int J Biol Sci. 2009;5(5):466–73.
17. Yamano T, Takayasu Y, Nakao N, Kubota A. Evaluation of hepatic toxicity following high-dose 5-FU arterial infusion chemotherapy: analysis of 42 cases of colorectal liver metastases. Nihon Igaku Hoshasen Gakkai Zasshi. 2000;60(3):94–102.
18. Stumpf C, Fan Q, Hintermann C, Raaz D, Kurfurst I, Losert S, Pflederer W, Achenbach S, Daniel WG, Garlichs CD. Anti-inflammatory effects of danshen on human vascular endothelial cells in culture. Am J Chin Med. 2013;41(5):1065–77.
19. Choi JG, Eom SM, Kim J, Kim SH, Huh E, Kim H, Lee Y, Lee H, Oh MS. A comprehensive review of recent studies on herb-drug interaction: a focus on Pharmacodynamic interaction. J Altern Complement Med. 2016;22(4):262–79.
20. Hu W, Kavanagh JJ. Anticancer therapy targeting the apoptotic pathway. Lancet Oncol. 2003;4(12):721–9.
21. Hanahan D, Weinberg RA. Hallmarks of cancer: the next generation. Cell. 2011;144(5):646–74.
22. Visconti R, Della Monica R, Grieco D. Cell cycle checkpoint in cancer: a therapeutically targetable double-edged sword. J Exp Clin Cancer Res. 2016;35(1):153.
23. Hao Y, Xie T, Korotcov A, Zhou Y, Pang X, Shan L, Ji H, Sridhar R, Wang P, Califano J, et al. Salvianolic acid B inhibits growth of head and neck squamous cell carcinoma in vitro and in vivo via cyclooxygenase-2 and apoptotic pathways. Int J Cancer. 2009;124(9):2200–9.
24. Orr GA, Verdier-Pinard P, McDaid H, Horwitz SB. Mechanisms of Taxol resistance related to microtubules. Oncogene. 2003;22(47):7280–95.
25. Kohno K, Kikuchi J, Sato S, Takano H, Saburi Y, Asoh K, Kuwano M. Vincristine-resistant human cancer KB cell line and increased expression of multidrug-resistance gene. Jpn J Cancer Res. 1988;79(11):1238–46.
26. Long BH, Wang L, Lorico A, Wang RC, Brattain MG, Casazza AM. Mechanisms of resistance to etoposide and teniposide in acquired resistant human colon and lung carcinoma cell lines. Cancer Res. 1991; 51(19):5275–83.
27. Beretta GL, Gatti L, Perego P, Zaffaroni N. Camptothecin resistance in cancer: insights into the molecular mechanisms of a DNA-damaging drug. Curr Med Chem. 2013;20(12):1541–65.

17

Astragalus membranaceus (Fisch.) Bunge repairs intestinal mucosal injury induced by LPS in mice

Yizhe Cui[†] ⓘ, Qiuju Wang[†], Rui Sun, Li Guo, Mengzhu Wang, Junfeng Jia, Chuang Xu[*] and Rui Wu[*]

Abstract

Background: *Astragalus membranaceus (Fisch.) Bunge* is one of the most widely used traditional Chinese herbal medicines. It is used as immune stimulant, tonic, antioxidant, hepatoprotectant, diuretic, antidiabetic, anticancer, and expectorant. The purpose of the study was to investigate the curative effects of the decoction obtained from *Astragalus membranaceus* root in intestinal mucosal injury induced by LPS in mice. An LPS-induced intestinal mucosal injury mice model was applied in the study.

Methods: The mice were post-treated with *Astragalus membranaceus* decoction (AMD) for 4 days after 3 days LPS induction. ELISA kit was used to detect the content of tumor necrosis factor (TNF)-α, interleukin (IL)-1β, IL-4,IL-6 and IL-8 in the serum of each group mice. The morphological changes in intestinal mucosa at the end of the experiments were observed. Both VH (villus height) and CD (crypt depth) were measured using H&E-stained sections.

Results: There were significant differences in IL-1β, IL-4,IL-6, IL-8 and TNF-α levels in AMD-treated group on the 7th day compared to the controls group. The VH was lower in duodenum, jejunum and the ileum in LPS-treated mice compared to the control animals. Similarly, there was also decrease in V/C. Compared to the control mice, for AMD-treated mice, VH and CD had no significantly differences.

Conclusions: *Astragalus membranaceus* reduced intestinal mucosal damage and promoted tissue repair by inhibiting the expression of inflammatory cytokine.

Keywords: *Astragalus membranaceus* (Fisch.) Bunge, Decoction, Mice, Lipopolysaccharide

Background

Intestinal mucosa is a natural barrier against bacteria. It prevents viruses and other harmful bacteria from entering the blood [1]. Endotoxin is the lipopolysaccharide (LPS) in the cell wall of Gram-negative bacteria, which has a variety of biological activity and is decomposed and released in the process of bacterial metabolism or after death. LPS can stimulate the release of inflammatory mediators from macrophages and neutrophils and eventually lead to the imbalance of inflammatory and anti-inflammatory reactions and the occurrence of excessive systemic inflammation [2].

Astragalus membranaceus (Fisch.) Bunge (syn. *Astragalus propinquus* Schischkin) (AM), also known as Huangqi or milk vetch root in China, is an important medicine in traditional Chinese medicine. [3]. This herb possesses many common pharmacological activities, such as multiple organ protection [4, 5], antioxidant [6], hypoglycemic [7], antiviral [8] and so on, and has their own pharmacological properties and mechanisms. Studies have shown that *A. membranaceus* can enhance the contraction of the right ventricular myocardium in rats in a dose-dependent manner [9] and has recently been reported to be a potential promote tissue wound repair. The water extract of *A. membranaceus* is one of the main active preparations obtained from the root of this specie. However, there are not so many reports studies focusing on the decoction of AM. Some studies showed that gastric mucosa and atrophic pathological damage

* Correspondence: xuchuang7175@163.com; fuhewu@126.com
†Yizhe Cui and Qiuju Wang contributed equally to this work.
College of Animal Science and Veterinary Medicine, Heilongjiang Bayi Agricultural University, 2# Xinyang Road, New Development District, Daqing 163319, Heilongjiang, China

significantly reduced in rats after Huangqi intervention [10]. However, it is still not elucidated whether oral administration of *Astragalus membranaceus* decoction (AMD) could provide a repair effect during intestinal mucosal injury and what is the underlying mechanism. In this study, we explored the repair effect of AMD in LPS induced experimental intestinal mucosal injury in mice.

Methods

Drugs and reagents
LPS (*Escherichia coli* O55:B5) and all other chemicals were obtained from Sigma-Aldrich (St. Louis, MO, USA). Distilled water was filtered through a Milli-Q system from EMD Millipore Corporation (Billerica, MA, USA). LPS was suspended in physiological saline and stored as a 20 mg/ml stock. Dilutions prior to injection were into physiological saline. Animals were weighed prior to injection of LPS and stock LPS was diluted to the appropriate dose for each animal.

Plant material
Astragalus membranaceus was purchased from Fu Rui Bang Chinese Medicine Co., Ltd. (Daqing, China), then it was authenticated by Dr. Pengyu Jia and also deposited in Veterinary drug research and Development Center, Heilongjiang Bayi Agricultural University, Heilongjiang, China) according to Chinese Pharmacopoeia (The Pharmacopoeia Commission of PRC, 2010).

Animals
Male ICR mice weighing 22–25 g were purchased from the Animal Experiment Center of HARBIN MEDICAL UNIVERSITY (DAQING) [Certification no. SYXK (HEI) 2,014,005]. Mice were maintained on a standard light/dark cycle under controlled temperature (22 ± 2 °C) and humidity (50 ± 10%) with certified standard diet and water adlibitum. Mice were habituated to animal facilities for 1 week before the experiment. All the experimental procedures were approved by, and conducted in accordance with Principles of Laboratory Animal Care and according to the rules and ethics set forth by the Ethical Committee of Heilongjiang Bayi Agricultural University.

Extraction procedure
The general preparation procedure of *Astragalus membranaceus* decoction (AMD) is as follows [11]. Briefly, 100 g the root of *Astragalus membranaceus* was extracted by refluxing with water (1:8, *w/v*) for 1.5 h following sonicating for 30 min, then the extraction solutions were combined to be filtered and concentrated to 100 mL under reduced pressure. The concentrations of the residues were 1 g/mL for *Astragalus membranaceus*. Finally, the concentration be adjusted to the required with distilled water for intragastrical administration. After being autoclaved at 100 °C for 20 min, the stock solution was stored at 4 °C.

Grouping and treatment
In experiments, animals were randomized into three groups of ten individuals (Fig. 1). The control group, LPS-treated group and AMD-treated group. Mice in the LPS groups and the AMD group, were intraperitoneally injected with LPS (*Escherichia coli* 055:B5, 5 mg/kg; Sigma) for 3 days. The chosen dose of LPS was based on Die Dai's study and preliminary experiments [12]. AMD-treated groups were given *Astragalus membranaceus* decoction by intragastric administration once daily and treatments lasted for 4 days after 3 days LPS induction. Briefly, 1 ml syringe with No. 12 gavage needle was used in intragastric administration. The volume of gavage was usually 0.1 ml/10 g body weight. Mice in control group were received physiological saline for 7 days. After euthanizing the mice by carbon dioxide, blood was obtained by cardiac puncture on the 7th day. On collection, blood samples were centrifuged at 5000 rpm for 10 min, and were subsequently stored at − 80 °C before metabolomics analysis. Survivals were recorded for 72 h.

Determination of inflammatory cytokine levels
Cytokine levels in serum were determined by ELISA by using commercially available kits (Endogen, Cambridge,MA). For each assay, serum was serially diluted to ensure that values obtained were within the linear range of the standards provided with each kit. Each sample was done in duplicate, and data from individual mice were averaged.

Histopathology
Specimens of the intestinal wall of the duodenum, jejunum and ileum were prepared for histological examination by fixing in 4% formaldehyde-buffered solution, embedding in paraffin, and sectioning. Paraffin sections were cut into slices of 4 μm and stained with H&E staining solution. Finally, the stained sections were observed and photographed under a light microscope (with 100× magnification). Villous height and the associated crypt depth were evaluated using the Image Pro plus 4 analysis software (Media Cybernetics, Baltimore, MD, USA) processing and analysis system. For each intestinal sample, at least 10 well-oriented were measured and the mean value was calculated. The method was the same as described by Nabuurs et al. [13].

Data analysis
Data were presented as mean and standard deviation (SD). One-way ANOVA showed significant differences among groups. A level of $P < 0.05$ was considered statistically significant. Analysis was performed with the software SPSS version 16.0 (SPSS Inc., USA).

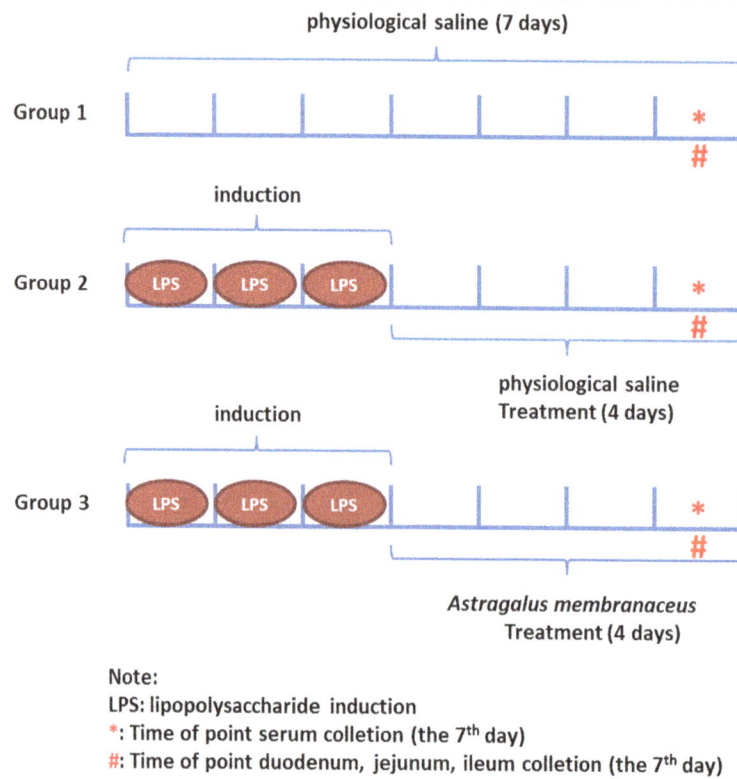

Note:
LPS: lipopolysaccharide induction
*: Time of point serum colletion (the 7th day)
#: Time of point duodenum, jejunum, ileum colletion (the 7th day)

Fig. 1 Experimental design and sampling schedule

Results

Serum concentrations of cytokine

The serum levels of IL-1β, IL-4,IL-6, IL-8 and TNF-α are important biochemical markers for evaluating intestinal mucosal structure and function [14]. In this experiment, the induction of LSP caused significantly higher levels ($P < 0.05$) of IL-1β, IL-4,IL-6, IL-8 and TNF-α in model group on the 7th day compared to the control group (Table 1). Compared with LPS group, the level of inflammatory cytokines decreased significantly ($P < 0.05$) in AMD group. Meanwhile, there were no significant differences of IL-1β, IL-4,IL-6, IL-8 and TNF-α levels in AMD-treated group on the 7th day compared to control group, though the level of IL-4 and IL-1β was higher in AMD group than that in control group, there was no

significant differences. The results suggested that AMD had no effect on the immunity of the body, moreover curative treated AMD was effective in ameliorating LPS-induced intestinal mucosal damage.

Histopathological changes in intestinal tissue

Pathological examinations of the intestinal mucosal injury were carried out and the LPS-treatment and AMD-treatment are shown in Fig. 2. Compared with the control animals, the pathological changes were obvious, LPS-treated groups caused significant mucosal damage, that is, epithelial shedding, villi fracturing, mucosal atrophy, edema and the villus had shortened on the 7th day after LPS injection (Fig. 2). However, as time goes on, the intestinal mucosa damage begins to recover slowly in the AMD-treated groups on the 7th day. These observations showed that AMD has obvious beneficial effects against intestinal mucosal damage.

Histomorphological analyses

The VH and CD, which indicated intestinal villus's absorptive functions, were measured. The experiments showed that the VH was lower in duodenum, jejunum and the ileum in LPS-treated mice compared to the control animals. Similarly, there was decrease in V/C. Compared to the control mice, for AMD-treated mice, VH and CD had no significantly differences (Fig. 3).

Table 1 Serum levels of cytokines in LPS- and AMD-treated mice

Parameters	Controls	LPS	AMD
TNF-α (pg/mL)	15.64 ± 1.04	50.30 ± 8.26*	7.29 ± 1.12
IL-1β (pg/mL)	6.21 ± 0.45	9.36 ± 0.71*	7.26 ± 0.45
IL-4 (pg/mL)	3.47 ± 0.33	11.81 ± 0.39*	3.65 ± 0.43
IL-6 (pg/mL)	11.34 ± 0.21	14.25 ± 0.36*	8.96 ± 0.63
IL-8 (pg/mL)	9.51 ± 1.07	11.86 ± 0.66*	7.93 ± 1.13

The data are expressed as the mean ± SD ($n = 10$ per treatment group).
*Statistically different from the control group; *$P < 0.05$. Tumor necrosis factor (TNF)-α, interleukin (IL) IL-1β, IL-4,IL-6 and IL-8

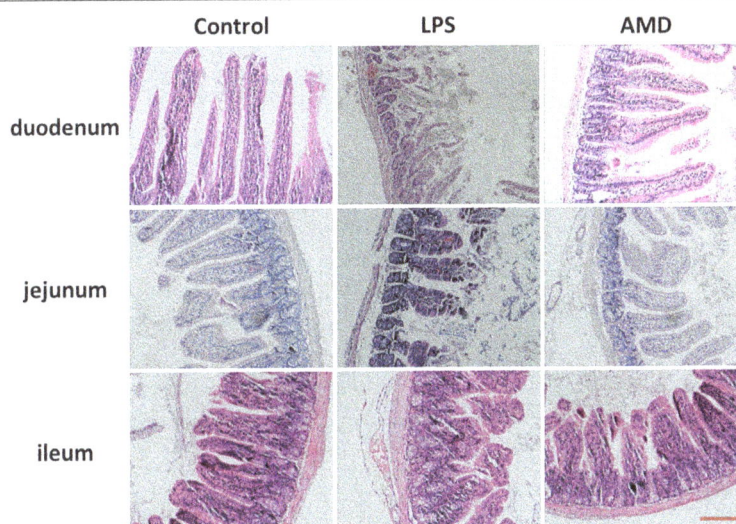

Fig. 2 Histomorphometric analyses of intestinal mucosa time changes. Histological appearance of mice intestinal mucosa after haematoxylin and eosin (H&E) stain (original magnification 100×). Scale bars: 50 μm

Discussion

Intestinal mucosal injury is associated with intestinal inflammation [15]. We investigated whether AMD could ameliorate the inflammatory response in mice induced by LPS. A large number of studies suggest that the intestinal ischemia/reperfusion injury, LPS challenge, and intestinal inflammatory diseases can induce the expression of inflammatory cytokines in humans and animals [16]. Both in vitro and in vivo studies show that over-secretory of inflammatory cytokines can have a negative effects on intestinal mucosal integrity, permeability and epithelial function of the intestinal mucosa [17]. The imbalance of cytokine and chemokine secretion plays an important role in mucosal defense. IL-8 is produced by macrophages and epithelial cells. It can chemotaxis and activate neutrophils, which leads to mucous edema, leukocyte infiltration, increased vascular damage and permeability, resulting in immune inflammatory lesions [18]. IL-4 can play a role in pro-inflammatory factors alone in the gut of mice, which can trigger inflammation [19]. The study showed that LPS was identified by Toll like receptor 4 (TLR4) to release TNF-α, IL-1 beta and IL-6 and other cytokines, which mediate and promote the occurrence of inflammatory bowel disease (IBD) [20]. Intraperitoneal injection of LPS can cause intestinal mucosal inflammation, which is characterized by increased inflammatory and anti-inflammatory cytokines. TNF-α plays a major role in causing intestinal inflammation, and its role is to accumulate inflammatory cells to the local tissues of the inflammation, cause edema, activate coagulation cascade, and form granuloma [21]. The common way to treat IBD in clinic is to inhibit TNF-α by using TNF-α antagonist to improve and alleviate IBD symptoms. In this experiment, the mice were intraperitoneally injected with LPS to establish a model of intestinal injury in mice. LPS challenge increased the level of TNF-α, IL-1β, IL-4, IL-6 and IL-8 in the serum (Table 1). Importantly, AMD reduced the concentrations of TNF-α, IL-1β, IL-4, IL-6 and IL-8 in the serum, compared to LPS-challenged mice. These findings indicate that the AMD has beneficial effects in reducing intestinal mucosal inflammation. AMD may inhibit intestinal immune damage, reduce intestinal mucosal edema and promote intestinal mucosal repair by downregulating the expression of cytokine.

The structural characteristics of the small intestinal mucosa are circular folds, intestinal villi and microvilli. These characteristics greatly expand the surface area of the small intestine and make the nutrients fully digested and absorbed in the small intestine. The complete structure of the small intestine is the physiological basis of its digestion and absorption function, and its morphological and structural changes directly affect the surface area of villi, thereby affecting the body's ability to absorb nutrients [22]. The integrity and height of the intestinal villi determine the absorption area of the small intestine, the absorption of nutrients and the growth of the animals [23]. Therefore, the increase of the villi height, the ratio of the villi/crypt or the decrease of the depth of the recess is related to the improvement of the digestion and absorption of nutrients [24]. Compared with the LPS group, AMD increased the villus height and villus/crypt ratio of the duodenum, as well as the villus height and chorionic ratio of the jejunum and ileum. Crypt depth was significantly reduced in the duodenum and the jejunum, compared with the LPS group. The expression of inflammatory cytokines was consistent with the

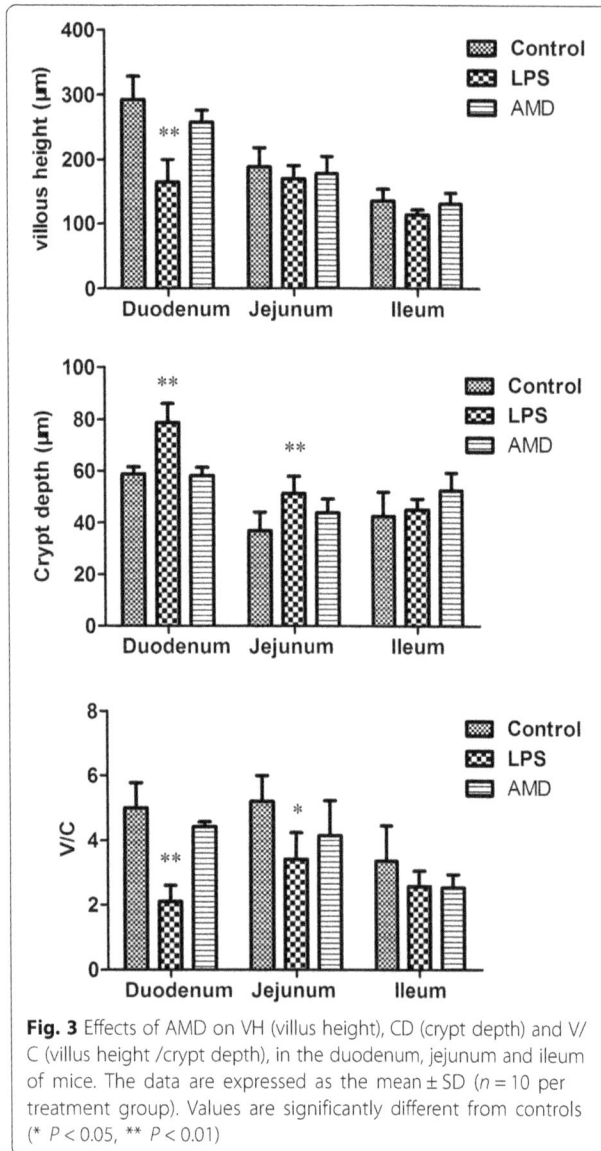

Fig. 3 Effects of AMD on VH (villus height), CD (crypt depth) and V/C (villus height /crypt depth), in the duodenum, jejunum and ileum of mice. The data are expressed as the mean ± SD ($n = 10$ per treatment group). Values are significantly different from controls (* $P < 0.05$, ** $P < 0.01$)

colon weight index, and reducing macroscopically and histological scores [32], which is similar to the results of this experiment.

Conclusions

Astragalus membranaceus treatment can protect small intestinal mucosa against LPS injury. Also, *A. membranaceus* promotes tissue repair by inhibiting the expression of inflammatory cytokine. These findings indicate that *A. membranaceus* can partly reduce small intestinal mucosa injury induced by LPS. Further studies of *A. membranaceus* are necessary to develop a new effective plant-derived therapeutic modality for intestinal mucosal injury.

Funding
This work was supported by Natural Science Foundation of Heilongjiang Province (C201444), China Scholarship council (201508230118), Postdoctoral Program Foundation of Heilongjiang Bayi Agricultural University of China (601038), Doctoral Program Foundation of Heilongjiang Bayi Agricultural University of China (XDB-2016-10) and China Postdoctoral Science Foundation (2017 M620124; 2018 T110320).

Authors' contributions
YC and QW contributed equally to this work. YC, QW, CX and RW designed the research; YC, RS, LG, YC performed the research; MW, JJ analyzed the data; and YC and QW wrote the paper. All authors read and approved the final manuscript.

Competing interests
The authors declare that they have no competing interests.

References
1. Vancamelbeke M, Vermeire S. The intestinal barrier: a fundamental role in health and disease. Expert Rev Gastroenterol Hepatol. 2017;11(9):821–34.
2. Waseem T, Duxbury M, Ito H, Ashley SW, Robinson MK. Exogenous ghrelin modulates release of pro-inflammatory and anti-inflammatory cytokines in LPS-stimulated macrophages through distinct signaling pathways. Surgery. 2008;143(3):334–42.
3. Guo K, He X, Lu D, Zhang Y, Li X, Yan Z, Qin B. Cycloartane-type triterpenoids from Astragalus hoantchy French. Nat Prod Res. 2017;31(3):314–9.
4. Wang XQ, Wang L, Tu YC, Zhang YC. Traditional Chinese medicine for refractory nephrotic syndrome: strategies and promising treatments. Evid Based Complement Alternat Med. 2018;2018:8746349.
5. Kim GD, Oh J, Park HJ, Bae K, Lee SK. Magnolol inhibits angiogenesis by regulating ROS-mediated apoptosis and the PI3K/AKT/mTOR signaling pathway in mES/EB-derived endothelial-like cells. Int J Oncol. 2013;43(2): 600–10.
6. Li H, Wang P, Huang F, Jin J, Wu H, Zhang B, Wang Z, Shi H, Wu X. Astragaloside IV protects blood-brain barrier integrity from LPS-induced disruption via activating Nrf2 antioxidant signaling pathway in mice. Toxicol Appl Pharmacol. 2018;340:58–66.
7. Cui K, Zhang S, Jiang X, Xie W. Novel synergic antidiabetic effects of Astragalus polysaccharides combined with Crataegus flavonoids via improvement of islet function and liver metabolism. Mol Med Rep. 2016; 13(6):4737–44.
8. Wang Y, Chen Y, Du H, Yang J, Ming K, Song M, Liu J. Comparison of the anti-duck hepatitis a virus activities of phosphorylated and sulfated Astragalus polysaccharides. Exp Biol Med. 2017;242(3):344–53.

alteration in the structure of intestinal villi (Table 1). Based on these results, we concluded that AMD protected the intestinal mucosa from the LPS-induced injury.

AM is a well-known medicinal herb for reinforcing Qi (the vital energy) in traditional Chinese medicine [25]. *Astragalus* polysaccharides has the characteristics of antioxidation [26], immunomodulation [27], antiviral, antitumor activities [28] and cardiovascular protection [29]. AM and its active components have been proved to be effective in the treatment of a variety of diseases, such as diabetes mellitus [30] and cardiovascular disorders [31]. In recent years, astragal's polysaccharides effectively reduced the mucosal damage of experimental colitis in mice by shortening colonic length, reducing

9. Cao Y, Shen T, Huang X, Lin Y, Chen B, Pang J, Li G, Wang Q, Zohrabian S, Duan C, et al. Astragalus polysaccharide restores autophagic flux and improves cardiomyocyte function in doxorubicin-induced cardiotoxicity. Oncotarget. 2017;8(3):4837–48.

10. Zhu X, Liu S, Zhou J, Wang H, Fu R, Wu X, Wang J, Lu F. Effect of Astragalus polysaccharides on chronic atrophic gastritis induced by N-methyl-N'-nitro-N-nitrosoguanidine in rats. Drug Res. 2013;63(11):597–602.

11. Cho CH, Mei QB, Shang P, Lee SS, So HL, Guo X, Li Y. Study of the gastrointestinal protective effects of polysaccharides from Angelica sinensis in rats. Planta Med. 2000;66(4):348–51.

12. Dai D, Gao Y, Chen J, Huang Y, Zhang Z, Xu F. Time-resolved metabolomics analysis of individual differences during the early stage of lipopolysaccharide-treated rats. Sci Rep. 2016;6:34136.

13. Nabuurs MJ, Hoogendoorn A, van der Molen EJ, van Osta AL. Villus height and crypt depth in weaned and unweaned pigs, reared under various circumstances in the Netherlands. Res Vet Sci. 1993;55(1):78–84.

14. Xiao K, Cao ST, le F J, Lin FH, Wang L, Hu CH. Anemonin improves intestinal barrier restoration and influences TGF-beta1 and EGFR signaling pathways in LPS-challenged piglets. Innate Immun. 2016;22(5):344–52.

15. Blikslager AT, Moeser AJ, Gookin JL, Jones SL, Odle J. Restoration of barrier function in injured intestinal mucosa. Physiol Rev. 2007;87(2):545–64.

16. Liu Y, Huang J, Hou Y, Zhu H, Zhao S, Ding B, Yin Y, Yi G, Shi J, Fan W. Dietary arginine supplementation alleviates intestinal mucosal disruption induced by Escherichia coli lipopolysaccharide in weaned pigs. Br J Nutr. 2008;100(3):552–60.

17. Oswald IP, Dozois CM, Barlagne R, Fournout S, Johansen MV, Bogh HO. Cytokine mRNA expression in pigs infected with Schistosoma japonicum. Parasitology. 2001;122(Pt 3):299–307.

18. Reddy KP, Markowitz JE, Ruchelli ED, Baldassano RN, Brown KA. Lamina propria and circulating interleukin-8 in newly and previously diagnosed pediatric inflammatory bowel disease patients. Dig Dis Sci. 2007;52(2):365–72.

19. Chen J, Gong C, Mao H, Li Z, Fang Z, Chen Q, Lin M, Jiang X, Hu Y, Wang W et al: E2F1/SP3/STAT6 axis is required for IL-4-induced epithelial-mesenchymal transition of colorectal cancer cells. Int J Oncol 2018;53(2): 567–78.

20. Liu HM, Liao JF, Lee TY. Farnesoid X receptor agonist GW4064 ameliorates lipopolysaccharide-induced ileocolitis through TLR4/MyD88 pathway related mitochondrial dysfunction in mice. Biochem Biophys Res Commun. 2017; 490(3):841–8.

21. Allocca M, Bonifacio C, Fiorino G, Spinelli A, Furfaro F, Balzarini L, Bonovas S, Danese S. Efficacy of tumour necrosis factor antagonists in stricturing Crohn's disease: a tertiary center real-life experience. Dig Liver Dis. 2017; 49(8):872–7.

22. Collins JT, Bhimji SS: Anatomy, Abdomen, Small Intestine. In: StatPearls. edn. Treasure Island (FL); 2017.

23. Greig CJ, Cowles RA. Muscarinic acetylcholine receptors participate in small intestinal mucosal homeostasis. J Pediatr Surg. 2017;52(6):1031–4.

24. Hou Y, Wang L, Yi D, Ding B, Yang Z, Li J, Chen X, Qiu Y, Wu G. N-acetylcysteine reduces inflammation in the small intestine by regulating redox, EGF and TLR4 signaling. Amino Acids. 2013;45(3):513–22.

25. Lin HQ, Gong AG, Wang HY, Duan R, Dong TT, Zhao KJ, Tsim KW. Danggui Buxue tang (Astragali Radix and Angelicae Sinensis Radix) for menopausal symptoms: a review. J Ethnopharmacol. 2017;199:205–10.

26. Huang WM, Liang YQ, Tang LJ, Ding Y, Wang XH. Antioxidant and anti-inflammatory effects of Astragalus polysaccharide on EA.hy926 cells. Exp Ther Med. 2013;6(1):199–203.

27. Du X, Zhao B, Li J, Cao X, Diao M, Feng H, Chen X, Chen Z, Zeng X. Astragalus polysaccharides enhance immune responses of HBV DNA vaccination via promoting the dendritic cell maturation and suppressing Treg frequency in mice. Int Immunopharmacol. 2012;14(4):463–70.

28. Dang SS, Jia XL, Song P, Cheng YA, Zhang X, Sun MZ, Liu EQ. Inhibitory effect of emodin and Astragalus polysaccharide on the replication of HBV. World J Gastroenterol. 2009;15(45):5669–73.

29. Yang M, Lin HB, Gong S, Chen PY, Geng LL, Zeng YM, Li DY. Effect of Astragalus polysaccharides on expression of TNF-alpha, IL-1beta and NFATc4 in a rat model of experimental colitis. Cytokine. 2014;70(2):81–6.

30. Zhang K, Pugliese M, Pugliese A, Passantino A. Biological active ingredients of traditional Chinese herb Astragalus membranaceus on treatment of diabetes: a systematic review. Mini Rev Med Chem. 2015;15(4):315–29.

31. Sun S, Yang S, Dai M, Jia X, Wang Q, Zhang Z, Mao Y. The effect of Astragalus polysaccharides on attenuation of diabetic cardiomyopathy through inhibiting the extrinsic and intrinsic apoptotic pathways in high glucose -stimulated H9C2 cells. BMC Complement Altern Med. 2017;17(1):310.

32. Zhao HM, Wang Y, Huang XY, Huang MF, Xu R, Yue HY, Zhou BG, Huang HY, Sun QM, Liu DY. Astragalus polysaccharide attenuates rat experimental colitis by inducing regulatory T cells in intestinal Peyer's patches. World J Gastroenterol. 2016;22(11):3175–85.

18

Network pharmacology-based strategy to investigate pharmacological mechanisms of Zuojinwan for treatment of gastritis

Guohua Yu[1], Wubin Wang[1], Xu Wang[1], Meng Xu[1], Lili Zhang[1], Lei Ding[1], Rui Guo[1] and Yuanyuan Shi[1,2*]

Abstract

Background: Zuojinwan (ZJW), a classic herbal formula, has been extensively used to treat gastric symptoms in clinical practice in China for centuries. However, the pharmacological mechanisms of ZJW still remain vague to date.

Methods: In the present work, a network pharmacology-based strategy was proposed to elucidate its underlying multi-component, multi-target, and multi-pathway mode of action against gastritis. First we collected putative targets of ZJW based on TCMSP and STITCH databases, and a network containing the interactions between the putative targets of ZJW and known therapeutic targets of gastritis was built. Then four topological parameters, "degree", "betweenness", "closeness", and "coreness" were calculated to identify the major targets in the network. Furthermore, the major hubs were imported to the Metacore database to perform a pathway enrichment analysis.

Results: A total of 118 nodes including 59 putative targets of ZJW were picked out as major hubs in terms of their topological importance. The results of pathway enrichment analysis indicated that putative targets of ZJW mostly participated in various pathways associated with anti-inflammation response, growth and development promotion and G-protein-coupled receptor signaling. More importantly, five putative targets of ZJW (EGFR, IL-6, IL-1β, TNF-α and MCP-1) and two known therapeutic targets of gastritis (CCKBR and IL-12β) and a link target NF-κB were recognized as active factors involved in the main biological functions of treatment, implying the underlying mechanisms of ZJW acting on gastritis.

Conclusion: ZJW could alleviate gastritis through the molecular mechanisms predicted by network pharmacology, and this research demonstrates that the network pharmacology approach can be an effective tool to reveal the mechanisms of traditional Chinese medicine (TCM) from a holistic perspective.

Keywords: Zuojinwan, Network pharmacology, Gastritis

Background

Gastritis is an acute or chronic, diffuse or focal inflation of the lining of the stomach [1]. It is brought on by many factors, including infection by *Helicobacter pylori*, drug induced such as aspirin, Non-Steroidal Anti-Inflammatory Drugs (NSAIDs), corticosteroids and alcohol consumption [2]. The most frequent symptoms of gastritis include upper abdominal pain, heartburn, nausea, and vomiting [3, 4]. Gastritis is believed to affect about half of people in the world and it generates considerable costs to society [5]. Although current therapies, including antacids, H-2 blockers, proton pump inhibitors and antibiotics can alleviate some major symptoms of gastritis, these medications have also triggered a series of serious side effects like abdominal pain (or stomach pain), constipation, and diarrhea. Therefore, it is still necessary to find novel and safe prevention strategies.

Traditional Chinese medicine (TCM) is a comprehensive medicinal system that plays an important role in health maintenance for Asian people, and has gradually gained popularity in western countries due to the reliable therapeutic efficacy and fewer side effects [6, 7]. Based on the theory of traditional Chinese herbal

* Correspondence: yshi@bucm.edu.cn
[1]School of Life Sciences, Beijing University of Chinese Medicine, No.11 East road, North 3rd Ring Road, Beijing 100029, China
[2]Shenzhen Hospital, Beijing University of Chinese Medicine, No. 1 Dayun road, Sports New City Road, Shenzhen 518172, China

medical science, TCM offers bright prospects for the prevention and treatment of complex diseases such as gastritis in a systematic way [8].

Zuojinwan, which consists of *R. coptidis* and *E. rutaecarpa* powder in the ratio of 6: 1(*w*/*w*), is a famous Chinese medicine prescription used for treatment of gastric diseases [9, 10]. ZJW was first recorded in a famous ancient medicine treatise *Danxi Xinfa* in Yuan Dynasty of Chinese history (1271 AD–1368 AD), and has been approved by the China Food and Drug Administration (CFDA). From the bench to the bedside, previous researches on ZJW for gastric diseases could be mainly documented into two sections: (1) Clinical practices show that ZJW has been widely used for treating gastric diseases. (2) Basic researches indicate that ZJW exerts a range of pharmacological activities, including anti-inflammation, anti-ulcer and anti-acid activities and inhibitory effect on the growth of *Heliobacter pylori*. Although well-practiced in clinical medicine, very little is known about the active substances and specific molecular mechanisms of ZJW acting on gastritis.

Similar to other TCM formulas, ZJW is a multi-component and multi-target agent that achieves its specific therapeutic efficacy through active components that regulate molecular networks within the body. Therefore, it is hard to investigate the pharmacological mechanisms of ZJW in the treatment of gastritis. With the rapid progress of bioinformatics, systems biology and polypharmacology, network pharmacology-based approaches have been proven to be a powerful way for compatible and mechanistic exploration of TCM formula [7, 11, 12]. For example, Yu et al. used a network pharmacology method to analyze the synergistic mechanism of Yin-Huang-Qing-Fei capsule acting on chronic bronchitis [13]. Yue et al. developed an integrated system pharmacology approach, combined a number of network-based computational methods and algorithm-based approaches to clarify the mechanisms of Danggui-Honghua for treatment of blood stasis syndrome [14].

In this work, we aim to use a comprehensive network pharmacology-based approach to investigate the mechanisms of how ZJW exerts the therapeutic effects on gastritis. The flowchart of the experimental procedures of our study was shown in Fig. 1.

Methods
Data preparation
Chemical ingredients database building
To determine the chemical ingredients of the two herbs contained in ZJW, we performed a search by Traditional Chinese Medicine Systems Pharmacology Database [15] (TCMSP, http://lsp.nwu.edu.cn/tcmsp.php, updated on May 31, 2014) and Chinese Academy of Sciences

Chemistry Database [16] (CASC, http://www.organc hem.csdb.cn/scdb/main/slogin.asp, updated on February 11, 2018) and related literatures using "*R. coptidis*" and "*E. rutaecarpa*" as the queries. TCMSP is a unique systems pharmacology database of Chinese herbal medicines which captures the herbs, chemicals, targets and drug-target networks [17]. CASC, one of the most comprehensive chemical databases in the world, can provide the chemical information of traditional Chinese herbs and natural products [13].

The prediction of known therapeutic targets acting on gastritis
We collected gastritis targets from two sources. One was the DrugBank database [18] (http://www.drugbank.ca/, version 4.3), which is a unique bioinformatics and cheminformatics resource that combines detailed drug data with comprehensive drug target information. The keyword "gastritis" was used and only drug–target interactions for drugs approved by the Food and Drug Administration (FDA) for treating gastritis and human gene/protein targets were selected. The other resource was the Online Mendelian Inheritance in Man (OMIM) database [19] (http://www.omim.org/, updated on May 4, 2018). The OMIM database catalogued all known diseases with a genetic component and linked them to the relevant genes in the human genome and provided references for further research and tools for genomic analysis of a catalogued gene [19]. We searched the OMIM database with the query "gastritis" as well.

The prediction of putative targets of the ingredients within ZJW
The integrative efficacy of the ingredients in ZJW was determined by analyzing the ingredients and targets interactions obtained from TCMSP Database and STITCH DataBase [20] (http://stitch.embl.de/, ver. 4.0) with the species limited as "*Homo sapiens*". STITCH was a database to explore known and predicted interactions between chemicals and proteins. Only the proteins which had direct interactions with each chemical in ZJW were selected as the putative targets.

Protein–protein interaction data
Protein–protein interaction (PPI) data were derived from eight major existing public PPI databases, namely, String [21], Reactome [22], Online Predicted Human Interaction Database (OPHID) [23], InAct [24], Human Protein Reference Database (HPRD) [25], Molecular Interaction Database (MINT) [26], Database of Interacting Proteins (DIP) [27], and PDZBase [28]. The eight open databases covered the majority of known human protein-protein interactions information. Detailed information about these PPI databases was provided in Additional file 1: Table S1. All the data were merged after removing redundant entries and

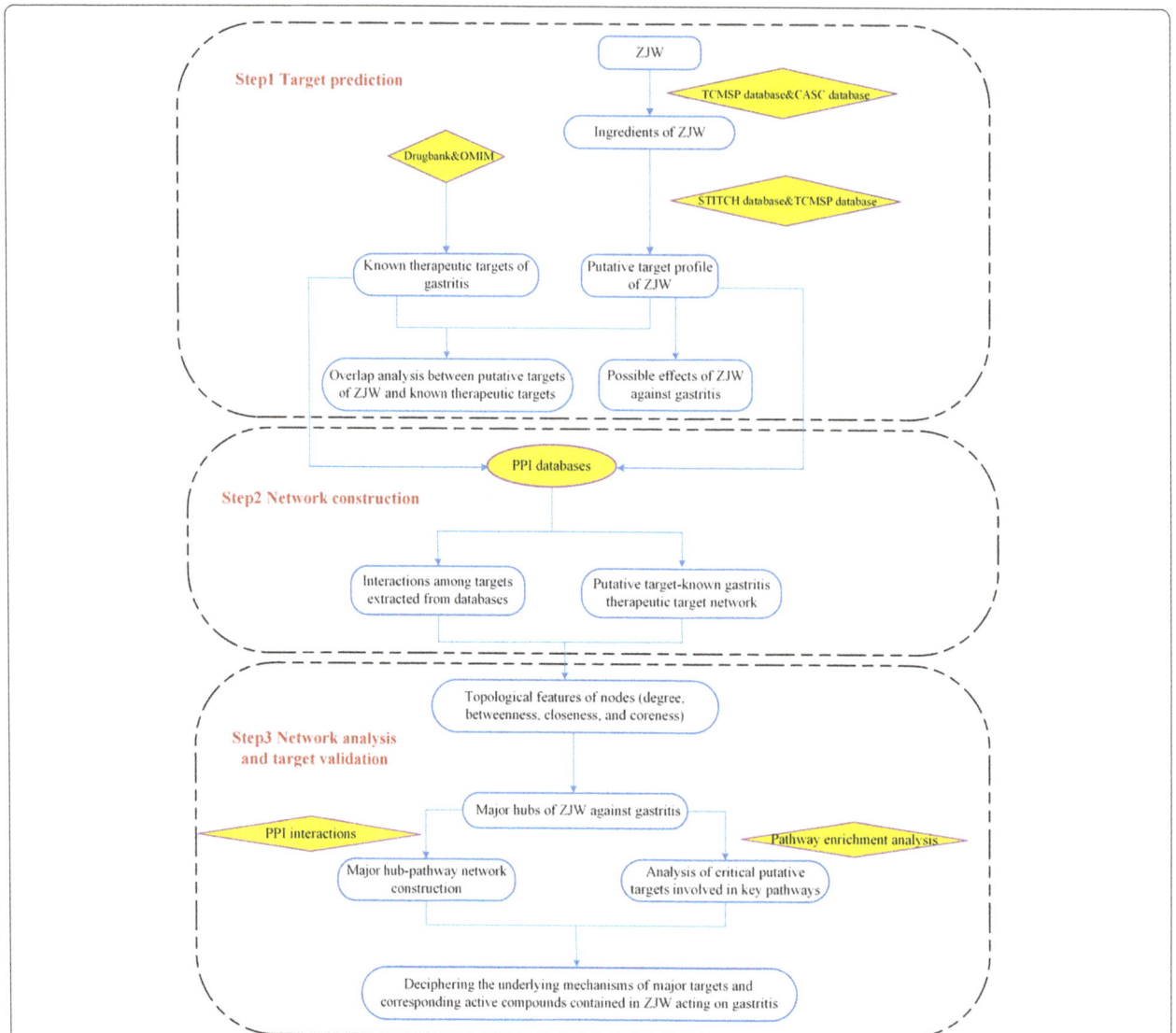

Fig. 1 The flowchart of network pharmacology-based strategy for deciphering the mechanisms of ZJW acting on gastritis. Abbreviations: ZJW, Zuojinwan; TCMSP, Traditional Chinese Medicine Systems Pharmacology; CASC, Chinese Academy of Sciences Chemistry; OMIM, Online Mendelian Inheritance in Man; PPI, protein–protein interaction

the differing ID types of the proteins were converted to UniProt IDs.

Network construction

The putative targets of ZJW, the gastritis disease targets and interactional proteins were connected based on the protein-protein interactions derived from the eight public databases. Then the interactions between proteins of the putative targets of ZJW, known therapeutic targets for gastritis and interactional human targets were combined to construct putative ZJW target-known therapeutic targets of gastritis network. It can be applied to illustrate the relationships between putative targets contained in ZJW and known therapeutic targets of gastritis. The graphical interactions in this network was visualized

using Cytoscape software [29] (version 3.6.0, Boston, MA, USA). In addition, a null model was constructed to verify the significance of the putative ZJW target-known therapeutic targets of gastritis network.

Putative ZJW target-known therapeutic targets of the gastritis network

Based on the interactions between putative ZJW targets, known therapeutic targets of gastritis and interactional human proteins, the whole links of the network were established. According to previous reports [30–32], a node would be defined as a hub when the degree of the node was more than twofold the median degree of all the nodes in the same network. After selecting hubs from the network, the direct interactions among hubs was constructed. Next, we used four topological parameters, "degree", "betweenness", "closeness", and "coreness" to evaluate the topological importance of the selected hubs. The definitions for each topological parameter mentioned above are given in 'Definitions of topological propertie' section. Only the hubs whose topological parameters were greater than the corresponding median values were considered as major hubs.

Definitions of topological properties

As for each node i in the networks, the definitions of four measures for evaluating its topological properties were shown as follows. 'Degree' is defined as the number of links to node i. 'Node betweenness' represents the number of the shortest paths between pairs of nodes that ran through node i. The concept of 'Node closeness' is the inverse of the sum of distances from the node i to all other nodes. The closeness centrality can also be seen as a metric of the time it will take to sequentially spread information from node i to all the other accessible nodes. We usually use 'Degree', 'Node betweenness' and 'Node closeness centralities' to describe a protein's topological importance in the network. In other words, the relationship between these three topological parameters and importance of corresponding protein is direct proportional [33]. 'Coreness' is shell index of 'K-core' decomposition. K-core analysis is an iterative procedure in which the nodes are removed from the networks in descending degree order. The highest degree node was selected as the main core or the highest k-core of the network. After repeatedly deleting vertices from the network whose degree is less than k, a k-core sub-network of the original network forms. This process generates a series of sub-networks that uncover the main hierarchical layers of the original network step by step. On this basis, 'Coreness' is a parameter to measure the centrality of node i.

Null model construction

In order to validate the non-trivial structure of putative ZJW target-known therapeutic targets of the gastritis network, we constructed a null model in which all the nodes of the ZJW network were conserved as well as the number of links, but the nodes were rewired randomly in terms of the Erdös-Rényi model. We also used the corresponding topological parameters to screen out the major hubs in the null model.

Pathway enrichment performance

To cluster the biological functions of the major hubs, they were uploaded to MetaCore™ [34] (https://portal.g enego.com) as Gene Symbol style to run pathway enrichment analysis. MetaCore online database delivers high-quality biological systems content as well as essential data and analytics, including sophisticated integrated pathway and network analysis for multi-omics data. First the list of major hubs was input into the Metacore database as a new event, we selected the new event in the online database and clicked on the icons with "protein functional annotation and enrichment analysis" and "network construction and analysis" successively to obtain the main pathways and network distribution involved in the functional regulation. Then the results could be analyzed in the next step. Also, we calculated and evaluated significant pathways assisted by Database Visualization and Integrated Discovery system [35] (DAVID, http://david.abcc.ncifcrf.gov/home.jsp, version 6.7) and the Kyoto Encyclopedia of Genes and Genomes database [36] (KEGG, http://www.genome.jp/kegg/, updated on April 18, 2016). Then we compared the generated results with a null model to assess the statistical significance.

Results

Composite ingredients of ZJW

A total of 170 chemical ingredients (Additional file 2: Table S2) of the two herbal medicines in ZJW were retrieved from TCMSP and CASC and related literatures, including 29 ingredients in *R. coptidis* and 141 ingredients in *E. rutaecarpa*.

Known therapeutic targets acting on gastritis

In total, 75 known therapeutic targets for gastritis were collected from DrugBank database. And 15 known therapeutic targets for the treatment of gastritis were acquired based on OMIM database. After eliminating the redundancy, a total of 90 known therapeutic targets in the treatment of gastritis were collected in this study. The details were described in Additional file 3: Table S3.

Putative targets for ZJW

According to the target prediction system in TCMSP and STITCH databases, the quantity of putative targets for *R. coptidis* and *E. rutaecarpa* was 175 and 348, respectively. There were 106 putative targets of the two herbs overlapped, which was suggestive of potential interactions between *R. coptidis* and *E. rutaecarpa* in the course of treatment. Detailed information about putative targets is provided in Additional file 4: Table S4.

Network and pathway analysis

To shed light on the potential mechanisms of ZJW acting on gastritis, the putative ZJW target-gastritis related target network consisting of putative ZJW targets, known therapeutic target for gastritis and interactional human proteins was constructed based on PPI databases. As a result, the network was composed of 5559 nodes and 21567 edges. For detailed information about this network, see Additional file 5: Table S5.

A hub target in a network is regarded as a crucial node and used to measure the essence of the whole network. It has been reported that [37], nodes will be defined as hubs if their degree is greater than twofold the median degree of all nodes in the network. In this network, we used the twofold median value of node degree (two) as a cutoff point primarily. After removing the targets whose degree was less than or equal to two, 2654 nodes were encoded as hubs. Then four topological features, "degree", "betweenness", "closeness", and "coreness", of selected hubs were calculated to screen the major hubs in the network. Only the hubs with higher values of "degree", "betweenness", "closeness", and "coreness" (above the median value of all the network nodes) were identified as the major hub targets. To focus on the further enrichment analysis of crucial hubs, we discarded some targets which might play unimportant roles in the network according to the topological features. Therefore, we kept proteins with "degree" >4, "betweenness" > 0.0002, "closeness" >0.3919 and "coreness" >5 as major hubs. Eventually, 118 major hubs were picked out for further study, of which 59 targets were from putative targets of ZJW and 12 targets were derived from known therapeutic target of gastritis. The details were shown in Additional file 6: Table S6.

To clarify the biological actions of these hubs, a pathway enrichment analysis was performed based on Metacore database. We fed MetaCore a gene list of major hubs, generating relevant pathways which might have an important influence on the biological process for ZJW treating gastritis. Only pathways with P-value<0.05 were considered as significant pathways. The full list of significant pathways was shown in Additional file 7: Table S7. We analyzed the data and relevant biological processes, choosing top ten remarkable significant pathways according to the P value for further study. The top ten main pathways were shown in Fig. 2.

Modularity could be an important aspect of a network. Nodes highly interconnected within a network were usually participated in the same biological modules. In terms of the functional distribution of major hubs and main pathways, the interaction network of putative ZJW targets and gastritis-related targets and interactional targets was divided into three modules. The assortments of the main pathways and modules are shown in Fig. 3. The maximum module consisting of major hubs was associated with inflammation suppression and immune responses, and the second module was sorted as a progression of growth and development, while the minimum module was concentrated in G-protein-coupled receptor signaling.

We analyzed the null-model-network topology and performed pathway enrichment analysis in the same way as we interpreted the ZJW network, and no modules or pathways were found since just a few genes without any interaction were screened out. The details of the whole null-model-network were shown in Additional file 8: Table S8. The major hubs of null-model- network were also supplemented in Additional file 9: Table S9. The null-model-network topology (Fig. 4a) and the core structure of the random network after calculation of four topological properties (Fig. 4b) were shown in Fig. 4. By contrast with the null model, the significance of ZJW network was verified.

Potential mechanisms of ZJW in the treatment of gastritis

In the maximum module, cytokines and genes were enriched in inflammatory pathways including IL-11 signaling pathway via MEK/ERK and PI3K/AKT cascades, IL-18 signaling pathway, GM-CSF signaling pathway, histamine signaling in dendritic cells and gastrin in inflammatory response. Most of these pathways contain PI3K/AKT signaling pathway and NF-κB mediated signaling pathway, and both play important roles in

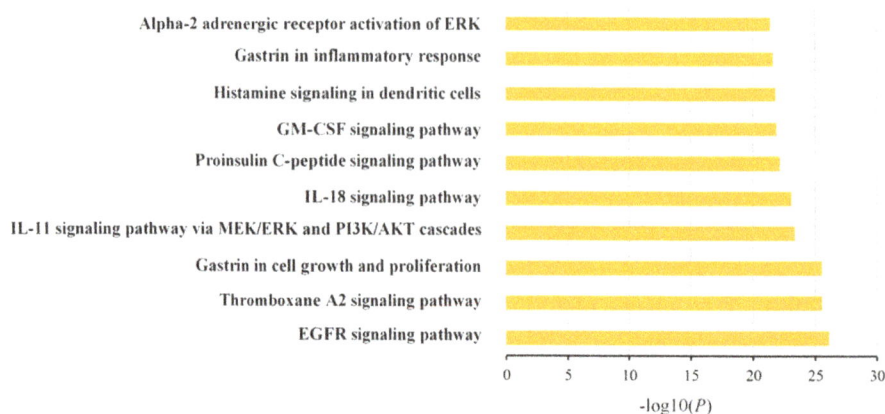

Fig. 2 Main pathways enriched by major hubs from Metacore database. The top 10 pathways measured by counts were selected to demonstrate the crucial biological actions of major hubs. The abscissa stands for target counts in each pathway; and the ordinate stands for main pathways

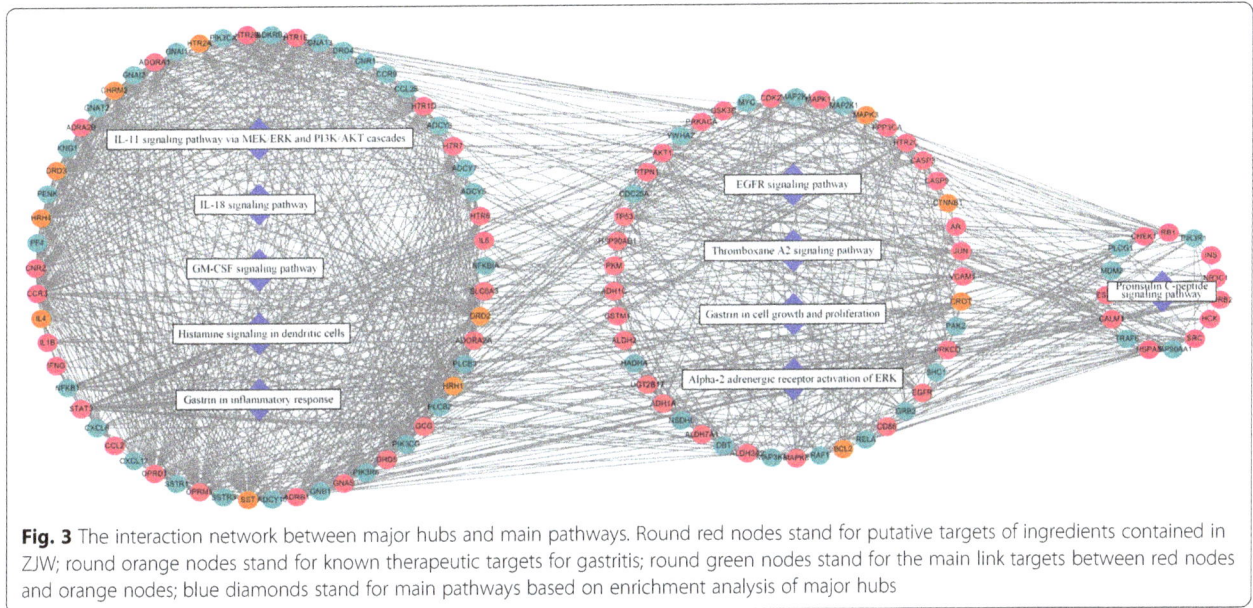

Fig. 3 The interaction network between major hubs and main pathways. Round red nodes stand for putative targets of ingredients contained in ZJW; round orange nodes stand for known therapeutic targets for gastritis; round green nodes stand for the main link targets between red nodes and orange nodes; blue diamonds stand for main pathways based on enrichment analysis of major hubs

inflammatory response as well as cell proliferation. Usually, the extracellular cytokine binding to its corresponding receptor leads to a series of activation of downstream molecules, and sequentially PI3K/AKT signaling pathway or NF-κB mediated signaling pathway can be activated, resulting in transcription of relevant transcription factors and secretion of some inflammatory factors participating in the process of inflammation.

EGFR signaling pathway occupied a leading position in the second module. The epidermal growth factor receptor (EGFR) is a cell surface protein that binds to epidermal growth factor. Binding of the protein to an extracellular growth factor ligand induces receptor dimerization and tyrosine autophosphorylation and leads to diverse biologic responses, including cell proliferation, differentiation, cell motility and survival [38]. EGFR dimerization and tyrosine autophosphorylation can activate several intracellular signaling pathways, such as PI3K/AKT signaling pathway, JUK signaling pathway. These pathways play an important role in cell growth and proliferation. As well, EGFR signaling pathway is partly involved in those main growth and development-related pathways including thromboxane A2 signaling pathway, gastrin in cell growth and proliferation, alpha-2 adrenergic receptor activation of ERK.

Proinsulin C-peptide signaling pathway composed a part of the minimum module. One of the putative receptor for proinsulin C-peptide was supposed to be a specific GPCR linked to the G-protein alpha-i family [39–41], which could stimulate PI3K/AKT and NF-κB. And then transcription of inflammatory genes and anti-apoptotic genes was activated by proinsulin C-peptide-stimulated NF-κB. A series of biological functions of inflammatory response and immune actions would be initiated. Furthermore,

proinsulin C-peptide also participated in regulation ERK. And the binding of proinsulin C-peptide and GPCR triggered ERK signaling via PLC-beta-dependent stimulation of PKC or PI3K-dependent pathway [42]. These biological reactions contributed a lot to cell proliferation.

Discussion

Gastritis can be caused by various factors, and some remarkable alterations of the stomach mucosa including epithelial damage and mucosal inflammation will appear once patients suffer from gastritis [43]. NF-κB mediated signaling pathway is activated while gastritis occurs. NF-κB can promote the expression of pro-inflammatory cytokines genes such as IL-1β, TNF-α, IL-12β, IL-6, IL-8 [44–49]. These cytokines are attributed to the inflammation of gastric epithelial cells. It has been reported that the injury of gastric mucosa barrier has a close relationship with gastritis, and long-playing activation by inflammatory factors will induce the severe lesion in gastric glandular tissues when the gastric mucosa is not well regenerated [50]. EGF is one of the most important factors in gastric tissue repair and cell regeneration, showing its effects through the combination with its receptor (EGFR) located in gastric epithelial basal or bilateral membrane. The level of the expression of EGFR can be highly detected in the damaged gastric barrier and perfused epithelia while it is rarely found in normal epithelial cells. It is also found that EGFR expressed more highly in the surface mucosal layer than the deep and muscle layers of stomach, implying its effects on the promotion of the growth and recovery of damaged gastric epithelial cells [51]. However, excessive expression of EGFR can induce malignant growth in gastric epithelial cells and may cause canceration to some extent [52, 53].

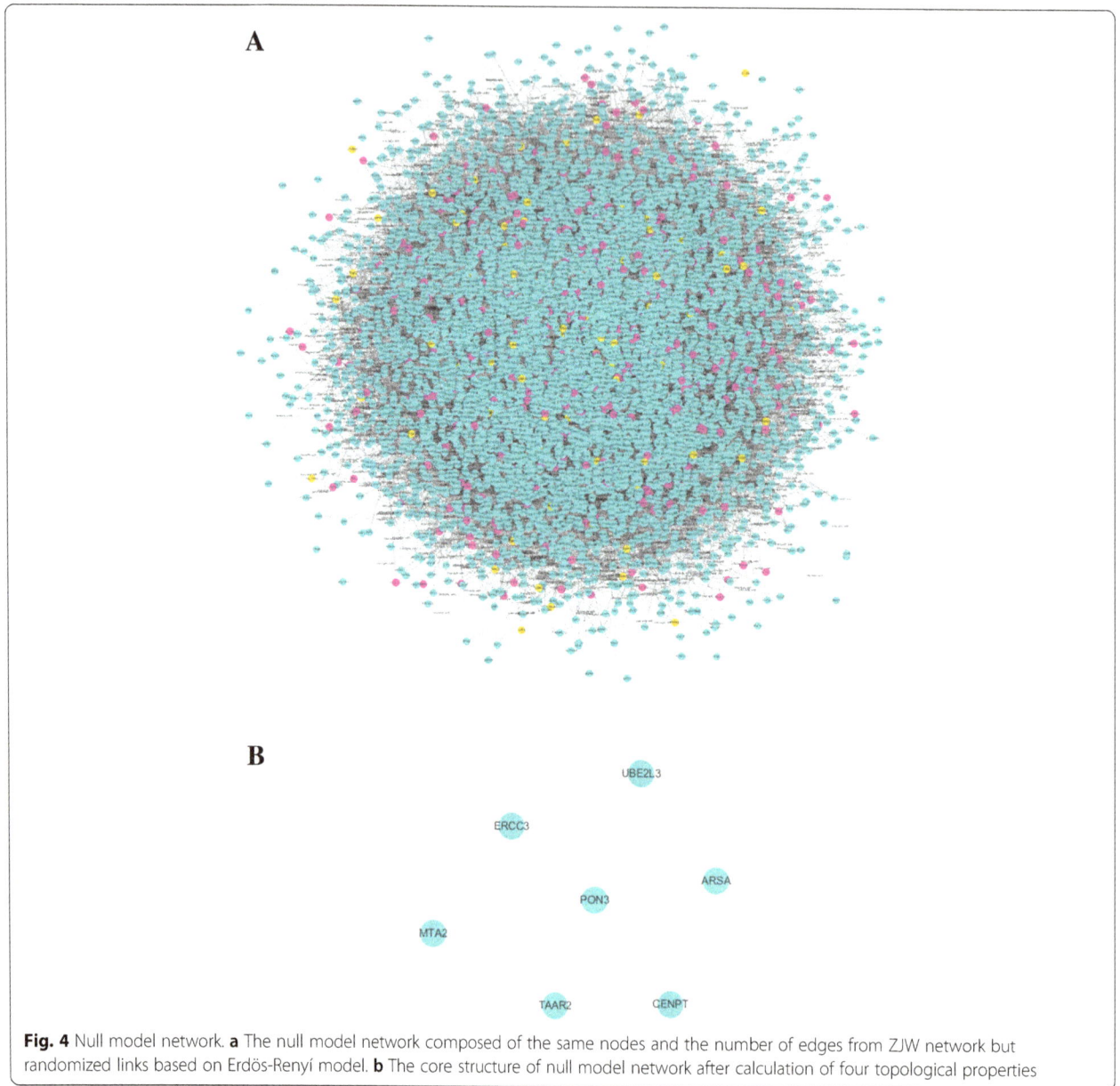

Fig. 4 Null model network. **a** The null model network composed of the same nodes and the number of edges from ZJW network but randomized links based on Erdös-Renyí model. **b** The core structure of null model network after calculation of four topological properties

Therefore, to regulate the balance of the expression of EGFR is very pivotal in gastric mucosa development and repairment. Besides, as a multifunctional gastro-intestinal hormone, gastrin is secreted by G cells in the gastric antrum and plays important roles in stimulating acid secretion, cell growth and mucous regeneration [54, 55]. As a result of increase of serum concentration of gastrin accompanying with increased grades of atrophic gastritis, the serum gastrin level is taken as a significant biomarker for evaluating the status of gastric inflammation [56, 57]. It is also evident that gastrin is a growth factor which can induce gastric carcinogenesis [58, 59].

The pathological processes of gastritis are closely related to inflammatory response and cell development. Five putative targets of ZJW (interleukin-6[IL-6], IL-1β, tumor necrosis factor [TNF]-α, monocyte chemotactic protein [MCP]-1 and EGFR), and two known therapeutic targets of gastritis (cholecystokinin-B receptors[CCKBR] and IL-12β) and a link target between ZJW and disease NF-κB are shown to be the most active factors that participate in these key pathways, which are implied an important role in the occurrence and promotion of gastritis. The main biological processes are shown in Fig. 5.

Cytokines and chemokines can be produced when a signaling cascade is activated during the progression of lesion in the stomach, inducing chronic inflammatory response. Gastric epithelium can secret a series of chemokines including interleukin (IL)-6 and IL-1β, which are chemotactic for neutrophils and mononuclear cells. With the recruitment of neutrophils and macrophages

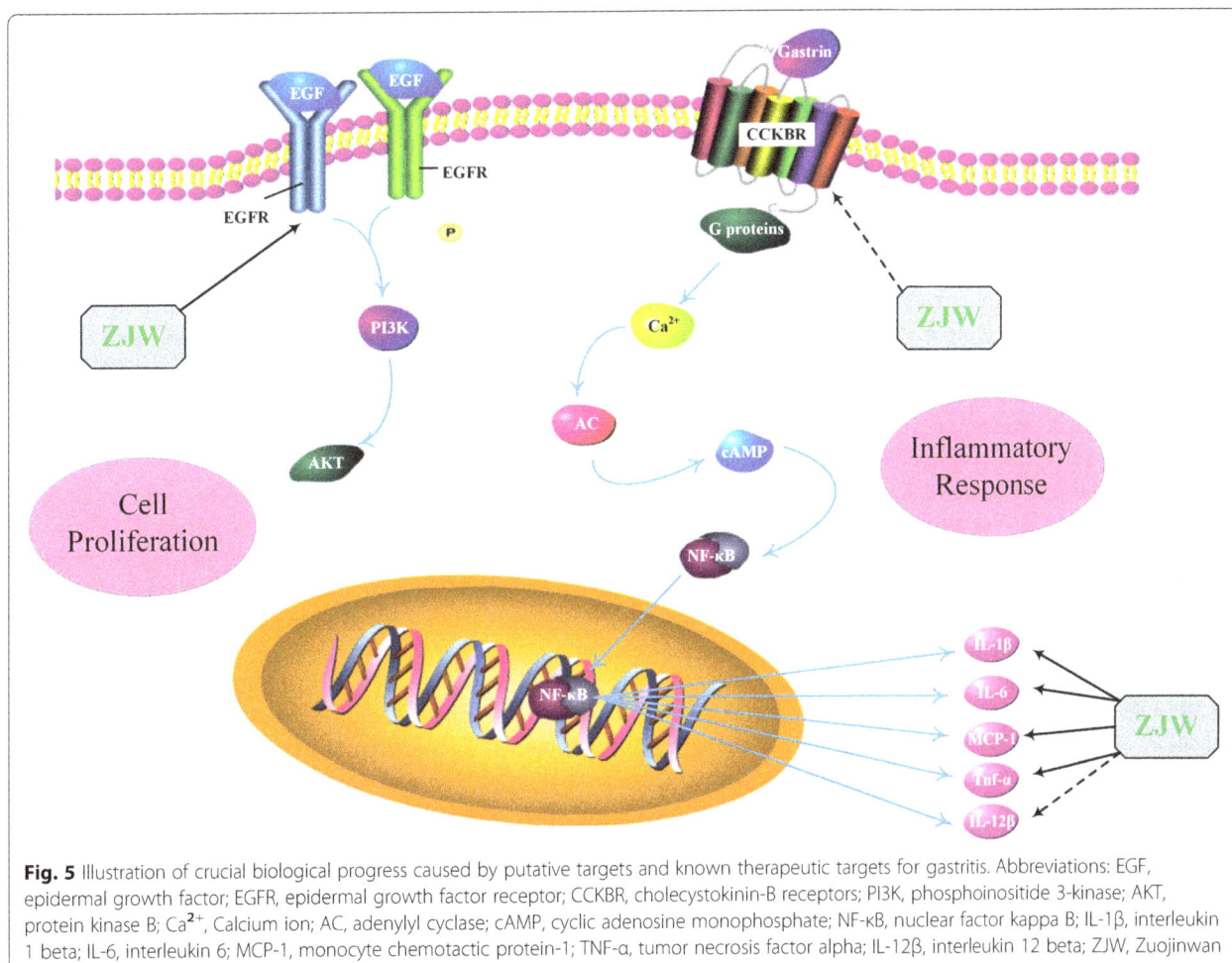

Fig. 5 Illustration of crucial biological progress caused by putative targets and known therapeutic targets for gastritis. Abbreviations: EGF, epidermal growth factor; EGFR, epidermal growth factor receptor; CCKBR, cholecystokinin-B receptors; PI3K, phosphoinositide 3-kinase; AKT, protein kinase B; Ca^{2+}, Calcium ion; AC, adenylyl cyclase; cAMP, cyclic adenosine monophosphate; NF-κB, nuclear factor kappa B; IL-1β, interleukin 1 beta; IL-6, interleukin 6; MCP-1, monocyte chemotactic protein-1; TNF-α, tumor necrosis factor alpha; IL-12β, interleukin 12 beta; ZJW, Zuojinwan

in the mucosa of stomach, the infiltration is the main factor of a chronic gastritis. Expect neutrophils and mononuclear cells, dendritic cells and T and B cells can also form infiltration and then activate the production of monocyte chemotactic protein (MCP)-1, tumor necrosis factor (TNF)-α, IL-12 and so on [60]. IL-6 can be produced by T cells and macrophages that gives rise to immune response during infection or after injury which induces inflammation in the gastric mucosa or other tissues [61]. It is also a pleiotropic cytokine associated with the growth and differentiation of immunocyte as well as the expression of some other cytokines [62]. Furthermore, IL-6 has been reported as a significant marker in the process of inflammation-related canceration [63, 64]. And there is evidence that in an inflammation-induced tumor model, IL-6 deficiency could relive the promotion of tumor development [65, 66]. MCP-1, known as CC-chemokine ligand 2 (CCL2), is a micromolecular potent chemoattractant for leukocytes to gather on the position where tissue is injured and inflammation or tumor are triggered [60, 67]. Studies have demonstrated that many tumor cells can express CCL2, suggesting its

role in the course of cancer [68–71]. It is also reported that tumor samples from 68 gastric cancer patients highly expressed CCL2, implied that CCL2 may have a close relationship with gastric disease. Thus, CCL2 is considered to be a predictive molecule for gastric carcinoma [72]. Secreted by monocytes and macrophages, TNF-α stimulates the production of a series of cytokine and play an important part in gastritis. TNF-α is suggested to be a considerable immune mediator in inflammatory response which is initiated by infection and other factors [73, 74]. It has a positive influence on gastric mucosal apoptosis, and persistent apoptosis may cause extensive gastric mucosa damage like gastric ulcer [75, 76]. IL-1β is referred to be a pro-inflammatory cytokine that can be largely produced as a result of host defense against external invasion and tissue lesions [77]. It is found that high expression of IL-1β in the stomach of transgenic mice can activate spontaneous severe gastric inflammatory response [78]. Therefore, IL-1β is an important signaling mediator in the promotion of gastritis. It is also emphasized on the investigation that the polymorphisms of IL1B gene may be involved in the high risk of the generation of gastric cancer [79–81]. Moreover, it is demonstrated that in a IL-1β-deficient mice model, the infiltration of immune cells and gastric tumors are positively suppressed [82]. Gastrin is identified as the chief stimulant of gastric acid secretion which is produced by G cells in the gastric antrum [50]. Gastrin exerts its effects primarily through binding to cholecysto kinin-B receptors (CCKBR) on enterochromaffin-like (ECL) cells of the gastric mucosa [83, 84]. CCKBR, also known as cholecystokinin-2 receptors (CCK2R), is a seven transmembrane G-protein coupled receptor that is mostly expressed in gastric fundus [85]. The expression of gastrin-CCKBR indicates the atrophic changes in the stomach [54, 56]. Consequently, gastrin-CCKBR level is a vital standard for measuring the severity of gastritis [57]. In addition, the expression of CCKBR is regarded as a symbol that has a close relationship with gastric canceration. IL-12β is a pro-inflammatory cytokine that is produced by various immune cells [86, 87]. The expression of IL-12β can be remarkably increased when the inflammatory response occurs in the layer of gastric tissues [88]. And studies have demonstrated that its regulatory gene IL12B is the target gene of NF-κB [89]. Importantly, the activation of NF-κB is critically responsible for the secretion of cytokines including IL-6, IL-1β, TNF-α and so on [90]. It has been reported that the extract of ZJW could significantly reduce the activity of NF-κB as well as some pro-inflammatory cytokines [91]. As is reported in the previous studies, ZJW was found to be an effective inhibitor for IL-1β, IL-6 and TNF-α in a concentration-dependent manner in LPS-induced RAW 264.7 macrophages [92]. It is also validated that ZJW could relieve the inflammation by downregulating the levels of TNF-α and IL-1β in rats, reducing the expression of the gene TNFA and IL1B in gastric mucosa [93]. And reducing cytokine IL-6 is another effective way for ZJW to attenuate the infiltration of immune cells and injury area in the stomach of rats [94]. It is evident that ZJW can upregulate the expression level of EGFR in rats with gastric ulcer induced by acetic acid, promoting the restoration of damaged gastric mucosa [95]. The down-regulation of ZJW for MCP-1 has been inferred as a result of anti-inflammatory effects of ZJW. Moreover, ZJW may exert its therapeutic effects through inhibiting the expression of IL-12β and CCKBR, cutting down the opportunity of further deterioration of gastritis. In summary, blocking these pro-inflammatory factors and raising relevant growth factors may be the pharmacological mechanism of ZJW acting on gastritis.

Besides, stimulation of growth and development signaling (EGFR signaling pathway, Gastrin in cell growth and proliferation and so on) leads to cell growth and proliferation. Excessive or inappropriate cell growth and proliferation can be one of the major causes of tumor development [96, 97]. It has been reported that

excessive NF-κB activation was detected in human colorectal cancer tissues [98], and ZJW played a suppressive role in the expression of NF-κB [99]. Furthermore, an investigation concerning effects of ZJW on eight kinds of human cancer cell lines suggested that ZJW has significant anti-cancer activities due to up-regulation of pro-apoptosis proteins (caspase-3, caspase-9, Bax and Bak) and down-regulation of anti-apoptosis proteins (Bcl-2 and Bcl-xl) [100]. However, anti-cancer effects of ZJW in vivo and specific molecular mechanisms deserved to be deeply explored.

In addition, among the putative targets of ZJW, IL-6 is putative target of 2-Methoxy-4-vinylphenol and caffeine from *E. rutaecarpa*, IL-1β is putative target of alpha-humulene from *E. rutaecarpa*, TNF-α is putative target of hexanal, palmitic acid, rutaecarpine from *E. rutaecarpa* and quercetin from *R. coptidis*, EGFR is putative target of rutin from *E. rutaecarpa*, MCP-1 is putative target of quercetin from *R. coptidis*. These compounds are proposed to be the active constituents of ZJW in the treatment of gastritis.

However, there are also some limitations for the use of network pharmacology approach to predict active ingredients and potential mechanisms. (i) the active ingredients screened might be inconsistent with the ingredients actually absorbed in blood of the patients with gastritis; (ii) to distinguish inhibitory effects from activated effects of the targets could be a difficult problem; (iii) the predicted results might be impacted by possible biases to highly studied pathways/functions. Therefore, further experimental verification of the potential effective ingredients is demanded to validate theoretical predictions.

Conclusion

TCM, one of the most important parts of complementary and alternative medicine, markedly contributes to the therapeutic action of gastrointestinal diseases. This study uses a scientific approach to holistically decipher that the pharmacological mechanisms of ZJW in the treatment of gastritis may be associated with its involvement into inflammation suppression and immune responses, growth and development pathways. Among these crucial biological functions, eight targets were identified as key active factors involved in the related pathways. However, to enhance the reliability of the results, further experimental experiments were demanded to validate these hypotheses.

Additional files

Additional file 1: Table S1. Detailed information on eight existing protein-protein interaction databases. (XLSX 12 kb)

Additional file 2: Table S2. Ingredients of each herb contained in ZJW.

Additional file 3: Table S3. Known therapeutic targets for gastritis.

Additional file 4: Table S4. Putative targets of each herb contained in ZJW and overlap between the two herbs.

Additional file 5: Table S5. Interactions between putative targets of ZJW and known therapeutic target for gastritis.

Additional file 6: Table S6. Major hubs in the network.

Additional file 7: Table S7. Significant pathways.

Additional file 8: Table S8. The whole null model according to Erdös-Rényi model.

Additional file 9: Table S9. The major hubs of null-model- network.

Abbreviations
AC: Adenylyl cyclase; AKT: Protein kinase B; Ca^{2+}: Calcium ion; cAMP: Cyclic adenosine monophosphate; CASC: Chinese Academy of Sciences Chemistry; CCKBR: Cholecystokinin-B receptors; CCL2: CC-chemokine ligand 2; EGF: Epidermal growth factor; EGFR: Epidermal growth factor receptor; IL-12β: Interleukin 12 beta; IL-1β: Interleukin 1 beta; IL-6: Interleukin 6; MCP-1: Monocyte chemotactic protein-1; NF-κB: Nuclear factor kappa B; OMIM: Online Mendelian Inheritance in Man; PI3K: Phosphoinositide 3-kinase; PPI: Protein–protein interaction; TCMSP: Traditional Chinese Medicine Systems Pharmacology; TNF-α: Tumor necrosis factor alpha; ZJW: Zuojinwan

Acknowledgments
We would like to thank Zhiqiang Luo for image processing and Tao Lu for manuscript review in this research.

Funding
This study was supported by the Start-up fund from Beijing University of Chinese Medicine to Yuanyuan Shi (No.1000061020013).

Authors' contributions
SYY conceived and designed the experiments; YGH, WWB and WX performed the experiments and wrote the paper; XM, ZLL, DL and GR analyzed the data. All authors have read and approved the final manuscript.

Competing interests
The authors declare that they have no competing interests.

References
1. Paduraru G, Lupu W, Diaconescu S, Burlea M. Particular considerations on helicobacter pylori-associated chronic gastritis in child. Romanian J Pediatr. 2011;60(1):29–33.
2. Ali El Zahaby A, Abdel Alim A, Elsharawy A. Role of Rebamipide and \ or pantoprazole in preventing dexamethasone induced gastritis in senile male albino rats. Egypt J Hosp Med. 2017;67(2):789–505.
3. Jones L, Brooks D. Cash. Gastritis. In Digestive Disease, National Institute of Diabetes and Digestive and Kidney Diseases. https://www.niddk.nih.gov/health-information/digestive-diseases/gastritis. Accessed July 2015.
4. Rosen & Barkin's 5-Minute Emergency Medicine Consult (4 ed.). Lippincott Williams & Wilkins. 2015:447.
5. Ferri's Clinical Advisor 2013,5 Books in 1, Expert Consult - Online and Print,1: Ferri's Clinical Advisor 2013. Elsevier Health Sciences. 2016:417.
6. Li B, Xue X, Xia W, Hua Y, Li X, Tao W, et al. A systems biology approach to understanding the mechanisms of action of Chinese herbs for treatment of cardiovascular disease. Int J Mol Sci. 2012;13(10):13501–20.
7. Zhao F, Guochun L, Yang Y, Shi L, Xu L, Yin L. A network pharmacology approach to determine active ingredients and rationality of herb combinations of modified-Simiaowan for treatment of gout. J Ethnopharmacol. 2015;168:1–16.
8. Fang J, Wang L, Wu T, Yang C, Gao L, Cai H, et al. Network pharmacology-based study on the mechanism of action for herbal medicines in Alzheimer treatment. J Ethnopharmacol. 2016;196:281–92.
9. Rui Y, Yin W, Shen W, Liu Y, Xin D. Comparative pharmacokinetics of dehydroevodiamine and coptisine in rat plasma after oral administration of single herbs and Zuojinwan prescription. Fitoterapia. 2011;82(8):1152–9.
10. Zhao FR, Mao HP, Zhang H, Hu LM, Wang H, Wang YF, et al. Antagonistic effects of two herbs in Zuojin wan, a traditional Chinese medicine formula, on catecholamine secretion in bovine adrenal medullary cells. Phytomedicine. 2010;17(9):659–68.
11. Ming L, Yan CL, Liu HX, Wang TY, Shi XH, Liu JP, et al. Network pharmacology exploration reveals endothelial inflammation as a common mechanism for stroke and coronary artery disease treatment of Danhong injection. Sci Rep. 2017;7(1):15427.
12. Fang HY, Zeng HW, Lin LM, Chen X, Shen XN, Fu P, et al. A network-based method for mechanistic investigation of Shexiang Baoxin Pill's treatment of cardiovascular diseases. Sci Rep. 2017;7:43632.
13. Yu G, Zhang Y, Ren W, Dong L, Li J, Geng Y, et al. Network pharmacology-based identification of key pharmacological pathways of yin–Huang–Qing–Fei capsule acting on chronic bronchitis. Int J Chron Obstruct Pulmon Dis. 2017;2:85–94.
14. Yue SJ, Xin LT, Fan YC, Li SJ, Tang YP, Duan JA, et al. Herb pair Danggui-Honghua: mechanisms underlying blood stasis syndrome by system pharmacology approach. Sci Rep. 2017;7:40318.
15. Wang CH, Zhong Y, Zhang Y, Liu JP, Wang YF, Jia WN, et al. A network analysis of the Chinese medicine Lianhua-Qingwen formula to identify its main effective components. Mol BioSyst. 2015;12(2):606–13.
16. Wang SS, Xu HY, Yan M, Wang XG, Shi Y, Huang B, et al. Characterization and rapid identification of chemical constituents of NaoXinTong capsules by UHPLC-linear ion trap/Orbitrap mass spectrometry. J Pharm Biomed Anal. 2015;111:104–18.
17. Xu T, Li S, Sun Y, Pi Z, Liu S, Song F, et al. Systematically characterize the absorbed effective substances of Wutou decoction and their metabolic pathways in rat plasma using UHPLC-Q-TOF-MS combined with a target network pharmacological analysis. J Pharm Biomed Anal. 2017;141:95–107.
18. Sheng S, Wang J, Wang L, Liu H, Li P, Liu M, et al. Network pharmacology analyses of the antithrombotic pharmacological mechanism of Fufang Xueshuantong capsule with experimental support using disseminated intravascular coagulation rats. J Ethnopharmacol. 2014;154(3):735–44.
19. Hamosh A, Scott AF, Amberger J, Bocchini C, Valle D, Mckusick VA. Online Mendelian inheritance in man (OMIM), a knowledgebase of human genes and genetic disorders. Nucleic Acids Res. 2005;33(1):514–7.
20. Hong M, Li S, Tan HY, Cheung F, Wang N, Huang J, et al. A network-based pharmacology study of the herb-induced liver injury potential of traditional Hepatoprotective Chinese herbal medicines. Molecules. 2017;22(4):632.
21. Hsia CW, Ho MY, Shui HA, Tsai CB, Tseng MJ. Analysis of dermal papilla cell interactome using STRING database to profile the ex vivo hair growth inhibition effect of a vinca alkaloid drug, colchicine. Int J Mol Sci. 2015;16(2):3579–98.
22. D'Eustachio P. Reactome knowledgebase of human biological pathways and processes. Methods Mol Biol. 2011;694:49–61.
23. Brown KR, Jurisica I. Online predicted human interaction database. Bioinformatics. 2005;21(9):2076–82.
24. Kerrien S, Aranda B, Breuza L, Bridge A, Broackes-Carter F, Chen C, et al. The IntAct molecular interaction database in 2012. Nucleic Acids Res. 2012;40:841–6.
25. Prasad TSK, Kandasamy K, Pandey A. Human protein reference database and human Proteinpedia as discovery tools for systems biology. Methods Mol Biol. 2009;577:67–79.

26. Licata L, Briganti L, Peluso D, Perfetto L, Iannuccelli M, Galeota E, et al. MINT, the molecular interaction database: 2012 update. Nucleic Acids Res. 2012;40:857–61.

27. Lehne B, Schlitt T. Protein-protein interaction databases: keeping up with growing interactomes. Hum Genomics. 2009;3(3):1–7.

28. Beuming T, Skrabanek L, Niv MY, Mukherjee P, Weinstein H. PDZBase: a protein-protein interaction database for PDZ-domains. Bioinformatics. 2005; 21(6):827–8.

29. Shannon P, Markiel A, Ozier O, Baliga NS, Wang JT, Ramage D, et al. Cytoscape: a software environment for integrated models of biomolecular interaction networks. Genome Res. 2003;13(11):2498–504.

30. Guo Q, Zhong M, Xu H, Mao X, Zhang Y, Lin N. A systems biology perspective on the molecular mechanisms underlying the therapeutic effects of Buyang Huanwu decoction on ischemic stroke. Rejuvenation Res. 2015;18(4):313–25.

31. Zhang Y, Wang D, Tan S, Xu H, Liu C, Lin N. A systems biology-based investigation into the pharmacological mechanisms of wu tou tang acting on rheumatoid arthritis by integrating network analysis. Evid Based Complement Alternat Med. 2013;2013(1):548498.

32. Zhang Y, Guo X, Wang D, Li RS, Li XJ, Xu Y, et al. A systems biology-based investigation into the therapeutic effects of Gansui Banxia tang on reversing the imbalanced network of hepatocellular carcinoma. Sci Rep. 2014;4(2):4154.

33. Wang L, Tan N, Hu J, Wang H, Duan D, Ma L, et al. Analysis of the main active ingredients and bioactivities of essential oil from *Osmanthus fragrans* Var. thunbergii using a complex network approach. BMC Syst Biol. 2017;11(1):144.

34. Yang ES, Willey CD, Mehta A, Crowley MR, Crossman DK, Chen D, et al. Kinase analysis of penile squamous cell carcinoma on multiple platforms to identify potential therapeutic targets. Oncotarget. 2017;8(13):21710–8.

35. Dennis G, Sherman BT, Hosack DA, Yang J, Gao W, Lane HC, et al. DAVID: database for annotation, visualization, and integrated discovery. Genome Biol. 2003;4(5):3.

36. Research NA. KEGG: Kyoto encyclopedia of genes and genomes. Nucleic Acids Res. 1999;27(1):29–34.

37. Li S, Zhang ZQ, Wu LJ, Zhang XG, Li YD, Wang YY. Understanding ZHENG in traditional Chinese medicine in the context of neuro-endocrine-immune network. IET Syst Biol. 2007;1(1):51–60.

38. Marmor MD, Skaria KB, Yarden Y. Signal transduction and oncogenesis by ErbB/HER receptors. Int J Radiat Oncol Biol Phys. 2004;58(3):903–13.

39. Rigler R, Pramanik A, Jonasson P, Kratz G, Jansson OT, Nygren PÅ, et al. Specific binding of proinsulin C-peptide to human cell membranes. Proc Natl Acad Sci U S A. 1999;96(23):13318–23.

40. Zhong Z, Davidescu A, Ehrén I, Ekberg K, Jörnvall H, Wahren J, et al. C-peptide stimulates ERK1/2 and JNK MAP kinases via activation of protein kinase C in human renal tubular cells. Diabetologia. 2005;48(1):187–97.

41. Al-Rasheed NM, Willars GB, Brunskill NJ. C-peptide signals via Galpha i to protect against TNF-alpha-mediated apoptosis of opossum kidney proximal tubular cells. J Am Soc Nephrol. 2006;17(4):986–95.

42. Kitamura T, Kimura K, Jung BD, Makondo K, Okamoto S, Cañas X, et al. Proinsulin C-peptide rapidly stimulates mitogen-activated protein kinases in Swiss 3T3 fibroblasts: requirement of protein kinase C, phosphoinositide 3-kinase and pertussis toxin-sensitive G-protein. Biochem J. 2001;355(Pt 1):123–9.

43. Sgouros SN, Bergele C. Clinical outcome of patients with helicobacter pylori infection: the bug, the host, or the environment? Postgrad Med J. 2006; 82(967):338–42.

44. Alzahrani S, Lina TT, Gonzalez J, Pinchuk IV, Beswick EJ, Reyes VE. Effect of helicobacter pylori on gastric epithelial cells. World J Gastroenterol. 2014; 20(36):12767–80.

45. Posselt G, Backert S, Wessler S. The functional interplay of helicobacter pylori factors with gastric epithelial cells induces a multi-step process in pathogenesis. Cell Commun Signal. 2013;11:77.

46. Trepicchio WL, Wang L, Bozza M, Dorner AJ. IL-11 regulates macrophage effector function through the inhibition of nuclear factor-kappaB. J Immunol. 1997;159(11):5661–70.

47. Zimmerman MA, Selzman CH, Reznikov LL, Raeburn CD, Barsness K, Jr MIR, et al. Interleukin-11 attenuates human vascular smooth muscle cell proliferation. Ajp Heart Circ Physiol. 2002;283(1):175–80.

48. Trepicchio WL, Dorner AJ. Interleukin-11: A gp130 Cytokine. Ann N Y Acad Sci. 2010;856(1):12–21.

49. Yan D, Kc R, Chen D, Xiao G, Im HJ. Bovine lactoferricin-induced anti-inflammation is, in part, via up-regulation of interleukin-11 by secondary activation of STAT3 in human articular cartilage. J Biol Chem. 2013;288(44): 31655–69.

50. Wang LJ, Chen SJ, Chen Z, Cai JT, Si JM. Morphological and pathologic changes of experimental chronic atrophic gastritis (CAG)and the regulating mechanism of protein expression in rats. J Zhejiang Univ Sci B(Biomedicine & Biotechnology). 2006;7(8):634–40.

51. Ichikawa T, Endoh H, Hotta K, Ishihara K. The mucin biosynthesis stimulated by epidermal growth factor occurs in surface mucus cells, but not in gland mucus cells, of rat stomach. Life Sci. 2000;7(9):1095–101.

52. Kopp R, Ruge M, Rothbauer E, Cramer C, Kraemling HJ, Wiebeck B, et al. Impact of epidermal growth factor (EGF) radioreceptor analysis on long-term survival of gastric cancer patients. Anticancer Res. 2002;22(2B):1161–7.

53. Wang YL, Sheu BS, Yang HB, Lin PW, Chang YC. Overexpression of c-erb-B2 proteins in tumor and non-tumor parts of gastric adenocarcinoma--emphasis on its relation to H. pylori infection and clinicohistological characteristics. Hepato-Gastroenterology. 2002;49(46):1172–6.

54. Maddalo G, Spolverato Y, Rugge M, Farinati F. Gastrin: from pathophysiology to cancer prevention and treatment. Eur J Cancer Prev. 2014;23(4):258–63.

55. Shimoyama T, Chinda D, Matsuzaka M, Takahashi I, Nakaji S, Fukuda S. Decrease of serum level of gastrin in healthy Japanese adults by the change of helicobacter pylori infection. J Gastroenterol Hepatol. 2014;29(S4): 25–8.

56. Naito Y, Ito M, Watanabe T, Suzuki H. Biomarkers in patients with gastric inflammation: a systematic review. Digestion. 2005;72(2–3):164.

57. Ito M, Haruma K, Kaya S, Kamada T, Kim S, Sasaki A, et al. Serological comparison of serum pepsinogen and anti-parietal cell antibody levels between Japanese and German patients. Eur J Gastroenterol Hepatol. 2002; 14(2):123–7.

58. Henwood M, Clarke PA, Smith AM, Watson SA. Expression of gastrin in developing gastric adenocarcinoma. Br J Surg. 2001;88(4):564–8.

59. Watson SA, Grabowska AM, Elzaatari M, Takhar A. Gastrin - active participant or bystander in gastric carcinogenesis? Nat Rev Cancer. 2006;6(12):936–46.

60. Sun X, Glynn DJ, Hodson LJ, Huo C, Britt K, Thompson EW, et al. CCL2-driven inflammation increases mammary gland stromal density and cancer susceptibility in a transgenic mouse model. Breast Cancer Res Bcr. 2017;19(1):4.

61. Poll TVD, Keogh CV, Guirao X, Buurman WA, Kopf M, Lowry SF. Interleukin-6 gene-deficient mice show impaired defense against pneumococcal pneumonia. J Infect Dis. 1997;176(2):439–44.

62. Cohen T, Nahari D, Cerem LW, Neufeld G, Levi BZ. Interleukin 6 induces the expression of vascular endothelial growth factor. J Biol Chem. 1996;271(2): 736–41.

63. Hong DS, Angelo LS, Kurzrock R. Interleukin-6 and its receptor in cancer: implications for translational therapeutics. Cancer. 2007;110(9):1911–28.

64. Thong-Ngam D, Tangkijvanich P, Lerknimitr R, Mahachai V, Theamboonlers A, Yong P. Diagnostic role of serum interleukin-18 in gastric cancer patients. World J Gastroenterol. 2006;12(28):4473–7.

65. Grivennikov S, Karin E, Terzic J, Mucida D, Yu GY, Vallabhapurapu S, et al. IL-6 and STAT-3 are required for survival of intestinal epithelial cells and development of colitis-associated Cancer. Cancer Cell. 2009;15(2):103–13.

66. Bollrath J, Phesse TJ, Burstin VAV, Putoczki T, Bennecke M, Bateman T, et al. gp130-mediated Stat3 activation in enterocytes regulates cell survival and cell-cycle progression during colitis-associated tumorigenesis. Cancer Cell. 2009;15(2):91–102.

67. Deshmane SL, Kremlev S, Amini S, Sawaya BE. Monocyte chemoattractant Protein-1 (MCP-1): an overview. J Interf Cytokine Res. 2009;29(6):313–26.

68. Wang H, Zhang L, Zhang IY, Chen X, Fonseca AD, Wu S, et al. S100B promotes glioma growth through Chemoattraction of myeloid-derived macrophages. Clin Cancer Res Official J Am Assoc Cancer Res. 2013;19(14): 3764–75.

69. Harlin H, Meng Y, Peterson AC, Zha Y, Tretiakova M, Slingluff C, et al. Chemokine expression in melanoma metastases associated with CD8+ T-cell recruitment. Cancer Res. 2009;69(7):3077–85.

70. Arnold JM, Huggard PR, Cummings M, Ramm GA, Chenevixtrench G. Reduced expression of chemokine (C-C motif) ligand-2 (CCL2) in ovarian adenocarcinoma. Br J Cancer. 2005;92(11):2024–31.

71. Kirk PS, Koreckij T, Nguyen HM, Brown LG, Snyder LA, Vessella RL, et al. Inhibition of CCL2 signaling in combination with docetaxel treatment has profound inhibitory effects on prostate cancer growth in bone. Int J Mol Sci. 2013;14(5):10483–96.

72. Tao LL, Shi SJ, Chen LB, Huang GC. Expression of monocyte chemotactic protein-1/CCL2 in gastric cancer and its relationship with tumor hypoxia. World J Gastroenterol. 2014;20(15):4421–7.

73. Essadik A, Jouhadi H, Rhouda T, Nadifiyine S, Kettani A, Maachi F. Polymorphisms of tumor necrosis factor alpha in Moroccan patients with gastric pathology: new single-nucleotide polymorphisms in TNF-α−193 (G/a). Mediat Inflamm. 2015;2015:143941.

74. Takeuchi T, Miura S, Lin W, Uehara K, Mizumori M, Kishikawa H, et al. Nuclear factor-kappaB and TNF-alpha mediate gastric ulceration induced by phorbol myristate acetate. Dig Dis Sci. 2002;47(9):2070–8.

75. Nagata H, Akiba Y, Suzuki H, Okano H, Hibi T. Expression of Musashi-1 in the rat stomach and changes during mucosal injury and restitution. FEBS Lett. 2006;580(1):27–33.

76. Nakashita M, Suzuki H, Miura S, Taki T, Uehara K, Mizushima T, et al. Attenuation of acetic acid-induced gastric ulcer formation in rats by glucosylceramide synthase inhibitors. Dig Dis Sci. 2013;58(2):354.

77. Dinarello CA. Biologic basis for interleukin-1 in disease. Blood. 1996;87(6):2095–147.

78. Tu S, Bhagat G, Cui G, Takaishi S, Kurt-Jones EA, Rickman B, et al. Overexpression of interleukin-1beta induces gastric inflammation and cancer and mobilizes myeloid-derived suppressor cells in mice. Cancer Cell. 2008;14(5):408–19.

79. Yang J, Hu Z, Xu Y, Shen J, Niu J, Hu X, et al. Interleukin-1B gene promoter variants are associated with an increased risk of gastric cancer in a Chinese population. Cancer Lett. 2004;215(2):191–8.

80. Palli D, Saieva C, Luzzi I, Masala G, Topa S, Sera F, et al. Interleukin-1 gene polymorphisms and gastric cancer risk in a high-risk Italian population. Am J Gastroenterol. 2005;100(9):1941–8.

81. Kumar S, Kumar A, Dixit VK. Evidences showing association of interleukin-1B polymorphisms with increased risk of gastric cancer in an Indian population. Biochem Biophys Res Commun. 2009;387(3):456–60.

82. Shigematsu Y, Niwa T, Rehnberg E, Toyoda T, Yoshida S, Mori A, et al. Interleukin-1β induced by helicobacter pylori infection enhances mouse gastric carcinogenesis. Cancer Lett. 2013;340(1):141–7.

83. Dufresne M, Seva C, Fourmy D. Cholecystokinin and gastrin receptors. Physiol Rev. 2006;86(3):805–47.

84. Kopin AS, Lee YM, McBride EW, Miller LJ, Lu M, Lin HY, et al. Expression cloning and characterization of the canine parietal cell gastrin receptor. Proc Natl Acad Sci U S A. 1992;89(8):3605–9.

85. Mjønes P, Nordrum IS, Sørdal Ø, Sagatun L, Fossmark R, Sandvik A, et al. Expression of the cholecystokinin-B receptor in neoplastic gastric cells. Hormones Cancer. 2018;9(1):40–54.

86. Petkevicius V, Salteniene V, Juzenas S, Wex T, Link A, Leja M, et al. Polymorphisms of microRNA target genes IL12B, INSR, CCND1 and IL10 in gastric cancer. World J Gastroenterol. 2017;23(19):3480–7.

87. Pellicanò A, Sebkova L, Monteleone G, Guarnieri G, Imeneo M, Pallone F, et al. Interleukin-12 drives the Th1 signaling pathway in helicobacter pylori-infected human gastric mucosa. Infect Immun. 2007;75(4):1738–44.

88. Guiney DG, Hasegawa P, Cole SP. Helicobacter pylori preferentially induces interleukin 12 (IL-12) rather than IL-6 or IL-10 in human dendritic cells. Infect Immun. 2003;71(7):4163–6.

89. Staff TPO. The NOD-like receptor signalling pathway in helicobacter pylori infection and related gastric cancer: a case-control study and gene expression analyses. PLoS One. 2014;9(6):e98899.

90. Yin Y, Si XL, Gao Y, Gao L, Wang J. The nuclear factor-κB correlates with increased expression of interleukin-6 and promotes progression of gastric carcinoma. Oncol Rep. 2013;29(1):34–8.

91. Wang QS, Cui YL, Ding SL. Study on anti-inflammatory and antidepressant mechanisms of Zuojin pill ethanol extracts (ZJP). China Pharma Conf. 2011:10-9.

92. Wang QS, Cui YL, Dong TJ, Zhang XF, Lin KM. Ethanol extract from a Chinese herbal formula, "Zuojin pill", inhibit the expression of inflammatory mediators in lipopolysaccharide-stimulated RAW 264.7 mouse macrophages. J Ethnopharmacol. 2012;141(1):377–85.

93. Wang QS, Zhu XN, Jiang HL, Wang GF, Cui YL. Protective effects of alginate-chitosan microspheres loaded with alkaloids from Coptis chinensis Franch. and Evodia rutaecarpa (Juss.) Benth. (Zuojin Pill) against ethanol-induced acute gastric mucosal injury in rats. Drug Design Dev Ther. 2015;9:6151–65.

94. Zhou XY, Yue H, Li CY, et al. Effect of Zuojin pill on inflammatory factors, oxidative stress factors and apoptosis factors in rats with stomach heat syndrome. Pharmacy Clin Chinese Materia Medica. 2017;8(2):49–52.

95. Pan Y, Ran R, Weng K, Chen YJ, Zhou FF, Yu HF. Therapeutic effects of Zuojinwan and its ingredients on rat gastric ulcer induced by acetic acid and influence on EGFR expression of the gastric mucous. Chinese J Integr Tradit West Med Digestion. 2008;16(6):368–71.

96. Lo HW, Hsu SC, Xia W, Cao X, Shih JY, Wei Y, et al. Epidermal growth factor receptor cooperates with signal transducer and activator of transcription 3 to induce epithelial-mesenchymal transition in Cancer cells via up-regulation of TWIST gene expression. Cancer Res. 2007;67(19):9066–76.

97. Sharon B, Stuart T, Elizabeth B, Suzanne R, Filippo P, Izabela SK, et al. Bypassing cellular EGF receptor dependence through epithelial-to-mesenchymal-like transitions. Clin Exp Metastasis. 2008;25(6):685–93.

98. Hien TT, Kim HG, Han EH, Kang KW, Jeong HG. Molecular mechanism of suppression of MDR1 by puerarin from Pueraria lobata via NF-kappaB pathway and cAMP-responsive element transcriptional activity-dependent up-regulation of AMP-activated protein kinase in breast cancer MCF-7/adr cells. Mol Nutr Food Res. 2010;54(7):918–28.

99. Sui H, Pan SF, Feng Y, Jin BH, Liu X, Zhou LH, et al. Zuo Jin wan reverses P-gp-mediated drug-resistance by inhibiting activation of the PI3K/Akt/NF-κB pathway. BMC Complement Altern Med. 2014;14(1):279.

100. Xu L, Qi Y, Lv L, Xu Y, Zheng L, Yin L, et al. In vitro anti-proliferative effects of Zuojinwan on eight kinds of human cancer cell lines. Cytotechnology. 2014;66(1):37–50.

19

Post-marketing safety surveillance and re-evaluation of Xueshuantong injection

Chunxiao Li[1], Tao Xu[1], Peng Zhou[1], Junhua Zhang[2], Ge Guan[1], Hui Zhang[1], Xiao Ling[1], Weixia Li[1], Fei Meng[1], Guanping Liu[3], Linyan Lv[3], Jun Yuan[4], Xuelin Li[1*] and Mingjun Zhu[1*]

Abstract

Background: Traditional Chinese medicine injections (TCMIs) have been widely used to treat severe and acute diseases due to their high bioavailability, accurate curative effect, and rapid effect. However, incidence rates of adverse drug reactions (ADRs) of TCMIs have also increased in recent years. Xueshuantong injection (XSTI) is a commonly-used TCMI comprised of Panax notoginseng total sapiens for the treatment of stroke hemiplegia, chest pain, and central retinal vein occlusion. Its safety remains uncelar. Therefore, post-marketing safety of XSTI was studied in this research.

Methods: In present study, post-marketing safety surveillance and re-evaluation of XSTI were reported. Thirty thousand eight hundred eighty-four patients in 33 hospitals from 7 provinces participated in this study. Incidence rate, most common clinical manifestations, types, severity, occurrence time, and disposal of ADRs were calculated.

Results: Incidence rate of ADR of XSTI was 4.14‰ and the most common clinical manifestations were skin and its appendages damage. Type A accounts for 95.49% of ADRs of XSTI and most of them (41.41%) were occurred within 24 h after receiving XSTI treatment. Severities of most ADRs of XSTI were moderate reactions (86.72%). Main disposition of ADRs of XSTI was drug withdrawal and symptomatic treatment (54.69%).

Conclusions: Our data provide basis for improvement of instructions of XSTI and clinical safety of XSTI. Post-marketing surveillance of TCMIs in this study is a powerful tool to identify types and manifestations of ADRs to improve safety and effectiveness of drugs in clinical applications.

Trial registration: This protocol has international registration in China clinical trial registration center (ChiCTR~OPC~ 14,005,718) at December 22, 2014.

Keywords: Xueshuantong injection, Post-marketing, ADRs/ADEs, Traditional Chinese medicine injections

Background

Traditional Chinese medicine injection (TCMI) is made by modern technologies and scientific methods to extract and purify effective substances from herbs (or decoction pieces). Compared with other traditional Chinese medicine formulations, injection has advantages of high bioavailability, rapid, and accurate curative effect. Therefore, TCMI is widely used to treat many severe and acute diseases [1–7]. In recent years, with the widespread use of TCMIs, the incidences of adverse drug reactions (ADRs)/adverse drug events (ADEs) has gradually increased [8–10]. However,

safety profile of most TCMIs remains largely unknown currently.

Xueshuantong injection (lyophilized) (XSTI) is a standardized herbal preparation and has been collected by "2012 national essential drugs list" and People's Republic of China Pharmacopoeia, respectively. Notoginseng total saponins, isolated from the root and rhizome of *P. notoginseng*, is the main component of XSTI. XSTI is generally used for treatment of cardiovascular and cerebrovascular disease [11]. Total revenue of XSTI in Chinese market in 2013 was over $700 million [12]. Therefore, the enormous consumption requires stricter and accurate evidence on its safety. However, many reports on the ADRs of XSTI were case reports and there is still lack large sample and high level evidence-based basis for safety of XSTI. Till now,

* Correspondence: lixuelin450000@163.com; zhumingjun317@163.com
[1]The First Affiliated Hospital of Henan University of Chinese Medicine, Zhengzhou 450000, People's Republic of China
Full list of author information is available at the end of the article

evaluation on post-marketing safety of XSTI has not been reported. Therefore, ADRs/ADEs of XSTI were studied in this research using hospital centralized monitoring method.

Hospital centralized monitoring also known as real world study (RWS), is an observational research method by recording detailed ADRs of drugs within a certain range of a hospital or an area in a certain period of time. It is attracting more and more attention in field of global clinical epidemiology due to its broad range of inclusion and exclusion criteria, comprehensive coverage of population, and authenticity [13–15]. A new hospital centralized monitoring method based on hospital information system (HIS) system was established in. our previous study on post-market clinical safety evaluation of TCMI [16]. In present research, post marketing safety (including incidence rate, types, severities, and other information of ADRs/ADEs) of XSTI with 30,884 cases by employing an improved method of hospital-centralized monitoring. This research is the first post-marketing ADRs/ADEs study of XSTI with large scale and multi-center and can provide essential basis for safe clinical use of XSTI.

Methods

Inclusion and exclusion criteria

Inclusion criteria: patients who used XSTI.
Exclusion criteria: patients who did not use XSTI.

Subjects

A total of 30,884 in-patients received XSTI from 33 hospitals in 7 provinces participated in this study between January 1, 2015 and December 31, 2016.

Drug

All three product specification (100 mg、150 mg and 250 mg per bottle) of XSTI were manufactured by Guangxi Wuzhou Pharmaceutical Co., Ltd. (Wuzhou, Guangxi, China). All drugs used in this research were sold on the market and in conformity with the standard of Ministry of Public Health of China.

Method design

This study was not a randomized controlled trial but a centralized monitoring study in hospital and all data were collected from clinical daily treatment without any intervention. Thus this study was not designed entirely according to CONSORT guidelines. We designed the monitoring data collection and quality control method according to other hospital centralized monitoring methods [13–16].

Method of monitoring data collection

The monitoring data were from two parts: monitoring table and hospital information system / laboratory information management system (HIS/LIS). Information in front page of the medical record, doctor's orders and results of laboratory examination were extracted from HIS/LIS system after being approved by ethics committee. To ensure the safety of the patient's personal information all monitors have been trained on information confidentiality. Monitoring table consists of Table A (basic monitoring information including daily dose, frequency, drug combination, etc.) and Table B (ADR/ADE information). Table A was filled by pharmacists within 5 days after the end of medication by "face-to-face" observation. Monitoring Table B was filled once ADR/ADE, especially serious ADR/ADE such as anaphylactic shock, severe allergic reactions, severe mucocutaneous lesions, liver damage, renal damage, and death, was happened. Accordance to requirements of "National ADR Reporting and Monitoring Management Measures", all serious ADRs/ADEs were further investigated by a panel consisting of head of organizer of the project and staffs from sub center and manufacturing enterprise. "Adverse Drug Reaction / Event Report" was written and submitted to official website according to the rules of the CFDA. The overall data collection flow chart is shown in Fig. 1 and ADRs/ADEs processing process is shown in Fig. 2.

Method of monitoring quality control

In order to guarantee the objectivity and accuracy of ADR results, unified training on monitoring plan and ADRs/ADEs judgment was carried out for monitoring personnel and a three-grade evaluation of ADRs / ADEs and third party quality control were conducted in this study. The detailed monitoring process is shown in Fig. 2. Strict selection criteria were set for the screening of participating hospital. Primary quality control monitoring hospital included comprehensive hospital and traditional Chinese medicine hospital. Sub-center monitoring hospitals were all three grade hospital in China and have organized or participated in the evaluation of drug safety. All participating hospitals had a team of clinical pharmacists and collected at least 500 cases within 1 years. There were 7 sub centers in total, and each sub center was responsible for 5–6 hospitals. A contract research organization (CRO) company (Shanghai Yongzheng medical science and Technology Co., Ltd.), was employed to carry on quality management of the study (Fig. 3). Reliability of monitoring reports and research progress of each monitoring hospitals and monitoring centers regularly were judged by CRO company. The hospitals which couldn't complete the monitoring progress on time or their monitoring reports were judged as unqualified more than three times were refused to continue to participate into the research project. The sub center was eliminated when more than half of its monitoring hospitals were eliminated.

Correlation assessment between ADRs and ADEs

Correlation assessment between ADRs and ADEs was conducted according to method recommended by CFDA

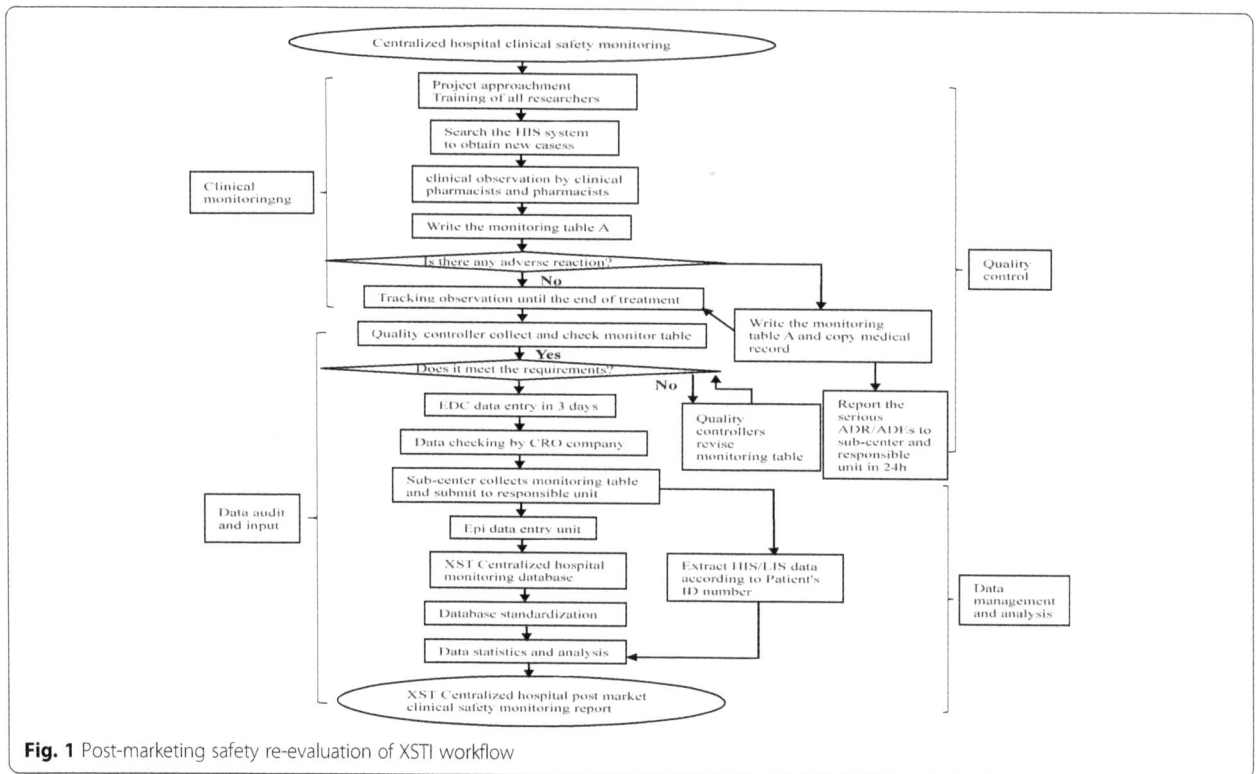

Fig. 1 Post-marketing safety re-evaluation of XSTI workflow

evaluation center of adverse reactions. All ADRs/ADEs were preliminarily classified on basis of their definitions, respectively. ADR is unrelated or unexpected adverse reaction to medication purpose when using approved drugs within normal dosage. It does not include reactions caused by accidental or intentional drug overdoses or improper medications. ADE refers to any injury occurred during drug administration period, whether or not drug usage is the cause of injury. ADR is a special type of ADE for which the causative relationship between drug usage and adverse reaction is identified. Relevance assessment is divided into 6 grades: (1) Certain: the sequence between medication and ADRs' occurrence is reasonable. ADRs could be stopped or quickly reduced or turn better after drug withdrawal. Alternatively, ADRs would be occured again or significantly worse when drug was re-administered. It could also be supported by literatures. Notably, primary disease and other factors should be ruled out. (2) Probable: there is no history of repeating medication, others are same as "Certain". If the investigated drug was administrated in combination with other drugs, the probability of ADR caused by combined drugs could be excluded. (3) Possible: there is close relationship between medication and ADEs' occurrence. It is coincided with common type of ADRs, but there is no reaction data after drug withdrawal, or there are more than one drug leading to ADRs/ADEs, or causative factors of primary disease could not be ruled out. (4) Unlikely: there was no close relationship between medication and ADEs' occurrence. The reactions do not link to ADRs/ADEs of the investigated

drug. Reactions during development of primary disease may display similar clinical manifestations. (5) Pending: There are missing contents of "Monitoring Information Form" and evaluation will not be completed until the supplementary specifications are provided. Thus, it is difficult to determine relationship between cause and effect due to absence in documentation. (6) Unassessable: many items in the "Monitoring Information Form" are unavailable. It is unable to analyze relationship between cause and effect because missing items could not be supplemented [2, 17, 18].

Results
Number of cases of XSTI in each hospital
In this study, a total of 30,884 cases received XSTI from 33 hospitals participated in the monitoring assessment. The number of ADE cases in 33 monitoring hospitals is shown in Table 1.

Association assessment of adverse reactions
In this study, 128 cases were grouped as "probable and possible ". Results of relevance evaluation were shown in Table 2.

Incidence rate and manifestations of ADRs
The ADR incidence of XSTI was 4.14‰. The clinical manifestations were 236 times. The most common clinical manifestations were skin and its appendages damage (52.97%), systemic injury (9.32%), and central and peripheral nervous

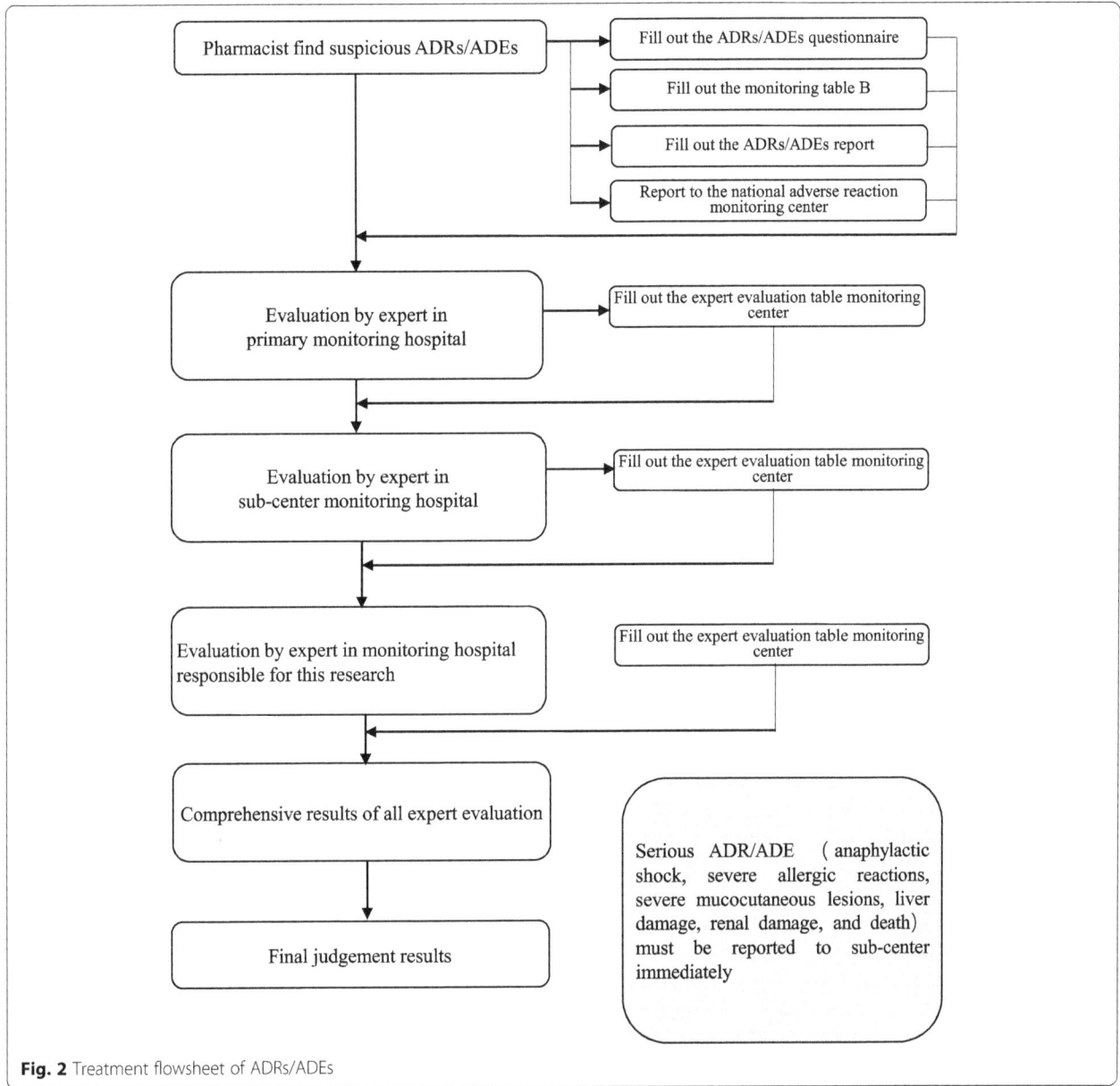

Fig. 2 Treatment flowsheet of ADRs/ADEs

system damage (8.90%). Statistics analysis were shown in Table 3 in detail.

Types of ADRs

ADRs are classified into three types (types A, B, and C) by WHO. Type A reaction caused by the enhancement of pharmacological effect of drugs is dose-related and able to be predicted. Type B reaction is abnormal reaction unrelated to normal pharmacological effect. It is not able to be detected by conventional toxicological screening and hard to make prediction. Type C reaction refers to abnormal reaction other than types A and B. According to above classification, all 128 cases of ADRs were divided into type A, B, and C, respectively as shown in Table 4.

Time of occurrence of ADRs

Time of occurrence of ADRs after injection of XSTI is shown in Table 5 and Table 6. According to the results, most ADRs of XST were occurred rapidly and nearly half cases of ADRs were appeared on the first day of injection (41.41%). There is 25.78% of ADRs were happened 2~ 4 days after injection.

Severity of ADRs

As shown in Table 7, severity of ADRs were classified into three grades: mild (symptoms or signs can be felt and stopping medication or special treatment is no necessary), moderate (symptoms and signs are tolerable and there is no effect on daily life but special treatment is necessary), and severe (symptoms and signs are intolerable and drug

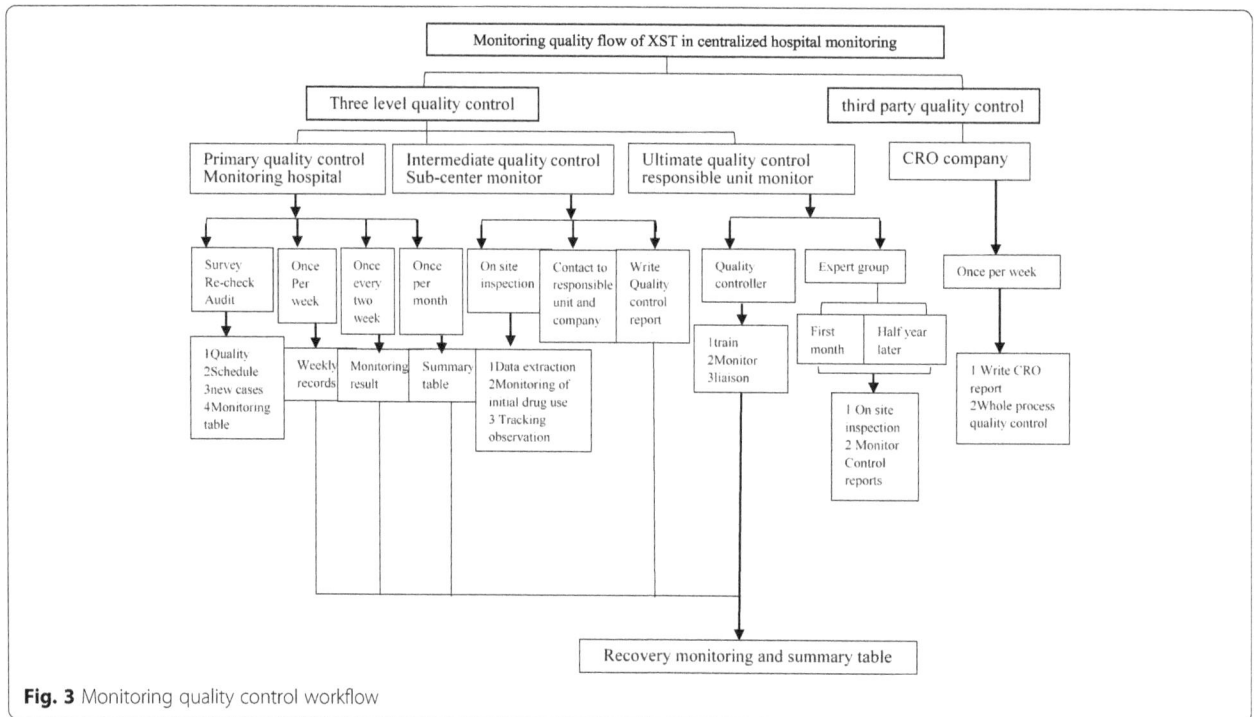

Fig. 3 Monitoring quality control workflow

withdrawal and special treatment are needed). Our results showed that most cases (86.72%) were graded into moderate reactions and 11 cases were classified as mild. In addition, among 6 cases with severe ADRs, 3 cases had severe symptoms, including rash, flushing, shivering, palpitation, high fever, dyspnea, and convulsions.

Disposal of ADRs

In most cases, ADRs need special treatments such as reducing times and dose of usage, withdrawal, symptomatic treatment, or combined together. Special treatments used in this study were listed as follows: withdrawal and symptomatic treatment (54.69%), withdrawal (30.47%), symptomatic treatment (7.03%) (Table 8). In addition, 1.56% of the ADRs did not get any special treatment.

Recovery of ADRs

Among of patients with ADRs, 80 cases were cured, 48 cases got improved, and there was no sequelae and death. Upon recovery time, 12, 26, 17, and 70 cases were improved within 1 h (9.38%), 1 ~ 6 h (20.31%), 6 ~ 24 h (13.28%), or over 24 h (54.69%), respectively. In addition, 3 cases were not recorded in detail.

Discussion

The incidence of ADRs of XSTI was 4.14‰, which was an "occasionally" "level and severe ADRs was 0.19 ‰, which was a "rare" grade and 95.49% of ADRs in this research were type A which can be predicted. 42.97% of ADRs were recovered in 24 h and there was no sequelae

and death. Therefore, XSTI is safe in clinical use according to the incidence, type and recovery of ADRs in this study. Most of ADRs were anaphylaxis which indicated that safety monitoring should be in progress promptly. In addition, ADRs of XSTI could happened throughout the whole course of treatment after administration which indicated that the whole process needs safety monitoring. So far, the description of the XSTI used in the study is not clear about ADRs. The results of this study make clear the manifestations of ADRs of XSTI, which provide a high level evidence-based basis for the improvement of the instructions. In this research, manifestations of ADRs were studied and the most common ADR manifestation of XSTI was skin and its appendages damages which were consistent with other published reports [19]. However, there is no suitable medicine to alleviate the ADRs of cutaneous systems. The main preventive measures by far is washing infusion tube before the injection of different injections to reduce the incidence of ADRs during the combined use of XSTI and other injections. It is generally believed that the skin and its appendages damages were caused by allergies. There is a study using P815 cell degranulation model to screen components of XSTJ [20]. Results showed that XSTI promoted the P815 cell degranulation and the effect may have related to Ginsenoside Rb1 and Rg1. Besides, impurities are difficult to remove in purification and refining processes due to the complex components in traditional Chinese medicine injections, which may also cause anaphylaxis [21–23]. However, few studies on the

Table 1 The number of ADE cases in 33 monitoring hospitals

Hospitals	Number of cases	Constituent ratio (%)
The First Affiliated Hospital of Henan University of TCM	2103	6.81
The Second Affiliated Hospital of Henan University of TCM	1006	3.26
Henan Province People's Hospital	1997	6.47
Luohe Central Hospital	697	2.26
General Hospital of Shenma medical group	1089	3.53
The First Affiliated Hospital of Guangxi University of TCM	1500	4.86
The First people's Hospital of Nanning	1011	3.27
The people's Hospital Guangxi Zhuang Autonomous Region	601	1.95
Nanning Hospital of TCM	607	1.97
The Jiangbin Hospital Guangxi Zhuang Autonomous Region	600	1.94
Wuzhou Red Cross Hospital	812	2.63
Wuzhou People's Hospital	802	2.60
The Second Affiliated Hospital of Tianjin University of TCM	1810	5.86
Peking University Binhai Hospital	515	1.67
Tianjin Huanhu Hospital	1203	3.89
Tianjin First Central Hospital	1213	3.93
Tianjin Hospital of ITCWM Nankai Hospital	802	2.60
Shuguang Hospital of Shanghai University of TCM	501	1.62
Tongji Hospital of Shanghai	501	1.62
Longhua Hospital of Shanghai University of TCM	502	1.63
People's Hospital of Pudong District of Shanghai	504	1.63
West China Hospital of Scichuan University	1504	4.87
Sichuan Cancer Hospital	1001	3.24
The people's Hospital of Dujiangyan	800	2.59
Affiliated Hospital of Chengdu University	603	1.95
Affiliated Hospital of Chengdu University of TCM	1034	3.35
Gansu Province Hospital of TCM	1223	3.96
The Second People's Hospital of Gansu	406	1.31
The People's Hospital of Gansu	807	2.61
Affiliated Hospital of Gansu University of TCM	635	2.06
The First Bethune Hospital of Jilin University	1830	5.93
Affiliated Hospital of Changchun University of TCM	502	1.63
The General Hospital of CNPC in Jilin	163	0.53
Total	30,884	100.00

Table 2 Results of correlation evaluation between ADRs and ADEs of XSTI

Results of correlation evaluation	Number of cases	Constituent ratio (%)
Certain	0	0.00
Probable	53	41.09
Possible	75	58.14
Unlikely	1	0.78
Pending	0	0.00
Unassessable	0	0.00
Total	129	100

Table 3 ADR manifestations of XSTI

Systems/organs	Number of cases/ incidence rate ‰	Constituent ratio (%)	Manifestations (number of cases/frequency‰)
Skin and its appendages	125/4.05	52.97	erythra (61/1.98), pruritus (50/1.62), maculopapule (8/0.26), hyperhidrosis (4/0.13), urticaria (4/0.13)
Systemic injury	22/0.71	9.32	fever (6/0.19), Shiver (6/0.19), edema (4/0.13), Chest pain (2/0.06), anaphylactoid reaction (1/0.03), periorbital edema (1/0.03), hot flush (1/0.03), acratia (1/0.03)
Central and peripheral nervous system damage	21/0.68	8.90	headache (9/0.29), giddy (6/0.19), paresthesia (4/0.13), lower limb spasticity (1/0.03), tremor (1/0.03)
Gastrointestinal system damage	14/0.45	5.93	sicchasia (4/0.13), vomit (2/0.06), hemorrhage of gastrointestinal tract (1/0.03), aggravation of gastrointestinal bleeding (1/0.03), dry lips (1/0.03), Stool discoloration (1/0.03), abdominal pain (1/0.03), discoloration of tongue (1/0.03), flatulence (1/0.03), toothache (1/0.03)
Respiratory system damage	14/0.45	5.93	Chest tightness (10), dyspnea (2), laryngeal spasm (1/0.03), epistaxis (1/0.03)
Extra cardiac vessel damage	10/0.32	4.24	flushing (9/0.29), phlebitis (1/0.03)
Medication site damage	10/0.32	4.24	local numbness (4/0.13), injection site pain (4/0.13), injection site numbness (1/0.03), injection site pruritus (1/0.03)
Urinary system damage	7/0.23	2.97	facial edema (6/0.19), hematuria (1/0.03)
Heart rate and arrhythmia	6/0.19	2.54	palpitation (5/0.16), tachycardia (1/0.03)
Nerve disorders	4/0.13	1.69	feel suffocated (3/0.10), insomnia (1/0.03)
Visual impairment	1/0.03	0.42	abnormal tears (1/0.03)
General cardiovascular system damage	1/0.03	0.42	Hypertension (1/0.03)
latelets and bleeding, coagulopathy	1/0.03	0.42	Gingival bleeding (1/0.03)
Total	236	100.00	

Incidence rate = number of adverse events *1000‰/ total number of cases

anaphylaxis mechanism of XSTI or panax notoginseng saponins and further investigation are needed to explore the ADR mechanism of XSTI. In addition, this study found some ADRs beyond instruction.

By comparison of four methods (hospital-centralized monitoring method, spontaneous reporting method, literature research method, and medical record review method) in our previous study on post-market clinical safety evaluation of TCMI and other reports, hospital centralized monitoring is a scientific, advanced, and feasible tool to assess clinical safety of TCM injection receiving approval [16]. In this study, monitoring method was improved on the basis of classic hospital-centralized monitoring. First, HIS/LIS system was utilized in the study. To analyze the impact factors of the ADRs/ADEs caused by XSTI, a large number of information associated with

ADRs/ADEs were collected. The data collected in the research were composed of general information, medication information and laboratory test data. The general information and medication information such as patients' ID number, gender, age, height, weight, admission diagnosis, allergic history, nationality, dosage, combined administration were mainly collected by monitoring table, while the laboratory test data such as blood routine, urine routine, faecal routine, liver function, renal function, thrombus and hemostasis and other inspection results were all extracted from HIS/LIS. Besides, the missing information in some of the monitoring tables were also supplemented by the HIS system. Secondly, majority of data collection and analyses in this study was performed by clinical pharmacists. Pharmacist plays important role in rational drug applications and improvement of life quality of patients. In one hand, clinical pharmacists are familiar with the treatment process of ADR/ADEs, on the other hand, they can put

Table 4 Comprehensive evaluation of occurrence types of ADR/ ADE

Type	Number of cases	Constituent ratio (%)
A	127	95.49
B	6	4.51
C	0	0.00
Total	133	100

Table 5 ADR Occurrence time of XSTI

	occurrence time (hours)				Total
	Day 1	Day 2~4	Day 5~7	>7 Days	
Number of cases	53	33	18	24	128
Constituent ratio (%)	41.41	25.78	14.06	18.72	100.00

Table 6 The time distance of ADR occurrence time and the last medication time of XSTI

	occurrence time (hours)				Total
	<0.5	0.5~1	1~12	12~24	
Number of cases	33	23	53	19	128
Constituent ratio (%)	25.78	17.97	41.41	14.84	100.00

more concentration on the research by comparison with clinician. Altogether, pharmacist is the best candidate for ADE surveillance. Last but not least, strict quality control method was designed in this multi-center research. Three-level quality control method used in this study has been successfully used in our previous post-marketing safety surveillance of Danhong injection. In order to strengthen quality control, third-party quality control, a contract research organization (CRO) company, was employed in this study. Because CRO companies has a large number of professional medical and pharmaceutical experts, they actively participate in many phase II or III clinical trials and undertake supervision as the third party, to guarantee the objectivity of the result in studies. Application of above working model in our study contributed greatly to improve objectivity of results and efficiency of research.

Our study has several shorter. We calculated the incidence, main types, main manifestations and severity classification of ADRs in this article, which reflect the safety of clinical use of XSTI in general, but the main influencing factors of ADRs were not studied in this article. However, all relevant data have been collected and are being analyzed. We will complete this part of study in following researches. In addition, the mechanism of the ADRs in the study is still unknown.

Conclusion

Post-marketing safety surveillance and re-evaluation of XSTI was carried out with 30,884 cases from 33 hospitals in 7 provinces. We obtained incidence rate, types, severities, as well as other information of ADRs/ADEs of XSTI. As far as we know, this research is the first study on the ADR of XSTI using large-scale hospital centralized monitoring method. The results in this study provide a high level

Table 7 The severity classification of ADR of XSTI

Severity classification	Number of cases	Constituent ratio (%)
Mild	11	8.59
Moderate	111	86.72
Severe	6	4.69
Total	128	100.00

Table 8 The disposal of ADR of XSTI

Disposal	Number of cases	Constituent ratio (%)
None	2	1.56
Reduce dripping speed (RDS)	7	5.47
Reduce dose	0	0.00
Drug withdrawal (DW)	39	30.47
Symptomatic treatment (ST)	9	7.03
RDS + DW + ST	1	0.78
DW + ST	70	54.69
Total	128	100.00

evidence-based basis for safety of XSTI. We further founded novel research system and mode of post-marketing safety surveillance and re-evaluation of TCMIs, which also provides a method to dramatically improve rationality and safety of clinical applications of TCMIs.

Acknowledgments
The authors want to thank all volunteers in our research team who participated in this study. We also thank academician Boli Zhang and researcher Weiliang Wong for guidance.

Funding
This work was supported by a grant from the National Science and Technology Major Projects for "Major New Drugs Innovation and Development" (2012ZX09101201).

Authors' contributions
C-XL, TX, PZ and GG were participated in this study as clinical pharmacists and all data were collected by them and C-XL wrote the manuscript. TX, J-HZ and HZ performed the analysis of the data. XL and W-XL were major contributors in writing the manuscript. FM, G-PL, L-YL, JY were major contributors in the data quality control. X-LL and M-JZ designed this research and were corresponding authors of this article. All authors read and approved the final manuscript.

Ethics approval and consent to participate
This study was an observational study. No medical intervention was conducted on the observed objects. The experiment protocol was approved by the Ethical Committee of the First Affiliated Hospital of Henan University of TCM (Approval number 2014HL~053). In addition, this protocol has international registration in China clinical trial registration center (ChiCTR~OPC~ 14,005,718). Written informed consents were obtained from all participants.

Competing interests
The authors declare that they have no competing interests.

Author details

[1]The First Affiliated Hospital of Henan University of Chinese Medicine, Zhengzhou 450000, People's Republic of China. [2]Evidence-based Medicine Center, Tianjin University of Traditional Chinese Medicine, Tianjin 300000, People's Republic of China. [3]Guangxi Wuzhou Pharmaceutical (group) Co., Ltd, Wuzhou 543000, People's Republic of China. [4]Shanghai Yongzheng Medical Science and Technology Co., Ltd, Shanghai 200000, People's Republic of China.

References

1. National Pharmacopoeia Committee, Chinese Pharmacopoeia. Part 1. Beijing: Chemical Industry Press; 2005: Appendix 13.
2. Ren D-Q, Zhang B-L. Clinical application guide of TCM injections, People's health publishing house. China: Beijing; 2011.
3. Li B, Wang Y, Lu J, et al. Evaluating the effects of Danhong injection in treatment of acute ischemic stroke: study protocol for a multicenter randomized controlled trial. Trials. 2015, 9;16:561.
4. Liu Y, Huang Y, Zhao C, et al. Salvia miltiorrhiza injection on pulmonary heart disease: a systematic review and meta-analysis. Am J Chin Med. 2014; 42(6):1315–31.
5. Yang H, Zhang W, Huang C, et al. A novel systems pharmacology model for herbal medicine injection: a case using Reduning injection. BMC Complement Altern Med. 2014, 4;14:430.
6. Luo J, Shang Q, Han M, et al. Traditional Chinese medicine injection for angina pectoris: an overview of systematic reviews. Am J Chin Med. 2014;42(1):37–59.
7. Fu S, Zhang J, Menniti-Ippolito F, et al. Huangqi injection (a traditional Chinese patent medicine) for chronic heart failure: a systematic review. PloS One. 2011, 6;6(5): 19604.
8. Guo XJ, Ye XF, Wang XX, et al. Reporting patterns of adverse drug reactions over recent years in China: analysis from publications. Expert Opin Drug Saf. 2015;14(2):191–8.
9. Liao X, Robinson N. Methodological approaches to developing and establishing the body of evidence on post-marketing Chinese medicine safety. Chin J Integr Med. 2013;19(7):494–7.
10. Wang L, Yuan Q, Marshall G, et al. Adverse drug reactions and adverse events of 33 varieties of traditional Chinese medicine injections on National Essential medicines list (2004 edition) of China: an overview on published literatures. J Evid Based Med. 2010;3(2):95–104.
11. Wang XM, Wang SX, Wang JX, et al. Neuroprotective effect of xueshuantong for injection (lyophilized) in transient and permanent rat cerebral ischemia model. Evid Based Complement Alternat Med. 2015;2015:134685.
12. Wang FJ, Wang SX, Chai LJ, et al. Xueshuantong injection (lyophilized) combined with salvianolate lyophilized injection protects against focal cerebral ischemia/reperfusion injury in rats through attenuation of oxidative stress. Acta Pharmacol Sin. 2017;36:1–14.
13. Zhao Y, Shi C, Huang P. Analysis of clinical use of post-marketing hospital centralized monitoring of Xiyanping injection. Zhongguo Zhong Yao Za Zhi. 2016;41(4):743–7.
14. Jiang JJ, Xie YM. Discussion on establishment of quality control system for intensive hospital monitoring on traditional Chinese medicine injections. Zhongguo Zhong Yao Za Zhi. 2012;37(18):2689–91.
15. Li X, Tang J, Meng F, et al. Study on 10 409 cases of post-marketing safety Danhong injection centralized monitoring of hospital. Zhongguo Zhong Yao Za Zhi. 2011;36(20):2783–5.
16. Li XL, Tang JF, Li WX, et al. Postmarketing safety surveillance and reevaluation of Danhong injection: clinical study of 30888 cases. Evid Based Complement Alternat Med. 2015;2015:610846.
17. Y.-Y. Wang, A.-P. Lv, and Y.-M. Xie. The key technologies of clinical re-evaluation of post-marketing traditional Chinese medicine, People's medical publishing house, Beijing, China,2011.
18. Baars E-W, Jong M, Nierop AF, et al. Savelkoul, "Citrus/cydonia compositum subcutaneous injections versus nasal spray for seasonal allergic rhinitis: a randomized controlled trial on efficacy and safety,". ISRN Allergy. 2011;2011:836051.
19. He GF, Dou WM. Zeng retrospective analysis on 697 cases of adverse drug reaction of Xueshuantong preparations. Chin J Pharmacoepidemiol. 2016; 11(25):715–8.
20. Li HC, Wu QY, Fu JT, et al. Study on screening method of allergenic ingredients of TCM injections. Pharmacol Clin Chin Mater Med. 2014;01(30):139–41.
21. Feng WW, Zhang Y, Tang JF, et al. Combination of chemical fingerprinting with bioassay, a preferable approach for quality control of safflower injection. Anal Chim Acta. 2018,20;1003:56–63.
22. Zhang L, Ma L, Feng W, et al. Quality fluctuation detection of an herbal injection based on biological fingerprint combined with chemical fingerprint. Anal Bioanal Chem. 2014;406(20):5009–18.
23. Ren Y, Zhang P, Yan D, et al. A strategy for the detection of quality fluctuation of a Chinese herbal injection based on chemical fingerprinting combined with biological fingerprinting. J Pharm Biomed Anal. 2011;56(2):436–42.

Permissions

The contributors of this book come from diverse backgrounds, making this book a truly international effort. This book will bring forth new frontiers with its revolutionizing research information and detailed analysis of the nascent developments around the world.

We would like to thank all the contributing authors for lending their expertise to make the book truly unique. They have played a crucial role in the development of this book. Without their invaluable contributions this book wouldn't have been possible. They have made vital efforts to compile up to date information on the varied aspects of this subject to make this book a valuable addition to the collection of many professionals and students.

This book was conceptualized with the vision of imparting up-to-date information and advanced data in this field. To ensure the same, a matchless editorial board was set up. Every individual on the board went through rigorous rounds of assessment to prove their worth. After which they invested a large part of their time researching and compiling the most relevant data for our readers.

The editorial board has been involved in producing this book since its inception. They have spent rigorous hours researching and exploring the diverse topics which have resulted in the successful publishing of this book. They have passed on their knowledge of decades through this book. To expedite this challenging task, the publisher supported the team at every step. A small team of assistant editors was also appointed to further simplify the editing procedure and attain best results for the readers.

Apart from the editorial board, the designing team has also invested a significant amount of their time in understanding the subject and creating the most relevant covers. They scrutinized every image to scout for the most suitable representation of the subject and create an appropriate cover for the book.

The publishing team has been an ardent support to the editorial, designing and production team. Their endless efforts to recruit the best for this project, has resulted in the accomplishment of this book. They are a veteran in the field of academics and their pool of knowledge is as vast as their experience in printing. Their expertise and guidance has proved useful at every step. Their uncompromising quality standards have made this book an exceptional effort. Their encouragement from time to time has been an inspiration for everyone.

The publisher and the editorial board hope that this book will prove to be a valuable piece of knowledge for researchers, students, practitioners and scholars across the globe.

List of Contributors

Quan Jiang, Xiao-Po Tang, Hong Xiao and Juan Jiao
Rheumatism Department, Guang'anmen Hospital, China Academy of Chinese Medical Sciences, No. 5 Beixiange Street, Xicheng District, Beijing 100053, China

Xian-Chun Chen
Pharmaceutical Department, Guang'anmen Hospital, China Academy of Chinese Medical Sciences, No. 12 Fuhai Street, Daxing District, Beijing 102628, China

Ping Liu
Clinical evaluation center, Guang'anmen Hospital, China Academy of Chinese Medical Sciences, No. 5 Beixiange Street, Xicheng District, Beijing 100053, China

Tianbo Zhang
School of Life Sciences, The Chinese University of Hong Kong, Shatin, N.T, Hong Kong, SAR 999077, People's Republic of China

Pang-Chui Shaw
School of Life Sciences, The Chinese University of Hong Kong, Shatin, N.T, Hong Kong, SAR 999077, People's Republic of China
Institute of Chinese Medicine and State Key Laboratory of Phytochemistry and Plant Resources in West China, the Chinese University of Hong Kong, Shatin, N.T, Hong Kong, SAR 999077, People's Republic of China
Li Dak Sum Yip Yio Chin R & D Centre for Chinese Medicine, The Chinese University of Hong Kong, Shatin, N.T, Hong Kong, SAR 999077, P. R. China

Mengjie Xiao
State Key Laboratory of Respiratory Disease, Guangdong Provincial Key Laboratory of Molecular Target & Clinical Pharmacology, School of Pharmaceutical Sciences and The Fifth Affiliated Hospital, Guangzhou Medical University, Guangzhou 510632, People's Republic of China
Guangzhou Institutes of Biomedicine and Health, Chinese Academy of Science, Guangzhou 510632, People's Republic of China

Huihui Ti
State Key Laboratory of Respiratory Disease, Guangdong Provincial Key Laboratory of Molecular Target & Clinical Pharmacology, School of Pharmaceutical Sciences and The Fifth Affiliated Hospital, Guangzhou Medical University, Guangzhou 510632, People's Republic of China
6HKU-Pasteur Research Pole, School of Public Health, Li Ka Shing Faculty of Medicine, The University of Hong Kong, Pok Fu Lam, Hong Kong, SAR 999077, People's Republic of China

Xin Zhao
State Key Laboratory of Respiratory Disease, Guangdong Provincial Key Laboratory of Molecular Target & Clinical Pharmacology, School of Pharmaceutical Sciences and The Fifth Affiliated Hospital, Guangzhou Medical University, Guangzhou 510632, People's Republic of China
Li Dak Sum Yip Yio Chin R & D Centre for Chinese Medicine, The Chinese University of Hong Kong, Shatin, N.T, Hong Kong, SAR 999077, P. R. China

Chun-Kwok Wong
Department of Chemical Pathology, The Chinese University of Hong Kong, Prince of Wales Hospital, Shatin, N.T, Hong Kong, SAR 999077, People's Republic of China
Institute of Chinese Medicine and State Key Laboratory of Phytochemistry and Plant Resources in West China, the Chinese University of Hong Kong, Shatin, N.T, Hong Kong, SAR 999077, People's Republic of China

Ka-Pun Chris Mok
HKU-Pasteur Research Pole, School of Public Health, Li Ka Shing Faculty of Medicine, The University of Hong Kong, Pok Fu Lam, Hong Kong, SAR 999077, People's Republic of China

Kai-Huan Wang, Jia-Rui Wu, Dan Zhang, Xiao-Jiao Duan and Meng-Wei Ni
Department of Clinical Pharmacology of Traditional Chinese Medicine, School of Chinese Materia Medica, Beijing University of Chinese Medicine, Beijing 100102, China

Chin-Chuan Tsai, Chi-Shiuan Lin, Chiu-Ming Chang and Li-Wei Lin
School of Chinese Medicine for Post-Baccalaureates, Chinese Medicine Department, I-Shou University and E-DA Hospital, Kaoshiung, Taiwan

Chun-Ru Hsu
Department of Medical Research, E-DA Hospital and School of Medicine, I-Shou University, Kaoshiung, Taiwan

I-Wei Chang
Department of Pathology, Taipei Medical University Hospital and School of Medicine, College of Medicine, Taipei Medical University , Taipei, Taiwan

Chih-Hsin Hung
Department of Chemical Engineering, and Institute of Biotechnology, I-Shou University, Kaoshiung, Taiwan

Jiun-Ling Wang
Department of Internal Medicine, National Cheng Kung University Hospital and College of Medicine,National Cheng Kung University, No. 138, Sheng Li Road, Tainan 70403, Taiwan

Shi Liu, Jia-Rui Wu, Dan Zhang, Kai-Huan Wang, Bing Zhang, Xiao-Meng Zhang, Di Tan, Xiao-Jiao Duan, Ying-Ying Cui and Xin-Kui Liu
Department of Clinical Chinese Pharmacy, School of Chinese Materia Medica, Beijing University of Chinese Medicine, Beijing 100102, China

Jielu Pan and Haiyan Song
Institute of Digestive Diseases, Longhua Hospital, Shanghai University of Traditional Chinese Medicine, Shanghai 200032, China

Guang Ji
Institute of Digestive Diseases, Longhua Hospital, Shanghai University of Traditional Chinese Medicine, Shanghai 200032, China
E-Institute of Shanghai Municipal Education Commission, Shanghai University of Traditional Chinese Medicine, Shanghai 201203, China

Yangxian Xu and Xiqiu Zhou
Department of General Surgery, Longhua Hospital, Shanghai University of Traditional Chinese Medicine, Shanghai 200032, China

Zemin Yao
Department of Biochemistry, Microbiology and Immunology, Ottawa Institute of Systems Biology, University of Ottawa, Ottawa, ON K1H 8M5, Canada

Chunjiang Tan, Jianwei Zeng, Yanbin Wu, Jiahui Zhang and Wenlie Chen
Chunjiang Tan and Wenlie Chen contributed equally to this work. Fujian Academy of Integrative Medicine, Fujian University of Traditional Chinese Medicine, Fuzhou, Fujian, China

Ning-hua Wu, Zhi-qiang Ke, Xiao-song Yang, Qing-jie Chen, Sheng-tang Huang and Chao Liu
Hubei Key Laboratory of Cardiovascular, Cerebrovascular, and Metabolic Disorders, Hubei University of Science and Technology, Xianning, China

Shan Wu
Xianning Maternal and Child Health Care Hospital, Xianning, China

Hwey-Fang Liang, Hsing-Chun Kuo and Chia-Hao Chang
Department of Nursing, Chang Gung University of Science and Technology, No.2, Sec. W., Jiapu Rd, Puzi City, Chiayi County 61363, Taiwan
Chronic Diseases and Health Promotion Research Center, Chang Gung University of Science and Technology, No.2, Sec. W., Jiapu Rd, Puzi City, Chiayi County 61363, Taiwan
Chang Gung Memorial Hospital, Chiayi, No.6, Sec.W., Jiapu Rd, Puzi City, Chiayi County 61363, Taiwan

Yao-Hsu Yang
Department for Traditional Chinese Medicine, Chang Gung Memorial Hospital, Chiayi, Taiwan
Health Information and Epidemiology Laboratory of Chang Gung Memorial Hospital,Chiayi, Taiwan
School of Traditional Chinese Medicine, College of Medicine, Chang Gung University, Taoyuan, Taiwan

Pau-Chung Chen
Institute of Occupational Medicine and Industrial Hygiene, National Taiwan University College of Public Health, Taipei, Taiwan
Department of Environmental and Occupational Medicine, National Taiwan University College of Medicine and National Taiwan University Hospital, Taipei, Taiwan

Ying-Hsiang Wang
Department of Pediatrics, Chang Gung Memorial Hospital, Chiayi, Taiwan

Kuang-Ming Wu
Department of Early Childhood Education, National Chiayi University, Chiayi, Taiwan

Xiaoni Liu, Shuang Wang, Jianji Xu, Buxin Kou and Dexi Chen
Beijing Institute of Hepatology and Beijing YouAn Hospital, Capital Medical University, No 8 Xi TouTiao, You An Men Wai, Feng Tai Qu, Beijing 100069, China

Yajie Wang and Xiaoxin Zhu
Institute of Chinese Materia Medica, China Academy of Chinese Medical Sciences, No 16 Nan Xiao Jie, Dong Zhi Men Nei, Dong Cheng Qu, Beijing 100700, China

Eun Suk Son, Sung Hwan Jeong and Jeong-Woong Park
Department of Internal Medicine, Gachon University Gil Medical Center, 21 Namdong-daero 774 beon-gil, Namdong-gu, Incheon 405-760, Republic of Korea

Young Ock Kim, Chun Geon Park and Kyung Hun Park
Department of Herbal Crop Research, National Institute of Horticultural and Herbal Science, RDA, Cheongju, Chungbuk, Republic of Korea

Se-Hee Kim
Gachon medical research institute, Gachon University Gil Medical Center, 21 Namdong-daero 774 beon-gil, Namdong-gu, Incheon 405-760, Republic of Korea

Jin Mo Ku, Se Hyang Hong, Soon Re Kim, Han-Seok Choi, Hyo In Kim, Dong Uk Kim and So Mi Oh
Department of Science in Korean Medicine, Graduate School, Kyung Hee University, Kyungheedae-ro 26, Dongdaemun-gu, Seoul 02447, Republic of Korea

Hye Sook Seo, Tai Young Kim, Yong Cheol Shin, Chunhoo Cheon and Seong-Gyu Ko
Department of Preventive Medicine, College of Korean Medicine, Kyung Hee University, Kyungheedae-ro 26, Dongdaemun-gu, Seoul 02447, South Korea

Ruijuan Zhou, Hongjiu Chen and Junpeng Chen
Department of Chest and Breast Surgery, Xiamen Hospital of Traditional Chinese Medicine, Fujian University of Traditional Chinese Medicine, 1739 Xianyue Road, Xiamen 361009, People's Republic of China

Xuemei Chen and Yu Wen
Department of Pharmacy, Xiamen Hospital of Traditional Chinese Medicine, Fujian University of Traditional Chinese Medicine, 1739 Xianyue Road, Xiamen 361009, People's Republic of China

Leqin Xu
Department of Science and Education, Xiamen Hospital of Traditional Chinese Medicine, Fujian University of Traditional Chinese Medicine, 1739 Xianyue Road, Xiamen 361009, People's Republic of China

Yue Wei, Xuemei Cheng and Changhong Wang
Institute of Chinese Materia Medica, Shanghai University of Traditional Chinese Medicine, The MOE Key Laboratory for Standardization of Chinese Medicines and The SATCM Key Laboratory for New Resources and Quality Evaluation of Chinese Medicine, 1200 Cailun Road, Shanghai 201203, China

Nan Zou
Institute of Chinese Materia Medica, Shanghai University of Traditional Chinese Medicine, The MOE Key Laboratory for Standardization of Chinese Medicines and The SATCM Key Laboratory for New Resources and Quality Evaluation of Chinese Medicine, 1200 Cailun Road, Shanghai 201203, China

Institute of Experimental Center for Scientific Technology, Shanghai University of Traditional Chinese Medicine, 1200 Cailun Road, Shanghai, China

Fenghua Li and Yang Yang
Institute of Experimental Center for Scientific Technology, Shanghai University of Traditional Chinese Medicine, 1200 Cailun Road, Shanghai, China

Yu Chen, Dong-jie Guo, Min-feng Wu, Ya-Nan Zhang, Su Li, Rong Xu, Jie Chen and Xing-xiu Jin
Department of Dermatology, Yueyang Hospital of Integrated Traditional Chinese and Western Medicine, affiliated with Shanghai University of Traditional Chinese Medicine, 110 Ganhe Road, Shanghai 200437, China

Fu-lun Li
Department of Dermatology, Yueyang Hospital of Integrated Traditional Chinese and Western Medicine, affiliated with Shanghai University of Traditional Chinese Medicine, 110 Ganhe Road, Shanghai 200437, China
Department of Dermatology, the Seventh People's Hospital of Integrated Traditional Chinese and Western Medicine, affiliated with Shanghai University of Traditional Chinese Medicine, Shanghai 200137, China

Hui Deng
The Sixth Hospital Affiliated with Shanghai Jiaotong University, Shanghai 200233, China

Qi Xu
School of Public Health, Shanghai University of Traditional Chinese Medicine, Shanghai 200433, China

Cheng-Yu Yang and Bo Peng
School of Dentistry, National Defense Medical Center, Taipei, Taiwan, Republic of China

Yuan-Wu Chen
School of Dentistry, National Defense Medical Center, Taipei, Taiwan, Republic of China
Department of Oral and Maxillofacial Surgery, Tri-Service General Hospital, No. 161, Section 6, Min-Chuan East Road, Neihu 114, Taipei 114, Taiwan, Republic of China

Cheng-Chih Hsieh
Department of Pharmacy Practice, Tri-Service General Hospital, Taipei, Taiwan, Republic of China

Chih-Kung Lin
Division of Anatomic Pathology, Taipei Tzu Chi Hospital, Taipei, Taiwan, Republic of China

Chun-Shu Lin
Department of Radiation Oncology, Tri-Service General Hospital, National Defense Medical Centre, Taipei, Taiwan, Republic of China
Graduate Institute of Clinical Medicine, College of Medicine, Taipei Medical University, Taipei, Taiwan, Republic of China

Gu-Jiun Lin
Department of Biology and Anatomy, National Defense Medical Center, Taipei, Taiwan, Republic of China

Huey-Kang Sytwu
Graduate Institute of Microbiology and Immunology, National Defense Medical Center, Taipei, Taiwan, Republic of China

Wen-Liang Chang
School of Pharmacy, National Defense Medical Center, Taipei, Taiwan, Republic of China

Yizhe Cui, Qiuju Wang, Rui Sun, Li Guo, Mengzhu Wang, Junfeng Jia, Chuang Xu and Rui Wu
College of Animal Science and Veterinary Medicine, Heilongjiang Bayi Agricultural University, 2# Xinyang Road, New Development District, Daqing 163319, Heilongjiang, China

Guohua Yu, Wubin Wang, Xu Wang, Meng Xu, Lili Zhang, Lei Ding and Rui Guo
School of Life Sciences, Beijing University of Chinese Medicine, No.11 East road, North 3rd Ring Road, Beijing 100029, China

Yuanyuan Shi
School of Life Sciences, Beijing University of Chinese Medicine, No.11 East road, North 3rd Ring Road, Beijing 100029, China
Shenzhen Hospital, Beijing University of Chinese Medicine, No. 1 Dayun road, Sports New City Road, Shenzhen 518172, China

Chunxiao Li, Tao Xu, Peng Zhou, Ge Guan, Hui Zhang, Xiao Ling, Weixia Li, Fei Meng, Xuelin Li and Mingjun Zhu
The First Affiliated Hospital of Henan University of Chinese Medicine, Zhengzhou 450000, People's Republic of China

Junhua Zhang
Evidence-based Medicine Center, Tianjin University of Traditional Chinese Medicine, Tianjin 300000, People's Republic of China

Guanping Liu and Linyan Lv
Guangxi Wuzhou Pharmaceutical (group) Co., Ltd, Wuzhou 543000, People's Republic of China

Jun Yuan
Shanghai Yongzheng Medical Science and Technology Co., Ltd, Shanghai 200000, People's Republic of China

Index